The Art of
Therapeutic
Communication

The Collected Works of
Kay F. Thompson

Edited by
Saralee Kane MSW and
Karen Olness MD

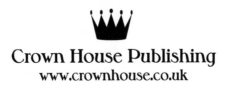

Crown House Publishing
www.crownhouse.co.uk

First published by

Crown House Publishing Ltd
Crown Buildings, Bancyfelin, Carmarthen, Wales, SA33 5ND, UK
www.crownhouse.co.uk

and

Crown House Publishing Ltd
P.O. Box 2223, Williston, VT 05495-2223, USA
www.CHPUS.com

British Library Cataloguing-in-Publication Data
A catalogue entry for this book is available
from the British Library.

ISBN 1904424287

LCCN 2004101977

Printed and bound in Wales by
HSW Print
Tonypandy
Rhondda

"When everything that can be done and should be done, has been done, there is no longer any reason to have the pain."

"What we are doing is taking our words to tap into the physiological substrate so the individual can control, not only his mind, but his body, his responses, and his behaviors."

"And you can become so entranced with knowing everything that you need to know about how the memory of that experience changed into something that it wasn't when it began, only because you hadn't thought about it being what you didn't think it was."

Kay F. Thompson

Saralee Kane

In memory of Kay Thompson and Marion, Lewis, Honey and Sol.

To all our teachers, including our children and grandchildren; to the teachings, and the willingness to listen and observe; to the qualities embodied by all of them: wisdom, compassion, integrity, generosity, courage and kindness.

With the deepest love and gratitude.

Karen Olness

To the memory of Kay Thompson on behalf of the many students and colleagues who were so profoundly and positively impacted by her life and teachings.

Contents

i

Acknowledgments

Saralee Kane

We wish to extend our gratitude and appreciation to all of the people who so generously helped in the production of this volume. There are several people we would like to especially acknowledge. First and foremost we would like to thank Ralph Krichbaum, Kay's husband, for making Kay's private papers and tapes available for our use, for his continuing support and encouragement and for writing a wonderful memoir.

Russ Scott, a dear friend and colleague of Kay's made a personal commitment to share his perspective on Kay's clinical legacy. He was very ill during the writing of his memoir and his dedication to this project is especially appreciated. To our great regret, he passed away on 14 February 2004. We also extend our special thanks to Learita Scott, Russ Scott's wife, for encouraging his participation and enabling him to continue despite his declining health.

We offer our thanks to Dan Kohen, Kay's close friend, for his significant contribution to this volume. Dan Kohen searched the archives of the Minnesota Society for Clinical Hypnosis, and generously copied tapes and videotapes for our review, many of which were eventually selected for inclusion in the present work.

We offer our special appreciation to all of the authors who so generously contributed to the *Collected Works*. Our special thanks to: Betty Alice Erickson, Roxanna Erickson Klein, Bernhard Trenkle, Camillo Loriedo, Dan Kohen, Akira Otani, James Auld, Alexander Levitan, Harold Golan, Peo Wikstrom, Sidney Rosen and Stanley Krippner. Their perspectives, at times both insightful and entertaining, on Kay's teaching and its impact on clinical hypnosis and their professional work is a critical addition to this volume. An additional thank you to James Auld for transcribing the dual inductions in this text. And we offer our special thanks to all the authors who, in their teaching vignettes, shared aspects of Kay's teaching which significantly affected their lives. The personalizing of this collected works through all of the efforts of the contributing authors adds a crucial dimension to the honoring of Kay's teaching legacy.

Our deepest appreciation is extended to the Erickson family, and the staff and Board of Directors of the Erickson Foundation whose congresses and meetings provided the forums where Kay participated as a lecturer, workshop presenter and panel member. The Foundation's dedication to preserving these contributions through edited collections of the congresses and audiotapes has made much of her work available to the public. Our special thanks to Jeff Zeig, Director of the Milton Erickson Foundation, whose energy and organizational skills helped to make all of this possible.

Harriet King, Kay's friend and former secretary, offered essential support during our review of Kay's private papers and tapes. Her ongoing help throughout the preparation of this text was of great value to our project. Roxanna Erickson Klein, a close friend of Kay's, not only produced an excellent chapter introduction and vignette, but also helped some of the contributing authors with their vignettes. Stacie Murrer, a former student and close friend of Kay's, was supportive and encouraging when the idea of a collected works was germinating, and introduced the co-editors, Saralee Kane and Karen Olness, to each other.

We wish to thank our publisher, Crown House Publishing, and their excellent staff for their consistent and professional support throughout this process. We especially thank Mark Tracten, Director of US Operations of Crown House Publishing, for his generous guidance, Pat Connolly for her incisive editorial assistance and Clare Jenkins for guiding the manuscript to publication.

We extend a very special appreciation to our families for their continuing interest and support during the long process of producing this volume. Their patience and encouragement allowed us to devote the time and energy necessary for its completion. A very special thank you to my husband, Mark Kane for his patience and support during this long process and to my sons, Adam and Seth, for their positive encouragement and insightful suggestions. I extend thanks to my close friends, Gale Nagao, Susan Harritt and Annette Sivak for their editing suggestions. We also thank our many friends for their continuing interest and support through this long process.

We thank everyone for joining us in honoring Kay's teaching legacy and are sure Kay is smiling on all of you.

Karen Olness

With many thanks to Saralee Kane for her hundreds of hours of loving labor to transcribe Kay Thompson's teaching tapes, to Ralph Krichbaum for his generous encouragement to us as we developed the ideas for this book, and to my husband, Hakon Torjesen, for his advice and assistance during the three-year process of completing this book.

Foreword

Crossing the Threshold with Kay Thompson

Terminus was the Roman god of boundaries but Mercury is better known for his ability to bypass conventional borders, restrictions and limitations. "Limen" is the Latin word for "threshold" and I am convinced that hypnosis is a "liminal phenomenon" because its use places both practitioners and their patients "betwixt and between" the ordinary distinctions of time and space, mind and body, and illusion and reality.

The use of imagination and altered states of consciousness for healing is one of humankind's oldest discoveries and traditions. Most cultures and indigenous societies throughout history have utilized some aspect of this remarkable human capacity, such as in yoga and the great meditative traditions. Shamanism is the most ancient lineage of this kind of healing, and modern therapeutic practices, such as hypnosis, that use imagination and altered states for healing and psychotherapy, can be traced back to these ancient traditions.

In many indigenous cultures, traditional healers were identified at early ages and were given rigorous training by advanced practitioners. A community was especially impressed if a young girl or boy remembered dreams frequently, had an affinity for animals, birds and other living creatures, and expressed empathy for people in the tribe who were suffering.

It has taken contemporary dentistry, medicine and psychotherapy many years to rediscover the wisdom of these ancient traditions, but hypnosis has been a more useful bridge than any other practice in re-establishing this venerable connection. In the indigenous societies I have visited, the role of the shaman is to serve as someone who can cross these boundaries in the service of his or her community and its members. Like Mercury, shamans are known as "tricksters" because they use paradoxical stories, employ confusion in their activities and deconstruct language to heal their clients, to mend broken relationships and to restore community solidarity. In other words, shamans were employing hypnotic-like techniques long before the days of Mesmer and Braid.

It is not surprising that in the Western world, there are some people who manifest a shamanic sensibility and intelligence, most typically among performing artists and in a variety of fields, including the healing arts. Milton Erickson would have been hailed as a shaman in an indigenous society, and the gifts of his student Kay Thompson would have been commended as well. Kay adored nature. She was a mountain climber and, with her husband, enjoyed canoe trips—on waters that were both calm and turbulent. Kay was close to animals; those who knew her well would conjecture that her "animal ally" would probably have been a dog.

Kay was also comfortable whenever she found herself in transpersonal realms, both experiencing and listening to patients undergoing experiences where boundaries between people seemed to melt, and where borders between the individual and the environment appeared to dissolve. Kay had no hesitation about using these transpersonal connections and spiritual experiences as vehicles for healing, even in the years when such practices were frowned upon. As usual, Kay was a pioneer, someone ahead of her time. Nowadays, some of the most popular books about psychotherapy deal with the role of spirituality in healing. But Kay's work went even further; as a gifted healer, she would often help her dying patients make a calm and peaceful transition.

I first met Kay at a meeting of the American Society of Clinical Hypnosis, a professional organization that elected her as its first female president in 1972. It was always a treat to have lunch or dinner with her, or to hear her presentations. Kay was a masterful teacher, and I still have a collection of notes from her lectures. I especially appreciated Kay's emphasis on ways to assess and enhance a patient's motivation, and her utilization of narrative and quasilogical explanations in this effort. Anthropologists who write about shamanism call these stories "trickster tales", and Kay's repertoire was both wild and extensive.

The role played by imagination is central to both indigenous healing rituals and hypnosis. This has been acknowledged by Division 30 of the American Psychological Association in its recent description of hypnosis as a procedure in which someone "is told that suggestions for imaginative experiences will be presented". Kay was a great practitioner of hypnosis because she understood the role played by imagination in helping her patients bypass pain, overcome phobias and change dysfunctional behavior patterns. It was appropriate that Kay was a dentist; one's teeth and one's oral cavity help form the boundary of the external and the internal worlds. They bring nurturance to the body, and prepare it for transformation. Shamans are known as "shape shifters" because they assume so many forms. The teeth transform food (and anything—or anybody—else they come into contact with) into a new format.

As in these greater traditions, when healers fall ill, they serve as role models for their community. After Kay's own rhinoplasty-dermabrasion surgery, her use of self-hypnosis became part of her legend and her legacy. During her terminal illness, Kay conducted herself with grace and dignity, again modeling the way in which an enlightened being makes his or her passage.

Hypnosis is a multifaceted phenomenon requiring explanation at multiple levels. Some investigators and practitioners have missed the importance of the social or interpersonal context in which hypnosis occurs, while others have come close to destroying the most interesting and useful hypnotic phenomena under the guise of objectivity. Kay understood these limitations and was persistent in her teaching that there is a difference in personal experience between the "experimental trance" and the "clinical trance". Despite the similarities in induction, there are several phenomenological differences that keep knowledgeable practitioners from confusing the two, and from making simplistic extrapolations from one to the other. Kay never lost contact with either end of the spectrum.

Kay was aware of the liminal nature of hypnosis and knew that all of its various aspects and facets had to be honored. The contributors to this book, and Kay's words themselves, attest to her knowledge regarding not only the use of hypnosis in dentistry and medicine, but in hypnotically facilitated psychotherapy as well. Novices in the field, as well as seasoned practitioners, will find value and wisdom in these pages. Kay always wanted to write a book of her own; this marvelous volume, because of its multidimensionality and because of the integrity of its contributors, will serve the purpose and grant Kay her final wish.

Stanley Krippner PhD

Introduction

Kay Thompson is acknowledged as one of the great hypnotherapists of the 20th century. She was renowned for her linguistic brilliance, as an international teacher of hypnosis, and as one of the most gifted students of the legendary psychotherapist, Milton Erickson. She lectured widely on the therapeutic use of language, the importance of motivation, pain management and pain control, the effect of language on physiology, and the use of hypnosis in dentistry, including the psychological importance of the oral cavity. Through her unique and extraordinary abilities with language, she entranced listeners throughout the world.

Her original contribution in articulating the importance of motivation is seminal in the field of psychotherapy and she played a significant role in the creation of the dual induction, one of the most innovative additions to the field of hypnosis. As importantly, she expanded the ways in which words and language, and thus metaphor, could be used in clinical hypnosis and psychotherapy. She was a genuine artist, capable of crafting complex, poetic and effective multilevel therapeutic messages, which inspired students and colleagues wherever she taught.

> "My words are the chisels, the brushes used to attempt to reach the inner block of material, the canvas of the individual, modifying the story as the cues demand, and waiting for the message that change is ready, leaving the creation to be interpreted by the patient, the one who commissioned the vision in the beginning." (Chapter Twenty-six.)

Equally impressive were her determination and ability to motivate others to learn these skills and to systematically teach them the "what and how" of her therapeutic communications. Her teaching presence, as an authentic model of everything she taught, was especially inspiring. All of her contributions are among the underpinnings of contemporary clinical hypnosis and are important resources for modern psychotherapy.

She began her professional career as a dentist and she also had a profound impact on the field of dentistry. Through her recognition of the psychological importance of the oral cavity, her teaching, political activities and mentoring of young dentists, especially women dentists, she has been described as having "as much of an impact on dentistry in the United States as Amelia Earhardt had on aviation". (1998)

It is of central importance to an understanding of Thompson's work to know that her dental practice was the impetus for her interest in learning about hypnosis. Since childhood, she had wanted to become a dentist, because she was both fascinated by her father's dental practice and impressed by the help he offered his patients. With her father's encouragement and support she applied to dental school and was the youngest student and, at one time, the only female student in her dental school; after graduation in the early 1950s she became the first woman to practice dentistry in Pittsburgh. Overcoming gender barriers, especially in professional politics, became a lifelong process.

Local dentists sent her their difficult patients, thinking that a woman would be gentler and more understanding. In order to help meet the needs of these patients, she began to explore different therapeutic modalities, and in the course of that process attended a hypnosis seminar in 1953 with Milton Erickson MD. By that time, Erickson, a brilliant psychotherapist, had published numerous articles on clinical hypnosis and was considered by many to be one of the most important influences, if not the most important influence, on the resurgence of modern hypnotherapy. He was an independent, uncommonly creative, and nontraditional therapist; only many years later would his ideas and work be credited for significantly influencing the course of modern psychotherapy.

After Thompson's first hypnosis course, she did an emergency root canal without any anesthesia on a pregnant patient and was amazed by her patient's ability to use hypnosis for what was normally one of the most intensely painful dental surgeries. Her lifelong passion for learning hypnosis had begun. After attending numerous hypnosis seminars, she was selected by Erickson for more advanced study, eventually becoming one of his closest friends and colleagues. Her father and Erickson were probably the most significant personal and professional mentors in her life.

In many ways, Kay Thompson was a pioneer, perhaps because she was willing to be really in the present, by truly seeing and listening, outside the many cultural trances and belief structures which usually organize our perceptions of reality. She observed, observed and observed. She "knew" from a deep experiential understanding, and wasn't afraid to teach what she saw and experienced and understood, but couldn't yet explain. When her clinical experience contradicted what she "thought she had known" she noticed, acknowledged with curiosity, and was open and willing to change her mind. Her approach was phenomenological and generative, not ideological.

Thompson emphasized the crucial importance of motivation in clinical hypnosis, an idea that is relevant to all kinds of psychotherapy. Through highlighting the significance of the client's motivation in a therapeutic situation, and by encouraging therapists to accept responsibility for motivating their clients, she espoused a view that was and still is far ahead of accepted norms of therapy practice. It is interesting to note that intention, which is very similar to motivation as it was conceived in the late 1970s and early 1980s, when Thompson was initially emphasizing its crucial significance, has recently become a core issue in modern therapeutic practice.

Throughout her career, Thompson was vehement in her repeated emphasis on the profound difference between clinical and experimental trance."I refuse to restrict myself and the patient to their ability to learn based on some artificial criteria determined by somebody, when the individuals who established those criteria really didn't have any motivation to go into trance." (Chapter Fourteen.)

Drawing from her clinical experience, she lectured about the power of belief and its potential effect on physiology, and demonstrated her understanding in her pioneering work with pain control and mind-body communication, again far ahead of her time. In 1972 (Chapter Seventeen), she confronted the accepted views about pain by showing a film depicting her own surgery at a Society for

Experimental and Clinical Hypnosis meeting (SECH), to force the attention of the established order.

At that time, there was a controversy among hypnotherapists about whether people actually learned to turn off pain with hypnosis or somehow denied the pain they were experiencing. All agreed, however, that skin is sensitive and that procedures involving trauma to skin really do hurt. This film forced many of the prominent teachers in the field to admit that they couldn't explain how Thompson could have undergone that kind of surgery by merely denying pain.

Thompson used suggestion and motivation to direct her clients in therapy; if necessary she used quasi-logical explanations to convince her patients to do the "impossible" things she knew they could do with their bodies.

In the following clinical vignette, Thompson describes an unusual healing event.

Many years ago, when I was teaching a course in dental school, one student said his girlfriend had been a volunteer patient for one of his buddies, and his buddy had gotten an unintentional mechanical exposure of the nerve with the drill, and did I think anything could be done. And I went over [while she was in trance] and said she could deposit secondary dentin around the opening into that nerve and she could keep the nerve from being infected and I said, "I know you can do this!"

When we finished and she came out of trance, she said that when the other two (her boyfriend and his buddy) were talking to her, there was no conviction there. The difference was that I said, "I *know* you can do this!" and that she heard me, she believed me, and understood that it was something she could do. Fortunately, I have some follow-up on that, because six weeks later, we took an X-ray of that particular tooth, and the calcification had taken place over that exposed nerve. You can't do that, but you see she didn't know you couldn't do that, and she did it and they didn't need to have to do a root canal in that tooth (Chapter Six).

Thompson was passionate about the necessity for engaging clients' beliefs in their healing, years before many of the fascinating aspects of body-mind communication were generally accepted. Her equally insistent emphasis on not giving negative suggestions was far ahead of the very recent publications on the "nocebo" effect—the ability of negative beliefs and expectations to actually cause harm (Barsky et al., 2002). "Your best patients have all the worst things happen because you told them they would. Do you have the right to do that to your patients? I don't think you do. I know I don't." (Chapter Twenty-five.)

In a variety of poignant clinical stories, Thompson described how some of her terminally ill clients used hypnosis to choose when they were ready to die, empowering their control and dignity at a time when they were typically deprived of these fundamental resources (Chapter Fifteen). It is too early, even now, to know whether her understanding and teaching in this area will eventually become accepted in modern clinical practice.

Although she was pleased to "see" some of her clinical experiences verified by experimental research, she didn't let the lack of verifiable evidence limit her understanding of what she saw and dealt with on a daily basis. She observed that patients could "conceptually" control pain, outside of neurological and physiological pathways, and although she did not understand the mechanisms involved, she continued to help people manage their pain by asking them to do what they had the potential to do.

No one had ever given them permission before to do the wonderful things their bodies could do, she claimed. "We don't know what the limits (of body–mind communication) are," she often taught. However, she believed, because of her clinical experience, that some day these processes would be scientifically explained. Her courage lay in speaking the truth as she understood it, from her own personal exploration, clinical observation and experience.

However, Thompson followed significant research in her field and frequently discussed its importance.

I think that Candace Pert[1] made it clear that we are having an explosion of knowledge and understanding of the biochemical basis of

---

[1] Candace Pert, PhD, a research professor, is best known for her discovery of opiate receptors in the brain and as the author of *Molecules of Emotion*.

emotion and the body-mind connection. She demonstrates that we can, through hypnosis, imaging and suggestion, influence the immune system. There are a lot of us that have been saying this for forty years but nobody had ever given us scientific proof (Chapter Six).

Thompson's direct and implied emphasis on balance and self-regulation was fundamental in all her teaching and clinical work, and paralleled several humanistic and transpersonal therapies of her time. Her intuitive sense of what the client was lacking or needed provided the template for her clinical work.

Kay Thompson was dedicated to awakening the potential in others, and she used whatever keys were necessary to fit the locks she found. "I hold everything that they can be, not just who they are now. Otherwise, how will they grow?" she taught. She believed in the capacity of each person to awaken to his or her full potential, but understood what a "disturbing" understanding that could be. As she said repeatedly in her lectures, "I know that everybody *can* do these wonderful things, but whether they will or not is up to them."

However, she didn't wait patiently to see if they would. Instead, she placed part of the "willing" on the therapists' shoulders, teaching therapists how to motivate patients to "will" change, to truly *want* to change, and it then became the therapist's responsibility to encourage clients to draw from their wellspring of potential.

In the same way that her father and Erickson had patiently and lovingly nurtured her personal and professional development, she eagerly assumed that role with many people, including clients, students and colleagues. Just as importantly, she facilitated their access to unconscious process and their unlimited potential and challenged their belief systems about reality, so that new and more positive realities could emerge. It is not surprising that she played a prominent role in so many people's lives.

Although her work was presented within a humanistic framework and Ericksonian tradition, the transformational aspects of her work are akin to the process of some meditative or spiritual traditions. Several discussions by Thompson are found throughout this text about the similarities between hypnotic trance and meditative states, and she consistently defines the difference as a function of the purpose or motivation for the trance or state.

Thompson was very knowledgeable about the transpersonal[2] realm of consciousness, and she accepted transpersonal states as normative experiences that any serious hypnotherapist might encounter while exploring self-hypnosis. Through defining transpersonal experiences as just another kind of "learning experience", she encouraged clients and students to explore the wisdom and opportunities they offered and not become distracted by any "special" identification with them. When they occurred in client sessions, they were important suggestions or communications for utilization, always in the interest of helping the client. Through providing a "container" for her clients' and students' explorations and transformational journeys, she was also ahead of her time.

Through personally integrating her teaching, Thompson went further than many teachers and therapists were and are willing to go. The integrity of her being, as Betty Alice Erickson notes in her introduction to Part I, was a significant reflection of all her teaching. Other contributing authors have also illustrated numerous ways in which Thompson embodied her teaching. Modeling is profoundly inspiring and requires students to actively learn on many levels, including through unconscious awareness. Perhaps, through modeling, Thompson was actively entraining[3] her students' unconscious learning processes. In this way, as in so many others, Thompson was a pioneer.

Kay Thompson developed her unique and resourceful capacities through painstaking practice and dedication. She had an unusual ability to establish rapport with almost any client and was remarkably perceptive. Equally impressive was her capacity to be fierce, loving, playful and encouraging, according to the needs of her clients or audience, and to easily and quickly shift among these different positions.

---

[2] "[S]hared aspects of consciousness, which extend beyond the usual boundaries of body and ego and beyond the limitations of time and space"(Grof, 1988).

[3] "Entraining" is defined as "influencing or synchronizing with" (Rossi, 1996).

Her fierceness was reflected in her courage, determination and ethical integrity, and through tirelessly fighting in both clinical and political circles for everything she believed in. Her folksy sense of humor and frequent laughter transmitted a joy and pleasure in the moment for those lucky enough to share them with her. And those moments felt as though they were the most important moments for her at that time. She was totally present.

Thompson was primarily a clinician and master teacher. Her profound and lasting influence in the field of clinical hypnosis was through her teaching and its effect on practitioners in the field, many of whom went on to also become teachers. It is well known that she always credited Milton Erickson for being her mentor; however, it is beyond the scope of the present discussion to discern what aspects of her teaching were continuations of Erickson's legacy.

Her untimely death in May 1998 caught most of her students and colleagues by surprise. She lived less than a year after her diagnosis of cancer; a year spent teaching hypnosis throughout the world, fulfilling her obligations as a trustee of the American Dental Association (ADA), and managing her disease and pain. Prior to her diagnosis, she had mentioned to several people that she might write a book about her work with hypnosis, but this was not to be.

We cannot know what Kay Thompson would have included in a book about her clinical work, and this is in no way an effort to accomplish that task. She alone could have written that book. Our purpose is quite simple—to honor her legacy by collecting her most important teachings and providing them as a resource to colleagues and students of hypnosis and psychotherapy throughout the world.

We began that process through carefully examining all of her published articles, private papers, and her personal collection of both workshop and clinical tapes, and reviewing a wide selection of teaching tapes available from many different sources. It became evident during this review that Thompson's range of clinical expertise was often best exemplified during teaching workshops and panel discussions, and in her spontaneous answers to the wide range of questions posed by students and colleagues in these forums.

In order to make this available in written form, we transcribed tapes from those sources which we believe contain her most important teaching and have included numerous question-and-answer segments, which present teachings not included elsewhere in the text. As a result, this edition of her collected works contains what we consider to be both her most significant published articles and oral teachings.

Most of the material in this volume has not been previously available in print, and some material has never been available to the public, outside of the particular workshops where they were presented. This is the first time that Thompson's teaching legacy, both published and oral, has been collected for publication.

By the 1980s, she had already given more than 400 lectures and teaching workshops throughout the world. In order to cover the breadth of her teachings, we have included a wide range of subject matter, an extensive collection of her favorite metaphors, inductions, stories, and clinical vignettes, and a representative sample of her clinical demonstrations. As a result, this volume can serve as a general clinical guide to hypnosis and suggestion, the art of therapeutic communication and the use of hypnosis to control pain.

Kay Thompson's original lectures and workshops come alive with her inimitable spirit and extraordinary use of language. Excerpts have been chosen which reflect the depth of her experiential knowledge, her particular emphases, orientation and approaches, her dynamic and forceful personality and her playful hypnotic communications, as in: "You can become so entranced with really knowing all there is that you need to know about how to make the memory of that experience change into something that it wasn't when it began, only because you hadn't thought about it as being what you didn't think it was."

Insightful clinical discussions, discerning responses to questions, ingenious hypnotic suggestions and examples of verbal gymnastics for speaking to the unconscious process represent part of the large spectrum of Kay Thompson's abilities with language. However, her vocabulary was purposefully both simple and general in order that a broad spectrum of listeners could interpret her teaching and use it for whatever they needed to learn or know at that time. For example, the words *feeling* and *pain* were often subjects of Thompson's thoughtful communications, as in, "Feeling in itself need not be painful. You can use real pain to hide painful feelings. When you learn you can utilize feelings other than having to have painful ones, than you don't need to have so much real pain"(Chapter Sixteen).

Thompson's passionate zeal in conveying what she considered to be key ideas in hypnotherapy is reflected in the variety of ways they are offered for the reader's consideration. Her teachings are presented both directly with explanation and example, and indirectly, woven throughout her workshops and lectures in stories, clinical vignettes, metaphors and demonstrations.

When reading this text, one can "hear" her enthusiasm while teaching about her vast repertoire of therapeutic interventions, such as challenging limited realities, deconstructing language and meaning, doing the unexpected, suggesting new perspectives, evoking child's play and imagination when anything can become anything, and then waiting patiently for the mystery to unfold and for horizons to expand.

Kay Thompson utilized every part of herself in her work, using her voice to embody her messages by means of changes of tone, inflection, emphasis, phrasing and rhythm, engaging audiences worldwide. Hypnosis is an oral art and Thompson's performances were among the most sophisticated in the field.

Her "live" presentation was such an important part of her teaching, that we have created a CD as an accompaniment to this volume. It would be impossible to claim that this was a collected works without having also collected her spoken voice. Some of her most memorable teaching has been included for the readers' learning and enjoyment (see Appendix II).

Just as Thompson encouraged her students to study with a variety of teachers, we feel that it is important that readers have access to multiple perspectives about the impact of her work. As a close friend once remarked, "Kay was *art*." In order to provide a variety of perspectives on her work and offer examples of her "living art" for the reader's interest, we have invited close colleagues and students to participate in this volume. Respected colleagues introduce some of her teaching, comment on her influence on their work, and discuss her contributions to clinical hypnosis.

Kay Thompson's teachings have been arranged into general sections in this volume to create a basic organizational structure. However, her multilevel communications make some of these categories hazy, at the very least. Thompson was renowned for weaving suggestion, motivation and utilization into most of her teaching and therapeutic communications, and the majority of material in this volume is infused with these therapeutic messages.

Many chapters in this volume could be perceived on a metalevel as containing a series of ideas and suggestions, followed by metaphors or analogies as examples, and then motivating messages and reinforcing directions. Even brief comments are often presented within a similar structure, as in: "Why is this important to you? Because you are a healer. Because you constantly have the potential to influence other people. This is what you want to do. This is what you *chose* to do."

Both the complexity of her messages and their beguiling simplicity, and the poetic manner in which they are presented, offer the reader a unique opportunity to savor this text, as a collection of art whose depth and richness continue to expand with each visit.

Betty Alice Erickson and Bernhard Trenkle introduce Part I, "Hypnotherapy: The Basic Principles of Therapeutic Practice", which opens with a general introduction to hypnosis, followed by four of Thompson's most outstanding articles, which form the corpus of her conceptual teachings.

Camillo Loriedo and Dan Kohen introduce Part II, "The Language of Hypnosis". The two chapters in this section "Language to Effect Change" and "Metaphor, Analogy and Word Play Development", derive from workshops and contain a wide collection of Kay Thompson's inspired teaching about the language of hypnosis.

Part III, "The Nature of Trance", contains an introduction by Akira Otani, important discussions about aspects of trance and wonderful illustrations of trance inductions, including a self-hypnotic technique, conversational trances and dual inductions. Roxanna Erickson Klein introduces Part IV, "Suggestion and Utilization". These critical subjects are explored through a variety of imaginative perspectives and illustrations, including an especially fascinating collection of Thompson's thinking about the nature of suggestion.

Part V, "Therapy with Pain", is introduced by Alexander Levitan and contains most of Thompson's key teachings on the use of hypnotherapy for working with pain. Part VI, "A Holistic Approach to Dentistry", has introductions by Harold Golan and Peo Wikstrom, and contains Thompson's seminal contribution on the psychological importance of the oral cavity and a thorough discussion of the utilization of hypnosis in dentistry.

Part VII, "Clinical Demonstrations", is introduced by Sidney Rosen and presents a unique collection of fascinating clinical demonstrations by Thompson. A selection of her key teaching on ethics from a variety of panel discussions comprises Part VIII, "Ethics in Caring".

Part IX, "The Personal Impact of Hypnosis", contains two chapters, a prepared lecture from Thompson's private papers on the impact of hypnosis on her life and personal reflections in "Why we should learn hypnosis".

The first appendix contains two fascinating narratives, followed by a collection of teaching vignettes. Ralph Krichbaum, Kay Thompson's husband, has written, a memoir, illustrating Kay Thompson's "living art", with an interesting collection of stories about her life. Russell Scott, PhD, one of Kay Thompson's closest friends and colleagues, publicly discusses her role as a clinical psychotherapist for the first time and shares a variety of intriguing stories about some of their professional "escapades".

Much of Kay Thompson's influence was a direct result of her masterful teaching. Students and colleagues whose lives were significantly impacted by her teaching were invited to share glimpses of her extraordinary presence and its effect on their work and lives. Their vignettes follow Karen Olness's introduction, "Kay Thompson: The Consummate Educator". Information about the selected tracks on the accompanying CD is listed in Appendix II.

The expected boundaries between patient, student, colleague and friend were blurred when working with Thompson, as with Erickson. Readers will note that many of her colleagues and friends were originally her students, and some were her patients, and that her mentoring and encouragement transformed these relationships over time into deep friendships.

Many of our contributing authors have commented about her "casual" teaching and therapy woven into a seamless generosity of giving, regardless of normative cultural boundaries. She was unobtrusively doing dual inductions at parties, giving hypnotic suggestions during all kinds of interpersonal interactions, working with students and colleagues at professional meetings until late at night; every moment seemed to be an opportunity for her to teach and help others.

Numerous stories of Thompson "tuning in" to others and selflessly offering her help, guidance and even "amazing" clinical expertise have been shared by the large group of colleagues, friends and students we have contacted; there is no way that we can possibly present or even allude to the range or extent of her boundless generosity. For example, in her vignette, Stacie Murrer tells about how Thompson helped a child who was losing her vision and comments that "Kay was involved daily in helping people achieve unusual events".

When the seeds she planted and nurtured in so many of us sprouted and grew and blossomed, she smiled with the pleasure of a mother who has given birth. But she always acknowledged the person's movement, achievement or growth as his or her own and identified herself as the "helper" or "guide".

We honor her with this collected edition of her teaching and with our commitment to continue her legacy, by opening doors for others.

Saralee Kane MSW

References

Barsky, A. J., Saintfort, R., Rogers, M. P. and Borus, J. F. (2002). "Nonspecific medication side effects and the nocebo phenomenon", *JAMA*, 287(5): 622–7.

Grof, S. (1988). *The Adventure of Self-discovery: Dimensions of consciousness and new perspectives in psychotherapy and inner exploration*, Albany, NY: State University of New York Press.

Memorial Service for Kay Thompson (1998). Quote from one of the speakers.

Rossi, E. L. (1996). *The Symptom Path to Enlightenment: The new dynamics of self-organization in hypnotherapy*, Pacific Palisades, CA: Palisades Gateway.

Thompson, K. (1998). "How I Got to Be What I Am Becoming", from Dr Thompson's private papers, for an address she gave to the American Society for Clinical Hypnosis in March, 1998.

Part I
Hypnotherapy

The Basic Principles of
Therapeutic Practice

Part I opens with discussions by Betty Alice Erickson and Bernhard Trenkle about Kay Thompson's contributions to hypnotherapy. In "Ericksonian at Heart", Betty Alice Erickson illustrates numerous ways in which Thompson continued Erickson's legacy through modeling and teaching its most important aspects, and then she relates a personal story about Thompson's elegant therapeutic intervention with her son. Bernhard Trenkle follows with a remarkable anecdote about learning the importance of motivation, one of Thompson's most passionate teaching themes.

In Chapter One, "An Introduction to Hypnosis", Thompson presents a fundamental structure for understanding hypnosis through exploring the mechanics of trance, hypnotic techniques and approaches, fallacies about hypnosis and different kinds of trance. Some of her favorite conversational trance inductions end the chapter.

The following four articles contain the corpus of Dr. Thompson's teaching about the principles of therapeutic practice. In Chapter Two, "The Curiosity of Milton H. Erickson, MD", Kay Thompson defines Erickson's innate curiosity and humanity as the heart of his therapeutic presence. His curiosity is expressed in really listening and observing and creatively intervening, while his humanity unfolds into a powerful and compassionate belief and respect in both the uniqueness and potential of each individual. With distinctive clarity, Kay Thompson describes what she learned from Erickson and shares a wealth of important insights about his work.

1

In Chapter Three, "Almost 1984", Kay Thompson discusses the misuse of Erickson's name and legacy and debunks some myths about Erickson's work. Change *is* the primary focus of therapy, and therapists must both do whatever is necessary to help their clients change, and be "all the someones needed at whatever times they are needed", according to Kay Thompson. Her ability to convey the intensity of her principled messages within a natural playfulness is especially evident in this article.

"Metaphor: A Myth with a Method" contains many of Kay Thompson's key contributions to the art of therapeutic communication. In this chapter she explores the many ways that language and metaphor can be used to elicit change, through bypassing conscious processes and accessing unconscious potential. She also illustrates how metaphor encourages clients to look at things differently and expand their options, and emphasizes how stories need to be matched to the individual's experiential life and understanding, so the resources can be retrieved that the person needs, to generalize learning to present and future experiences.

Chapter Five, "Motivation and the Multiple Levels of Trance", presents one of the significant contributions Kay Thompson has made to clinical hypnosis and psychotherapy in general—the importance of motivation in therapy. "Making the listener *want* to hear what needs to be said," is a very critical skill, according to Kay Thompson. Using a phenomenological approach, she delineates six types of trance and offers an important model for distinguishing types of trance, through looking at the purpose of the trance, and the motivation of the practitioner and the person entering trance.

Ericksonian at Heart

Betty Alice Erickson

Kay wasn't known so much for her writings—she put most of her energies into teaching and "being and doing". She was and is strongly identified with the "Ericksonian" movement, and in fact, she was central to the continuation and refinement of many approaches that have come to be identified as Ericksonian. Wise enough to know that what she had learned from Erickson had become her own, she also knew that what she identified as Ericksonian would influence others in a far-reaching way. This burden of responsibility, which she gracefully sought and accepted, was undertaken in ways which were far different from most of her contemporaries. She never attempted to mimic, define, describe, distill or even explain the effective yet elusive work done by a man whose work could not be defined or explained in words. Kay approached from a different direction—the experiential whole of simply being.

Originally, she only wanted to learn hypnosis from Erickson. But she found a loving sponsor, someone who recognized her potential, mentored her, encouraged her and helped her develop her own internal skills and strengths. Kay understood the depths of this process and development and dedicated herself to giving back to others and to the community as a whole.

In Kay, Erickson found a bright, energetic protégé who could carry his work forward as well as develop her own unique and considerable talents. He saw a woman of integrity, whom he could trust on both personal and professional levels. In breaking both political and professional gender barriers, Kay developed great internal strength. She used this formidable asset throughout her life to help her endure and overcome the problems and strife that inevitably accompany professional and organizational development.

Erickson mentored Kay's participation with the American Society of Clinical Hypnosis (ASCH), which he had founded. Both of them were aware that the long-term success of the ASCH depended on a successful transition from those who had fathered the organization to the new generation of professionals. With Erickson's confidence in her innate abilities and knowing that together they could accomplish more than either could individually, she became more and more involved. Erickson coaxed, guided, reassured, instructed and, at times, even emphatically told her how to proceed. Sometimes Kay listened to his counsel; sometimes she disagreed and argued vigorously. Always, she made her own decisions and always Erickson respected those decisions.

Kay became president of the ASCH in 1972 in a way that still inspires awe. She was not only the first female president, but she won on a write-in ballot! She then played a key role in moving the ASCH from a group dependent on the leadership and presence of Erickson, to a professional society standing on its own merits and going in its own direction.

Clearly, there was a great deal of turbulence and political strife during this transition. Without Kay's decisive and insightful leadership, the organization might not have risen to the position of international respect that it now holds.

The two worked harmoniously in many areas. Kay excelled as a protégé and Erickson deeply admired her abilities, especially in communication. Her intuitions, her innate playfulness, and her disciplined diligence allowed her to excel in giving therapeutic messages beyond what any other student of Erickson had done or has yet done.

After Erickson's death, she remained faithful by crediting him for what she had learned from him, and continued to build on her exceptional skill of teaching healing through hypnosis. She understood Erickson's dictums of "say only what is necessary" and "trust your patient's unconscious". She was able to do this much as Erickson did—in ways that cannot be captured within the limits of written words.

Though many learned from her in teaching settings, she refused to confine teaching to these arenas. Like Erickson, she saw every moment as yet another opportunity to teach and give. Those privileged to spend time in her company found it difficult to know where the "official" teaching began or ended and where friendly conversation began or ended.

When my son David was 5, he had been intentionally frightened and even threatened with a spanking by a dentist on his very first checkup. I asked Kay for help when she was visiting our family a few months later. I told her what had happened and she spent the whole evening talking with David, playing with him, and essentially ignoring the adults. At the end of the visit, she held David in her arms as she made her goodbyes. Almost as an afterthought, she looked directly into his eyes and asked, "Do you know what I do?"

This unusual question prompted an immediate trance in David and he waited, puzzled, for what she was going to say next. In measured tones she said, "I am a dentist." David, dumbfounded, continued to stare at her. "There are men dentists and lady dentists. There are good dentists and bad dentists." The two looked at each other for a moment while the little boy processed this new information.

Nothing more was ever said to him. He consciously forgot the interaction with Kay and the unfortunate encounter with the first dentist. Years later, after a mouth injury required considerable dental work, I told him I thought he was very brave. He looked surprised and repeated what Kay had told him so long ago: "There are good dentists and bad dentists." Then he added, "I've been lucky. I've always had good dentists." David's recollection that he "always had good dentists" illustrates the profound impact that Kay was able to make. Not only had the initial harm been compensated for, it was as if the trauma had never existed. In one evening's work, she provided David with a new foundation of strength from which to face the rest of his life.

The dictum, that the "dental work is inside your head" is the fundamental point from which she embarked on the important therapeutic work which she did—work which has become so integrated into standards of dentistry, that the time can hardly be remembered when it was not there.

Kay Thompson will live forever—in the hearts of those who knew her, in those who didn't know her but who have reaped the benefits of her work, and in the heart of Ericksonian work.

Motivation: One of the Deepest Trances
Bernhard Trenkle

A year after attending a hypnosis workshop that I sponsored, I contracted terrible tooth pain and needed a root canal. My dentist, who had also attended the workshop, asked me, "Do you want an injection or do you want to do it with hypnosis?"

That was a question of honor. On the one hand, I had motivated this dentist to attend the hypnosis workshop and tried to convince him that hypnosis was a helpful tool for dentists. On the other hand, I had no experience with hypnotic analgesia and was not sure it would work. I also was insecure that I could accomplish what was expected.

My pride won out. "I will do it with hypnosis," I nervously proclaimed. The dentist meant self-hypnosis, as I soon found out, and he started to work. I looked at the ceiling and found a little spot to focus on. Desperately, I hoped that my unconscious mind would know what to do. Soon I was in such a deep trance, that I heard my dentist saying to the nurse that the nerve of my tooth must be dead. He could not believe that someone could remain absolutely relaxed and motionless, with almost no visible breathing during the surgery.

When the treatment was over, I reoriented myself back from what appeared to be a very deep trance. After 20 years of experience with hypnosis, I can say that it was one of the deepest trances I have ever experienced.

I had learned experientially what Kay Thompson was teaching about motivation throughout her professional career. She continually emphasized the importance of understanding the relevance of the situation and how the motivation of the subject can lead to deeper hypnotic phenomena.

In her article on motivation, Kay explains that trance is an altered state of awareness and that such states are not discrete but exist on a continuum. Trance behavior, even in the same person, may vary from trance to trance. The differences can be understood by examining the purpose of the trance and the motivations of the practitioner and the patient.

Kay Thompson concludes, "The basic difference I see is motivation." Techniques and the type of the trance induction are less important than the motivations of the people involved. Kay Thompson critically explains, "We are often focusing on the vehicle, while the important aspect is the journey and even more important, the destination."

Kay was a very impressive person. She was one of those people I always impatiently looked forward to meeting again at the regular conferences. With her enormous heart and keen intelligence she reflected the best aspects of the development of the field of hypnosis. I remember our discussions in the early nineties about the fact that mostly men were teaching at the hypnosis conferences and that only a few exceptional women had been on the faculty of our International and European conferences. In one of our dialogues the idea was born to organize hypnosis conferences where only women were allowed to teach in order to motivate more women to teach and to share their wisdom and knowledge.

The conference in Germany took place in 1994; it was successful and gave a boost to the field. Now we have many more women teaching hypnosis here in Germany. This is only one of the many examples of how Kay was influencing the field of hypnosis and how her motivation so inspired others.

Chapter One
An Introduction to Hypnosis

History

In all countries, people have fallen into altered states of mind, more or less closely resembling the hypnotic state. This has understandably excited the wonder and curiosity of people who were looking at these states.

There is evidence that many aspects of trance were known and used by our ancestors. Some of the earliest allusions to suggestion can be found in Paleolithic bone carvings and cave paintings. One of these shows a picture of a deerlike individual standing over the body of a pregnant woman. The obvious interpretation is that the strength of the animal will pass through into the woman, so that she will be able to endure the difficulty of giving birth a little easier. That kind of sympathetic magic was understood and recorded something like 30,000 years ago. We have traditions of medicine men who treated people who were evidently in pain. They threw bones, breathed into the people's eyes and mouths, and the individuals would go into some kind of a trance or stupor and get better.

For many centuries, Persian magi produced self-induced trances by staring at precious stones. Temple sleep, popular in Egypt about 200 B.C., probably relied on the principles of trance and hypnotic suggestion. And from time immemorial, Indian yogis have utilized many autohypnotic-like skills to achieve astonishing physiological and meditative feats.

All kinds of forms of self-trance have been utilized throughout the years. It has only been more recently that we have begun to use the term *hypnosis*.

The probable forerunner of current hypnosis is the mesmerism of Franz Anton Mesmer, a Viennese physician active in the 1770s. He proposed that the influence of the heavenly bodies on the fluid forces in human beings could cause many maladies and that magnetism could reverse these processes, resulting in convulsions and miraculous cures.

He used his animal magnetism and his magnet, and over a period of time, his patient, who had migraines, was free from symptoms. As a result of the notoriety that his "animal magnetism" received, a commission appointed by the French Academy of Science investigated the phenomenon very carefully and came to the conclusion that imagination was everything and magnetism was nothing. But they didn't recognize what they were saying, that imagination is everything. They didn't pursue the idea of what happened with the magnetism or the imagination or suggestion.

It was the Marquis de Puysegur who, in 1784, discovered the somnambulistic state of hypnosis rather than the usual convulsion response. Other phenomena that we use today, including hypnoanesthesia, hallucinations and posthypnotic suggestions, quickly developed from this discovery. In 1837 the French Academy of Science witnessed the first recorded demonstration of hypnotic anesthesia when a dentist member, Dr. Oudet, extracted a tooth from a patient without any pain. Since anesthetics were unknown at that time, this was indeed a novel development.

In 1841, an English physician, Dr. James Braid, took hypnosis out of the realm of the charlatan with the recognition that hypnosis could be attained without a formalistic induction. It was he who coined the term *hypnosis*, from the Greek word *hypnos*, meaning sleep. Braid was responsible for giving us the theory of eye fixation. He held bottles above people's heads and recognized that hypnosis was a response to sensory stimuli, and people would respond by going into this quiet sleep state, which was really good.

During this same period, a Scottish physician, Dr. James Esdaile, was performing surgery in India using hypnoanesthesia. He recorded 261 operations with a startlingly low mortality rate of 5.5%. Since sterility was not yet recognized and mortality rates generally were 90% for surgical procedures, it appears that Esdaile's technique involved some control beyond simple anesthesia. The attention this report might have received was diverted because it appeared in 1837, the year that gas anesthesia was introduced. Since gas anesthesia was more reliable and more readily explainable than hypnosis, it quickly became more popular. Interest in hypnotism declined by 1850.

Early in the 1900s, Sigmund Freud and Joseph Breuer did some work with hypnosis but soon abandoned it. Freud was not comfortable using hypnosis. Also, when he developed and publicized the dynamics of free association, these techniques became so popular that hypnosis was eclipsed. Freud did comment, however, that group hypnosis would be the only possible method to use for mass psychotherapy.

Nothing further of note occurred until there was a resurgence of interest in hypnosis following World Wars I and II. This interest after World War I came about as the need for treating large numbers of shell-shocked victims increased and the time-consuming process of psychoanalysis fell short. Hypnosis offered an effective and more rapid method of treatment for what we now call posttraumatic stress disorder (PTSD).

Hypnosis was the best and most effective way to treat these people, who came back from the war with various neuroses. This was the beginning of the resurgence in hypnosis, both experimentally and clinically. Since the end of World War II, interest in hypnosis has been maintained by health care professionals in research, in both experimental and clinical situations. Dr. Clark L. Hull of Yale University is credited with classic experimental work in hypnosis in the 1930s. One of his students, Milton H. Erickson, became the individual most responsible for the current views regarding clinical hypnosis. He worked and published exhaustively on the subject for almost 50 years. He is credited with recognizing that trance is a natural capacity of the patient and that the unconscious potential of the individual can be tapped to assist in attitudinal changes.

Description

Hypnosis is an altered state of consciousness. How many of you hear the clock strike and recognize that you haven't been thinking

11

about anything for the last half-hour? How many of you hear a commercial on the radio and find out it's stuck in your head and can't get it out? When you listen to the radio, how many of you listen for the weather report and you hear, "the weather report is coming, here's the weather report," but you don't hear it because you have been in a trance? You have been in an altered state of consciousness. It's not new. We all do it. Hypnosis is simply learning to do it and to focus it a little bit better for your benefit. It taps into those behaviors about the commercial or the weather report you didn't hear.

The building blocks for hypnosis are verbal and nonverbal communication. The psychologist says, "How do you and your husband get along?" And the individual says, "Oh, yes, I love my husband very much," and the head is shaking side to side. Do you believe the nonverbal or the verbal? You have direct or indirect suggestions. You have a solitary cough in a room which sets off a lot of coughing. I could ask, "Please get me a glass of water," or grab my throat and cough and clear my throat. They are both giving the same message.

Hypnosis is a state of hyperacuity. Most people think about it being a detached, unaware kind of state. It's not. It is a highly focused state, wherein sensory and motor capacities are altered in order to initiate appropriate behavior. The term *appropriate* is the ringer there. In utilizing hypnosis, appropriate behavior may be simply relaxation. Or it may be the kind of state I'm in right now in order to keep my mind functioning, know what it is I want to talk about, think about what I'm going to say before I say it, and if it isn't appropriate, change my mind. That's every bit as much of a trance as the relaxed kind of zombie state people associate with trance.

Hypnosis is a natural, normal state that can be utilized in the doctor–patient relationship. The emphasis is on the natural and normal state that can be utilized. It is not an abnormal state of mind. It is not an unnatural state. It is something that people do all the time, particularly in the doctor–patient relationship, because in that doctor–patient relationship, you have a special stress develop. All hypnosis is autohypnosis. I have never hypnotized anyone except for myself. I cannot. I am a reasonably good teacher and have taught a lot of people how to go into trance.

Myths and Misconceptions

Hypnosis is not unconsciousness. Individuals can hear and remember trance. People thought that amnesia was a part of the trance. It is not necessarily a part of trance. That also means that if it is appropriate, it may be a part of the trance.

One common misconception is that only weak-minded, gullible persons can be "hypnotized". Actually, it takes effort, concentration, and intelligence to go into trance. The only people who cannot really learn how to go into trance are people who have a low IQ. The smarter you are, the better able you are to utilize hypnosis.

There is no surrender of will or loss of autonomy during the trance. Frequently, people suspect that if they go into trance, they will have to follow the orders of the person who is teaching them to go into trance. Erickson would instruct the patient that at some point when he asked them to do something, to deliberately not do it, so they would demonstrate to themselves that *they had control* over the trance. It is a normal, natural state of hyperacuity wherein your own best skills are enhanced and utilized. Surrendering your will or losing your autonomy certainly does not lend itself to that.

Hypnosis is not related to being asleep, even though one of its phenomena may be extreme relaxation that resembles sleep. The EEG of the patient in a trance more closely resembles his EEG when he is awake than asleep, as do blood pressure, pulse rate and other vital signs. The person is aware and can talk and function in any way necessary for his understanding of the situation.

Since the individual knows what is occurring, there is no possibility that he will reveal any secrets because of the trance. Many people are also concerned that if they are hypnotized, they will come out of the trance at the wrong time or not be able to come out of the trance at all. Since the individual is aware and responsible during the trance, there is no basis for this concern. The trance is easily terminated once the patient understands that it is time to do so and that the goal for which the hypnotic state was entered has been achieved.

13

The trance state is not a truth serum state. Dr. Lewis Wolberg[4] had a case where a woman brought in her husband to be hypnotized so she could question him about whether he was having an affair. The husband went into trance and he assured his wife that he loved only her and wasn't carrying on with the widow next door and besides there wasn't any time. Dr. Wolberg felt very good because he had saved the marriage. A couple of weeks later, Dr. Wolberg met the husband on the street who freely admitted that he was having an affair with the widow and thanked the doctor for getting his wife off his back.

Appropriate Use

Except for Christian Scientists and Seventh Day Adventists, every major religion has accepted the utilization of hypnosis in the health professions. The recognition of the self-control that hypnosis gives people, gives it religious acceptability. Some professionals work with hypnosis all the time, but don't use the name *hypnosis*. If all you are doing is medical relaxation, and you don't use the term, there's no problem with it.

Hypnosis gets blamed for the individuals manipulating this tool. If a surgeon does surgery and leaves a sponge in the patient, the surgeon gets blamed. If there is a problem with hypnosis, it isn't the dentist, the physician or the therapist that gets blamed, it's the hypnosis. That's one of the things that the public needs to understand. It is a tool, the same way as my instruments, the physician's scalpel, the anesthesiologist's IV is a tool. It is the person who utilizes the tool who must be ethical and responsible for what they do.

Hypnosis is not a panacea. It is not a cure-all. It should be utilized when it is appropriate, when it has the potential for helping the individual, and in a fashion when you and your patient are going to benefit from its utilization, as with your other tools. We do expect

---

[4] A former assitant clinical professor of psychiatry at New York Medical College, who authored numerous articles on hypnosis, including an extensive treatise on medical hypnosis in the 1940s.

that you are going to be able to do your medicine, dentistry and therapy better because you can help your patient accept what you have the training and skill to offer. That's what hypnosis can do for your practice, not to mention what it can do for you in your personal life.

Personally, hypnosis is probably the best thing that has happened to me in my life. If someone passed a law tomorrow and said, nobody can use hypnosis again, I would say, "Okay." But that wouldn't stop me from using it for and with myself. That aspect of it, if no other, if it didn't help my patients at all, would have made it worth the 40-plus years teaching and working with it.

My involvement as a dentist has a different kind of intensity. I can understand psychotherapy in terms of reframing and reorienting the individual. With surgery, it isn't just inside your head, it's inside your physiology that you have to change. Looking at those kinds of things that people are able to do, gives me such a respect for the tremendous ability of the person going into that trance. I have no end of wonder about what it is that people can do. Every operation that can be done has been done using hypnosis as the sole anesthetic. It has been used to control pain and bleeding and increase the speed of healing.

No, it isn't going to work with everybody or for everybody. When the need is there, people do the most wonderful things. And hypnosis is a way of enabling them to do that. That gives you a really good feeling when you can help somebody to do that.

Mechanics of Trance

The mechanics of trance include concentration, belief and motivation. This is the reason why the person who is mentally disabled has trouble. Yes, you can work with this kind of person, but you have to be very skillful and keep refocusing their attention so they can concentrate on the idea you want them to realize.

One principle of hypnosis is that when attention is concentrated on an idea, that idea tends toward realization. You are alone for the weekend and you've turned out lights, locked doors and have started upstairs to bed. You hear a noise and you stop and think about what that noise might be. You think about someone trying the door, somebody opening the window and every possible way an intruder could break into your home. You take a deep breath and go downstairs and find that a pen you left on the table has rolled off and fallen on the floor. While you were concentrating on whether an intruder was breaking into your house, every muscle, nerve and fiber of your being was focused on that, and you were really thinking about it or concentrating on it.

The second mechanical aspect of trance involves belief. Belief is a double-edged sword. The individual has to believe that something good can happen. You must understand that the patient can go into trance—whether they *will* or not is negotiable. It depends on their motivation, it depends on their concentration, it depends on whether they like the way you part your hair. The belief system has to be there for that patient, that *something different* can happen. In many of the experiments that are designed, that are standardized, you do not have that belief. In the experimental context, you have to be objective, and maybe even objective to the point that you put it on a tape recorder. The belief system is not there. The lack of belief on the part of the experimenter "trance-lates" itself for the person who is listening, and what they hear is a lack of conviction as though it doesn't work. That lack of belief on the part of the experimenter is a really difficult experience to get beyond in the experimental situation.

One of Erickson's favorite techniques, when he was teaching hypnosis, was to use a subject who could develop all of the phenomena of hypnosis. He would tell group A that she—the subject—was a really, really good subject, but she couldn't do anesthesia; group B that she was really, really good and could do all these neat things but couldn't do amnesia. They could try amnesia but it wouldn't work. And he'd tell group C that she was really, really good, could do amnesia and anesthesia but couldn't do positive hallucinations. After the practice, each group found she couldn't do what Erickson had said she couldn't do. Where did the inability to do anesthesia amnesia or hallucinations come from? It came from the conviction on the part of the individuals who were working with her.

We don't have the right to presume what the patient cannot do. We need to work with that patient with the expectation that they can do everything they need to do. Whether they will do it or not depends on our skill and their motivation. I firmly feel that motivation is the most critical factor in the utilization of hypnosis. If somebody comes in and says, "I have tried everything and I'm really desperate and I really need this," then I'm going to spend as much time as necessary to help that patient learn it. When the motivation is there, the individual can learn. Sometimes it will take longer than others. You learn to develop a sense of each individual's motivation.

You also learn how to *enhance* that motivation. That's part of our job as health professionals, to be able to make the individual recognize how valuable this tool will be for them and how much it can do for them. When they recognize that, that's really all that they need to do. There are different types of motivation and those are all valid. We need to identify them, work with them and enhance them, so the patient can be the very best that they have the potential to be.

Techniques

If you just talk at somebody, like in approaches with deep relaxation, how do you know if anything is happening? How do they know if anything is happening? There is no feedback, all you are doing is just talking. With structured approaches, you get the opportunity of physiological feedback. Levitation is one of the best techniques because something is happening that the patient isn't controlling. If that can happen, then maybe one of these other things can happen outside of their conscious control, like stopping smoking, losing weight or using hypnosis as anesthetic.

There are at least one hundred induction techniques. There are the permissive techniques, the authoritarian techniques, the imaginative and the startle. If you are permissive and try to be authoritarian, it's not going to go over very well. Your voice is an instrument, it's a tool. You need to recognize what you are comfortable with, then that particular approach is one that is good for you. Most authoritarian people don't like to admit they are authoritarian when working with hypnosis. How do you find out? You record your voice and hear what your voice is saying, and hear what the words mean. If there is a dissonance there, then you need to change it. Instead of saying, "I would like for you to ..." you say *"You will find ..."* Recognize that is okay. That's your personality, that's what you are comfortable with.

Develop techniques and verbalizations that fit with your approach. The imagination is something we all work with. There's something really nice about closing your eyes and being in a canoe on a lake rather than sitting in a dental office. If you are really canoeing, you can't be here in this dental office so you can ignore what I am doing. The startle is not used often, except on stage. It literally startles the individual to retreat into trance. I have used it once in all my years with a 2-year-old hysterical child who had a toothache. I didn't know what else to do, so I startled her. By doing that we broke up the hysteria and I gave her an instruction to go to sleep. She went to sleep because she was so surprised that I was giving her an avenue of escape. In general, it's not a technique that nice people like to utilize.

With informal approaches, you rely on your own knowledge of that individual. You rely on conversational or other indirect approaches to achieve trance. You need to understand where your clients come from. You need to know enough about them to be able to pique their curiosity, to get them to follow the story on both the conscious and the unconscious level so they can utilize it in a way that is going to be helpful for them.

Every time I work with someone, I learn something new. With every patient I see and with every class I teach, I am learning and refining and enhancing my own skills. You need a wealth of experience, knowing what the patient is communicating both verbally and nonverbally before you can go into the utilization of the indirect techniques. You need to write out your induction techniques, especially if you are going to use metaphor and analogy.

Hypnotic Phenomena and Depth of Trance

Sample hypnotic phenomena include relaxation, anesthesia, amnesia, regression, dissociation, time distortion, physiological controls and posthypnotic suggestion, like you *will* enjoy yourselves these next two days. When I made a reference to think about what I'm going to say next and to modify what I am saying, that is time distortion. It's a very useful phenomenon.

The depth of trance is the state necessary to achieve the desired response, affected by motivation and sophistication. There are some people who will only do whatever it is they need to do for that particular phase of their work and will not do anything else. There are some people who in a medium trance can demonstrate anesthesia. There are other people in a very deep trance who will never demonstrate anesthesia, because this is not something that is important to them.

Hypnoidal trance is kind of, well, maybe they are going to do something or maybe they're not. Light, medium, deep, somnambulistic and plenary are the ways that people identify different levels of trance. I really think I've only seen a couple of plenary trances, which is when the person is totally unresponsive because they are in their own self-controlled state. We have a past president of the ASCH who had to have a cardiac catheter and was quite concerned about it. We had done some talking ahead of time, and after the procedure, her sister called me and said she wouldn't come out of this state and wouldn't pay attention to anyone around her. I said, "You need to tell her that she needs to tell the physician that she's fine and there's nothing wrong, that they should let her alone, and that she'll be able to go home and plant her tomato seeds." Her sister told her this. This woman, who had been in her particular plenary trance for 48 hours, came out and said to her doctors: "For Pete's sake, leave me alone! Don't you understand I'm doing what I need to do and I am perfectly fine?" She went right back in the plenary trance and they let her alone. That's what she needed for her own well-being. We need to respect that in the individual.

Termination of Trance

Termination of trance isn't difficult; it just needs to be appropriate. The patient needs to understand that it's time for the trance to be over. Termination of trance occurs when it's understood that the trance is no longer necessary. It can be maintained for widely varied time spans.

One of the more impressive examples of trance I am aware of, was with someone who was born with a cleft palate and wanted to have it repaired. They swung a graft from his left arm into the roof of his mouth and he had to walk around like that for a few weeks, which is not an easy thing to do. He chose to do it in trance. They did not put a cast on his arm, which is the normal procedure. They put a piece of adhesive tape from his forehead to his forearm so he would remember to walk with his mouth open. It was better to sleep like that and he did it very, very well. The impressive thing was not only that he could do that for three weeks. It was when they cut him loose, he was able to regain full use of his hand and his arm mobility within that day. That was the thing that really impressed the team of doctors working with him.

Language about Relationship

We talk about an operator and subject in hypnosis. Why do we do that? "Operator" doesn't have a good connotation, because it has an association of someone who is kind of smooth and sleazy and not real nice. Why do we call the people who work with hypnosis, operators? Why do we call the patients who are utilizing hypnosis, their subjects? You are subject to the orders of the king, the laws of the land. Whenever you are a subject in an experiment, you are in a one-down position, aren't you?

Why do we use the terms *operator* and *subject* and put ourselves in a one-down position with the phenomena of hypnosis? Why do we say, "I hypnotized her", when the only person I have ever hypnotized is myself? Why do we say, "I put him deeper into trance" for precisely the same reason. Why do we do it? Because it's easier and because it's shorter and because we are lazy. With operator, it's a doctor, the therapists, the health professional, whomever. The subject is a patient, a client, most of all a person, not a subject. Instead of "I hypnotized her", use "I taught her how to go into trance". It takes longer and may raise questions you may have to answer. Because we are economical in our language we take the short cut. "He went deeper into a trance" is pretty obvious, but it's not what we learned. Learn to say the language this way, so the people can be more comfortable and less of a subject to you.

Motivation and Trance

I think that motivation is the most important part of this. Over a hundred states of consciousness have been identified by Charles Tart.[5] I have never quite figured out why people think that hypnosis is just one little bit on that continuum. I think that hypnosis should be able to occupy more than one space on the continuum. From the motivation situation, there are different trances: clinical, experimental, demonstration, entertainment, forensic, spontaneous and involuntary (different types of trances are discussed in Chapter Five).

The forensic trance is motivation for enhanced recall. It is not necessarily the truth. The answers are not necessarily valid or accurate. It gives enhanced recall and gives you the opportunity to pursue more information. I worked with a man accused of murder. There was no question that he was going to be convicted of murder one. He had no memory for a four-hour block of time involved with drugs and alcohol. His attorney asked us to work with him to see if we could get any additional information about that period of time. He was a very good hypnotic trance person and took us through that four hours, step by step.

That was not admissible in court but we didn't want it to be. What the attorney was looking for was additional information. It allowed

---

[5] Charles Tart, PhD, internationally known for his psychological work on the nature of consciousness, and author of *Altered States of Consciousness*, is one of the founders of the field of transpersonal psychology.

her to follow up on a number of other leads, find out that another person was involved and identify that other person. This particular person who had been accused ended up doing four years for some of the other things involved in this situation. He was not the murder perpetrator. Without hypnosis, he would not have been able to take us through that four-hour period of time and he would have been convicted. None of the hypnotic work came up in court. The only thing that it did was enhance his recall so the additional information could be found.

People in trance interpret very literally. The prosecuting attorney asked this man, when he was on the witness stand, "Where was your hand at that moment?" And the answer that came out of him was, "At the end of my arm." You say, "Your hand is getting lighter and lighter. Your hand is going to float up and touch your face." I'm sitting there thinking, why doesn't her hand go up and touch her face? She's thinking, if she wants me to get my hand to touch my face, she needs to get my arm light because my hand stops here. It's as light as it can get and she hasn't said, "arm" and I'm stuck. The understanding of what you are really saying to the person is what is so important.

Spontaneous trance occurs with clients who are really uptight. If you watch carefully, you'll recognize when they go into that trance. The motivation is self-help and self-control. I'm only going to allude to the involuntary trance because it is an external motivation and an external control. It generally goes by the name of brain-washing.

Utilization

The utilization of hypnosis encompasses ideas and work with words and involves teaching people how to use their minds in ways they haven't thought about before. If the worst thing that can happen is that nothing happens, then you have nothing to lose and everything to gain by working on these words you are going to learn that will create these magical responses.

That's what hypnosis is all about—taking the rainy, yucky, miserable evenings and turning them into the sunshine, daisy-filled meadows and good times. You can take the fantasies people have, the incredible fantasies they would like to fulfill and the things they would most like to be able to do; all you have to do is turn them upside down and turn them into reality. Fantasy to reality. That's what hypnosis is all about. It enables people to do things that they really would like to do. It gives you the best feeling in the world for being able to do that. Hypnosis taps into all these behaviors, and the language of trance can be the therapeutic tool for change.

We are into spring and I think that each spring is the end of another long winter. With spring comes the promise that every ending is a new beginning because that's what every spring is. And you can begin anew to observe and to appreciate the new ways to look at the old ways that you have been looking at things all your lives. And to absorb the curious integration of using the old in the new way you are going to learn. So that you can begin to broaden your base of experience and to understand, and to look at things in a way that will let you understand them in ways, that you've never been able to do before.

Louis Thomas[6] is someone I really like and I like to paraphrase from his books. He talks about this real amazement:

> We start out as one single cell, which splits to become two, and then those two become four and then those four become eight. And there emerges with all of this work, with all of this splitting, as the cells differentiate, one cluster which will have as its progeny, the human brain. The mere existence of these special cells should be the great astonishment of the earth.
>
> One group of cells is switched on to become the whole trillion-celled apparatus for thinking and imagining. Why does that one group of cells become the brain, and not the left big toe? Why does the little finger know that it's the little finger and not the left rib? How in that one cell is there enough knowledge and enough understanding? If there is in every one of those cells, that kind of understanding of all the other cells, then all the information

---

[6] Past President of New York Memorial Sloan-Kettering Cancer Center and author.

needed for learning to read and write, to play the piano, or the marvelous act of just putting your hand out and touching a tree; all of grammar, all of math, all of music, all unconscious learning, responding, and thinking are contained in that first cell. And that individual is capable of translating all of that information into every other cell (Thomas, 1974).

The mind is an absolutely amazing machine, when we look at it that way. We talk about computers being patterned after the mind. Some say that trance is merely mind over matter. Why should we be surprised about that because the mind should know what matters? When we trust ourselves, I think we find out what really matters. Is it mind over matter or matter over mind? Because what really matters in this matter is that we have two parts of our brain that make up our mind, one of which we call the conscious and the other we call the unconscious. What really matters is allowing those parts of the brain to function as if they know what is best and they know what really matters.

Just as you have two levels of consciousness, you also have two halves of your brain, the right half and the left half. What really matters when you think about it is that both halves are the right half. Because it's right to use the right half when that's the right half and it's right to use the left half when the left half is the right half. And what matters is that you know what it is that's right for you to use when that is what really matters. And your right can be your left or your left can be your right. But you need to know which it is and which it is going to be. And you find that your right cannot be your left but your left can be your right, when it's right for it to be so. Just as using the left hand is right for a left-handed person and the right hand is right for a right-handed person.

But if something happens to that right hand or that left hand, you learn that the other hand can become the right hand with which you write the right kinds of things for understanding the things that you begin to need to know. When you do that, it's easy to imagine how difficult it is for you to know which is always your right and which is always the one which is left on your left. You can understand and begin to appreciate that as you follow and you begin to think that the really difficult part of this is that you understand what it is that I am saying.

You recognize how easy it is to take that kind of thinking and make it into a convolution that both the conscious and the unconscious mind can learn to follow and learn to learn from. You can tap into the parts of consciousness that have been suppressed. You can permit the part of the unconscious that understands that it doesn't really matter what it is that matters, as long as you can trust the conscious and unconscious to be learning what is right from what it is you have left about the things you have been learning what's right about this evening.

And when you listen to it, it sounds as though I am playing games with words and I am. What I am also doing is appealing to that part of you that learned how to learn many years ago, by playing those games with words. With hypnosis, it's kind of a regression in the service of the ego. What you are really doing is tapping into this skill and this ability to learn and understand and think, and to *expand* into this knowledge that all of these cells that you have, have all of the understanding, all of the wisdom, all of the utilization that they need.

Hypnosis is simply a matter of permitting yourself to learn something new and potentially different and exciting. You can be pleasantly surprised about how curious you can be about what it is you are going to learn that you already know that you know. The words that you play with and the way you use them can intrigue the parts of your brain that have been kind of dormant and sleeping like sleeping beauty and along comes the prince. I think that the kiss is believing and understanding.

You can wake up and begin to enhance your own trillion celled apparatus that this body–mind system, that psychoneuroimmunology is telling us, can really give us the explanation for this magic that people have been able to do for such a long time. The vibrations we have and the intensity with which we work can share the wonder of the magic of the mind and the things that really matter. So the patients can do things that just really *explode* into this expansion of thought and being and feeling and organizing.

What happens is that you begin to understand that you have two options. One is that you can listen to the words and get into the playfulness of it and go along with it in your trance. Or you can

25

decide not to go along with it. The only way you can not go along with it is by going into your own trance to stay out of the trance that I am asking you to go into. Either way is a win-win situation. The idea is not for *me* to get you to go into trance but for *you* to learn the experience of trance. That's what this is all about—the experience of trance and being able to do it. And to have this super good feeling yourself is the part that is most important. Because then you *know* how good it is.

When that happens, it can become such a positive force for good and healing that the rest of the world is not going to be able to resist it. Then we are all going to buy into it and everybody is going to be better off. I think it's perfectly fine that I have my head way up there in the clouds as long as I keep both feet planted firmly on the ground. I make every effort to do that. That's why I give all this emphasis on structure and on practice and on learning and on say-ing the words and paying attention to them. Only when you have that foundation can you then be free to get rid of it.

Question: When you are working with a group, if you are doing group induction or group trance work, if someone has an abreaction or other adverse response, how do you deal with it?

T: You deal with it the same way you would deal with it if hypnosis was not being used. As a health professional you are trained to deal with these situations. That is not hypnosis; that is your own training, your own skill and understanding. In all my years of training, I have seen two people who have had these kinds of reactions. One of them was a valid interpersonal reaction and the other was getting even with the person doing the trance work. Lewis Wolberg examined 15,000 cases of individuals using hyp-nosis (Wolberg, 1967). He found that not one of those patients had substituted a problem of greater dynamic significance or that hypnosis had created other problems for the individuals. No matter what happens, we can handle it. The hypnosis is not what causes the abreaction. It's the circumstances surrounding it. That's where your own skill and understanding and knowledge come into play.

Question: What is levitation?

T: The ability of a part of the body to lift up in the air as if it were doing it by itself, as if the arm had a mind of its own. I really like it because it gives you such good feedback and it tells you exactly where the patient is. There's a levitation where the hand goes up and there's a physiological one where you hang a weight on the arm and the arm goes down.

Question: You commented that everybody can be hypnotized?

T: I have an obligation to go in believing that everyone can go into trance. Not everybody needs to or will, except for the mentally retarded because of their inability to concentrate. I work one day a week at a handicapped residential facility for the mentally retarded. Believe me, I have not been successful there. I really am convinced that under the right circumstances, that everybody [else] can and does use trance.

Erickson did not work with everyone who came to him. The man was *human*. Some of us may not believe that. He could not possibly have seen everybody who wanted to come to him. There were other people for whom he felt that hypnosis was not appropriate, so he didn't see them. He was selective whether or not you see that in the books. He did not believe hypnosis was a panacea. He referred a lot of patients as well.

Question: Helping someone go into trance is frequently helping someone concentrate?

T: Your ability and your responsibility to help someone to go into trance and helping them to concentrate is the same as your responsibility as a health professional to them in any other respect. It is a tool and you learn to utilize it with the same skill and practice as any other tools. I don't expect for you to use 100% hypnosis with everybody who comes in your office. You don't have sufficient practice. It doesn't have to be 100% successful. If it just helps 5%, if it helps them 10%, it's better than they would have been without it. If the root canal patient can be a little more comfortable when I put the xylocaine in or if the relaxation makes that local anesthetic be a little more effective, then that was worth doing. It can be an incremental kind of use and utilization.

Question: Is there a lower age limit or developmental stage for using hypnosis?

T: The youngest person I have ever done anything physiological with was 2 years old.

References

Thomas, L. (1974). *The Medusa and the Snail*, New York: Viking Press.

Wolberg, L. R. (1967). "Hypnosis in psychoanalytic psychotherapy", in J. E. Gordon (ed.), *Handbook of Clinical and Experimental Hypnosis* (pp. 260–80), New York: Macmillan.

Chapter Two
The Curiosity of Milton H. Erickson, MD

I learned a lot from Milton Erickson about the double bind, but my being here today may be, for me, the ultimate example of it. This tribute to him, with all his friends, but without his expected presence, just may be a magnificent demonstration of how he manipulates situations even by his absence. Many of us think that we must say something important here today, but all we can hope to do is contribute a little to something that began in 1901, and then rely on it to continue if it is meant to be.

This is not going to be a presentation for the lover of four-syllable words or erudition. Instead it is a statement of what I believe I've learned from Erickson, which I hope you will accept without interpreting it as religious fervor. There is a myth that if something is explainable in simple language, it is not valuable. The incestuous perpetuation of this myth mollifies the large group of people who need to convince themselves that they, their words and their works are highly complex and therefore superior. I do not believe that myth, and neither did Erickson. I will try, in the simplest way I can, to tell you some of what I've learned about and from Erickson, and then rely on you to use that knowledge in your own ways.

It is curious how he knew, and I believe he did know, when he chose some of us for special attention, that we would try in our own ways, not his, to carry on the work he started. He did not expect us to be like him, and so he cultivated each of us according to our own needs. These encounter sessions over the years taught me many things, many of which I do not yet know I know. I do know that the mellowing and seasoning process is an important enrichment, for it does take time to begin to understand what you know. The power and the magnificence of Erickson 25 years ago is something I was privileged to enjoy and be part of, and I am sad for those who did not have that opportunity and for those who did but did not understand what was given to them.

It is amazing that so many people who thought they learned from him missed so much of the learning. There are those people today who maintain that they can explain Erickson. There are even some among them who will try to capitalize on his death now that it is safe to quote and interpret him without fear of refutation. But they fall far short of understanding Erickson the man, the curiosity.

No one should presume to explain someone who had so many facets. If a number of people look at a diamond from different angles and describe the light they see, they may all be accurate and yet all see a different light, with none of them being able to describe the whole or the source. I suspect that Erickson would want each of us to see the light first in our own way, and then to accept that our view is not the complete vision, but rather a glimpse of what might be possible. He did not want us to replicate his light; he wanted us to develop our own.

There are those who came to him but could not learn because he demanded that they respond to him as individuals. They went away with the need to explain the change in them by explaining him. They went away knowing what they thought he taught. Yet, they missed so much of the man who treasured humanity, who was so curious because there was always a new problem to solve in a novel way, because his aim was to help people by always learning new ways. Yes, he was a curious curiosity, but his curiosity led many others to be quietly curious on their own.

To stimulate the imagination of each individual about what he might be able to do, and to demand the patient's recognition of his fullest potential were both in Erickson's repertoire for growth and health. He was a very human and sensitive man who could accept hostility and abuse from his purported colleagues, and who persevered because he knew his methods worked. He must have understood that gradually the healing professions would learn the techniques incorporated in his work and occasionally even acknowledge his pioneering leadership.

Like the many sides of a diamond, the devil has appeared in many guises; Erickson was frequently a devil's advocate with his Machiavellian maneuvers, his manipulative machinations and his occasionally outrageous therapy. But those behaviors were not

Erickson; they were an essence of his methodologies to help the patient. It remained for his patients, in many instances, to be the ones to know that when he was manipulative he also took responsibility for teaching them how to handle the results of the manipulation. Anytime he was Machiavellian, the situation required it. Anytime that he was brutal, it was because the patient could not use sympathy but needed prodding to break through the walls restraining him from achieving his potential.

One of Erickson's greatest satisfactions was to see an individual achieve that potential and know that he had had a significant role in opening that person's world. Although he was never content with anything less than the most, he knew and accepted that the limits of potential could vary widely. And always, along with his most outrageous behavior, there was respect and regard for the person. Gentleness and tenderness were always there. Many onlookers missed it, but his patients always knew, although sometimes only in retrospect. To be as vicious as he sometimes seemed to be, and to do it out of love, demands an infinite love for the individual, just because he is a human being!

Erickson helped people who had grown up intellectually to grow up emotionally. In doing so, he suited the treatment to the person, unorthodox though that might be. He was never afraid of behaving like a fool, because he did not rely on artificial dignity, and thus never was a fool. I wonder if that fear of foolishness is one which restrains so many therapists from reaching further than they do. He cared, and was not ashamed to care. Many therapists learn that they must remain objective and "uninvolved". But remaining objective need not exclude caring, and there are some people who can do both. Not so curiously, Erickson had this capacity for compassion. He taught the ability to accept caring: Patients could leave their wildest fantasies in his closet; he would provide a home for patients during therapy; he would keep a pet for them when apartment rules or travel regulations necessitated it; he went for drives with phobics; he went to dinner with people who didn't think they could; he did whatever was necessary without fanfare.

His teaching and his therapy were inseparable. One of his ways of preparing people to be receptive to change was to initiate confusion, to disrupt their conviction that any reality was fact, and to induce a shift in attention. He taught by parable, but often it would be years before the story would be recognized for the profound lesson it contained, even though previous to the recognition of Erickson's meaning the ideas had been implemented and accepted as the patient's own. Milton knew that the individual does not need to defend himself against stories, that he can listen to them as a child would, wondering and curious not only about the story, but also about why Erickson chose it especially for him.

At the same time, the unconscious is listening to the multilevel messages, picking up nonverbal cues, and lulling the unsuspecting conscious mind with the recognition that this is, after all, only a story, but the simplicity that Erickson seemed to present was the most deceptive thing for the people who came along in later years. It was the result of years of observation, learning, working, reformulating, practicing and trying again and again. He learned to learn much by asking little, by seeming to ask innocuous questions, and by allowing intolerable silences. His final simplicity makes it difficult for us. We want to do it without work; our arrogance arises because he made it seem so simple.

There's another amazing quality that I'm not sure many of us have recognized about Erickson. He needed no credit from the individual. He did not need the person to come back and say, "Thank you; you did this for me." He was content for people to say, "Of course I can do this now." Few people have so little desire for credit or gratitude; yet this was a man who would laugh about having the biggest ego in the world. When you think about it, though, the meaning of ego depends on your orientation. It wasn't ego. It was hubris, that's the word—insolence in the face of the gods! He had it. I think he earned it.

Some men climb mountains because they are there. Milton couldn't physically climb mountains, but he could help people to achieve the summit of their own private mountains. I realized this one day as I was sitting on top of an actual mountain. He taught me that it was only right to be myself, that I could dare to do whatever it was that I had inside me to do, that I could be the person I wanted to be. To dare is to risk the chance for change! Milton dared to challenge the present order, to wonder about the future possibilities, and to take action to make the potential into the real. He had a curiously appealing and overriding quality of a child-learned faith that the world ought to be right and fair. Since it had to be your turn sometime, why not now?

The man was a clinician, a practitioner! But he had a sense of glee, a glad-to-be-alive curiosity about life. There was always some new toy to explore or an old one to look at in a new way—always with the wonder of a child. He retained the naiveté, the lack of inhibition of the child, and merged these with the sophistication of the ultra-observant therapist, a disturbingly effective combination. He was always sincere as he communicated his wonder, his awe, surprise and delight when one accomplished some new learning, even though many others had done it before. Like a parent watching his child learn to walk, he took pride and satisfaction in the marvelous achievement of each person's trying and accomplishing a new skill. And, like children who delight in their parent's excitement, Erickson's patients recognized his infectious pride and mischievous curiosity about their activities.

Erickson played with mood and feeling the way the sun plays with light and shadow on the peaks and valleys of the mountains. It really did not matter to him why a person had difficulty: All that was important was that the person could change! Explanation was irrelevant. In this, he differed greatly from "orthodox" therapy of the time, but times have changed, and insight is less essential now. The concepts he developed grow in strange and curious ways, through unlikely people in unusual places, as demonstrated by the variety of backgrounds represented at the Erickson Congress.

As Erickson liked to explain, each oak tree spreads millions of seeds. Many will not grow, but enough will hit receptive soil to take root and grow tall and strong. I wonder whether anyone can guess how many of the thousands of seeds he planted will grow, each in its own way, none exactly like any one before it. Maybe this is why some of us were "allowed" to plant a tree for his seventy-fifth birthday. He knew we could not be like him, and did not wish us to be. He wanted to stimulate our thinking: to get us to wonder; to explore within our minds, without our minds, within our bodies, about our bodies; to be curious enough to want to learn. I wonder how many of us can permit ourselves to acknowledge what we began to learn from him. Too often we cannot give credit to those who gave us the glimmer of ideas, but I hope many of us can acknowledge the subtle learnings which originated with Erickson.

We can carry on the tradition of learning, of being open, of allowing each experience to be a new one that can enlighten. It can be done scientifically, if that is what some people need. But there will be those of us who go on in our own low-key way, learning to appreciate the people who permit us to teach them, and hoping that they will, in turn, teach others. So the third generation Ericksonians followed the second generation Ericksonians, and third generation people know whom they follow even though they may never have met him. I know one person who put off meeting Erickson during his later years. There were two possible reasons: first, the possibility that when he came face to face with Erickson, Erickson would see his inadequacies and frailties; and second, the possibility that when he came face to face with him, this person would see Erickson's inadequacies and frailties, and have to cry.

Back when I began my own experience with Erickson I could not have realized where I might be today. All I knew then was the fear, the sheer terror, the wonder and the curiosity, even then, of the enigma named Erickson. Ted Aston was the reason this particular mouse came back to the seminars on hypnosis. Ted was a nice, comfortable man who, unlike Erickson, did not scare me. I had tried to stay clear of those eyes that could see inside my head (the "ocular fix", as Jay Haley described it), but then he singled me out for special attention, and the changing process began.

Erickson had the skill of the master teacher, who let us think we had discovered things for ourselves. It's curious but natural that his memorial service was attended, not by the people from the learned institutions, but by the people whose lives he enriched by having taught them that life is a game to be played the best way possible. He did not teach us what to expect—he couldn't. He taught us that we could handle the *un*expected, and that we would always have a response available. It might not be the perfect response, but it would be a response we could live with. As one of the people close to him was told, "Happiness is the endowment with value of all the things you have."

I have learned much from Erickson. As I improved in what he taught me about observation, formal induction techniques have evolved for me into informal trance with an emphasis on the recognition of the language of communication. Anything communicated in the therapeutic situation contains many multilevel messages. When a word or behavior charges out at me, I take the energy it has and utilize that spark from the person's polarity, offering positive potential even though sometimes in an apparently negative way. Just as I can generate a case for "pain interferes with healing", so too can I amplify one for "pain stimulates healing", depending on the circuitry the patient needs.

I've learned so much from Erickson that I cannot consciously teach, so others must learn from watching me. I have said for years that one of the most important things I learned from Milton Erickson was to trust in and rely on my own unconscious. My unconscious is more perceptive at times than I allow myself to be at a conscious level. Unconsciously, I absorb communications and then broadcast responses. When I am enthusiastic with these vibrations and people pick up on the smaller things, it means they can generalize to the larger, more significant messages, if they are worth it! (And if you were really paying attention, you aren't sure what I meant, because "if they are worth it" may refer to the "things", or it may refer to the "people".)

Maybe the true dreamer is the only true realist. We learn very early that reality never is what we think it is going to be, and so the dreamer can adapt to the unreal reality without it destroying his dreams. When we find genuine satisfaction in the growth of the present, we must know that when we get where we are going, we will recognize it again. The warm, creative influence of the imagination lends sensitivity, perception and spontaneity to our vision. We are the momentary product of a lifetime of past memories and experiences. We are altered so that we can grow within the reflection of ourselves that we learn to see in our imagination, and because of this legitimate reflection of the dream, we are able to grow.

Milton was an actor who would do anything to accomplish his goal. His act was meticulously performed to enthrall his audience, to gain their attention, to get them caught up in the play. That a man so restricted physically could expand so many horizons for others was astonishing. He presented vivid proof that one need not accept any restriction, because restrictions need not exist in the mind. He would delight in defying the usual laws of order in order to break down the restrictions and patterns of life. He thought, he worked, he wrote, he practiced his lines and his movements for greatest effect, and then he threw himself into the performance like a director showing others how to act. His phenomenal sense of humor tempered the performance, keeping the melodrama from becoming too heavy, even when it was.

"Observation"—that was his philosophy. It's fun to wonder how he got started, out there on the farm. One might conjecture that his curiosity was one of the ways he compensated for all the things he did not have, and it led him to make better use of all the things he could develop. Instead of learning to look at colors, he looked at shades of people: He learned to distinguish subtle nuances of hue and saturation and what was apparent when no camouflage was possible. Since he could not hear any music in music, he distinguished people's tones as tunes, and learned to recognize "what the pitch was" in the voice and the inflection.

For a man who suffered so much pain, he was intimately in touch with muscle and nerve control, reading nonverbal movements with accuracy. His illnesses taught him patience. He also knew that you could overcome physical disabilities by freeing the mind. His capacities were intimidating. His patients had to confront that intimidation, but once they passed it, the release of their own potential came so powerfully that it overflowed. The patient was then left waiting, and wondering, and wanting more.

He knew that we could not be he, and that we could not really even be like him, no matter how much we liked him, but that perhaps it did not really matter, since that matter was not really matter. We would be what we must be, but we should be what we could be. He saw some seeds take root and grow, and he understood that people are beginning to understand, even though we stand under so many misunderstandings. When we stand away, we find that his standards stand alone. They only need to be, and to be used, and the effectiveness of the reality of their effect affects our own affectional effectiveness. He taught so that we were not always sure what we had learned, but so that we could use it. We go on, with the curiosity instilled in us still in us, to know where we go now, I wonder? Strange, or should I say curious, that those of us who are most curious about it are the ones who are most content to wait and see what the curiosity of that special curiosity that is Erickson will become. If I speak, as some say, the language of hypnosis, it is because he taught me how to get ready; how to listen to what the person is really saying; how to hear; and how, sometimes, to be able to communicate, to know that understanding is one of the greatest gifts we can give, even when we do not understand.

Solve your private puzzle, hear the puns, enjoy. George Santayana said, "Life is neither a spectacle nor a feast. It is a predicament." Erickson saw it as a challenge, a puzzle to be solved, so the pieces could begin to fit. He even died between two birthdays and an anniversary, leaving us the puzzle of whether he did not want to spoil those days, or whether, in his own pixielike fashion, he wanted that day to be all his own. He would smile, as his daughter Kristi said in a letter to me, and say, "Enjoy every day." He was unorthodox, innovative, creative, often in pain and lonely. He was also immersed in, and happy with, his family and extended family. There are those of us who miss him as a person, and that is all right, too. He was quite a guy! And all of that helped to accomplish some of this, so this and that mean that this is that, and that that is this, and that's that!

This poem is very special to me, and I wasn't sure I was willing or able to share it here. I offer it in the hope that those who do not understand may begin to see how we whose lives began to change from our encounters with Milton Erickson feel about what we have learned—that we can be. This poem, by Roy Croft (cited in Lofts, 1970), is what I think I thought he taught:

> I love you, not only for what you are,
> But for what I am when I am with you.
>
> I love you, not only for what you have made of yourself,
> But for what you are making of me.
>
> I love you for the part of me you bring out.
> I love you for putting your hand into my heaped up heart,

And passing over all the foolish, weak things you can't help
    dimly seeing there,

And for bringing out into the light all the beautiful belongings
That no one else had ever looked quite far enough to find.

I love you because you are helping me to make,
Of the lumber of my life, not a tavern, but a temple,

And of the words of my everyday,
Not a reproach, but a song.
I love you because you have done more than any creed could
    have done to make me good,
And more than any fate could have done to make me happy.

You have done it,
Without a word,
Without a touch,
Without a sign.

You have done it by being yourself.

Perhaps that is what being a friend means, after all.

From: Lofts, W. O. (1970). *Men Behind Boy's Fiction*, London: Howard Baker Co.

Chapter Three
Almost 1984

Time does pass. Milton Erickson has been dead for only four short years, but the changes that have taken place in the way his work has been interpreted and imitated make me wonder whether 1984 and beyond will be an Orwellian nightmare in which history, experience, individual thought and just plain hard work are replaced by the facile allure of newspeak and doublethink. As Orwell knew, it is all too tempting for people to take the easy way out, to rely on slogans, to speak in preset formulas, and to cover our lack of knowledge and understanding with a veneer of jargon which the unsuspecting accept as truth. I see this happening to Milton Erickson's work, and it frightens me.

The horror of Orwell's 1984 was the way the past was sanitized, condensed and edited until it was reduced to a series of maxims so simple, and so simpleminded, that they could be readily remembered but never understood. The complexity was lost. What was lost in quality was made up for in quantity. That which was left was repeated over and over so that it became "true" through the simple process of constant repetition. I'm sad and worried to say that I see much the same thing happening to Erickson's work in the past few years. The work that Milton Erickson did day in and day out as a practicing therapist has been largely pushed aside. The range, complexity and variety of therapeutic approaches that he worked a lifetime to develop and apply have been supplanted by a narrow, simplified view of his work as interpolated from the teaching seminars he conducted in his last few years. This substitution has narrowed and distorted his work and, more importantly, narrows and distorts the work that those who try to follow him are now able to do.

In most cases, but not all, this distortion has not been a deliberate attempt to destroy the record, but, more simply, the result of ignorance. Erickson worked as a teacher and therapist for more than forty years, but most of the people who claim to be his followers knew him only in the last few years when his strength was declining and when he presented his techniques to students in ways that were least taxing to him. Students who had never observed him working as a therapist assumed that the teacher and the therapist worked in identical ways. Erickson's work thus has been simplified and narrowed to the point that I am quite sure he would not recognize it as his own.

The problem that I see is not simply one of setting the record straight. The past is not important in and of itself. Erickson would be the last to want us to carve his life in stone and proclaim it as the new truth, the one and only truth. The past is important, however, as a source of knowledge and information. If we are to invest our time and efforts in developing successful therapeutic techniques, we need to understand the base from which we are starting. For that reason, I think it's important to examine what has happened in the past few years, to take stock of our stock, to examine our bonds, and to wonder about our options for future investments.

One thing that has clearly happened is that Erickson's name and some parts of his work have become widely recognized. Erickson would, I'm sure, be pleased and amused to see that Ericksonianism has changed from an endemic state to an epidemic one. He would not, however, be pleased to see the way his ideas have been formulized and promoted so that he has become a kind of Big Brother whose name and slogans are invoked to lend credence and authenticity to ideas that he himself would not have supported. When we use Erickson in this way, we dehumanize him, and, in the process, dehumanize ourselves as well. What Milton Erickson did can be talked about, but *how* he did it cannot be interpreted by anyone.

I guess I am forced to acknowledge that I found the endemic state much pleasanter, but I am also pleased to see how widespread recognition of Erickson has become. It may well be that those many people who have come to know Erickson's name, in whatever way, will become interested enough in the man and his work to delve, to inquire, to learn more about him and his techniques. If that happens, the confusion of the last few years may be worth the price. If it does not, we will find ourselves deluged with pseudo-Ericksonian ideas, which will do little harm to him but may do much harm to the practice of hypnotherapy in the future.

The deluge has already begun, and it is damaging to both those who promote it and those who come eager to learn. All of the people who have never known the person that Milton Erickson was as a therapist can now watch videotapes, motion pictures that capture a two-dimensional quality and a tiny bit of what he did. By freezing and repeating the same images over and over, these tapes foster the false belief that they represent all of Erickson's work and all of his therapeutic techniques. This view oversimplifies and edits reality in much the same way that the TV news editor leaves all but a few selected segments of film on the cutting room floor. You have only to think of the difference in perception and learning that occurs when you witness an event yourself, when you read about it in detail in the newspaper, and when you watch it summarized in 30 seconds on the 11:00 p.m. news, to see how little one film or tape, no matter how good or accurate in itself, can teach us about a lifetime of work and ideas.

The videotapes are not, of course, the whole story. Those who seek to know something about Erickson can listen to audiotapes, read volumes of voluminous books and take copious crash courses in how to understand and interpret Milton Erickson from the people who affirm that they know the essence of the man and his work. It would be really convenient if we could put the essence of Erickson in a bottle to be taken as needed. Like hypnosis, marketing is a fine art. The imitators take apart the real heart of the fragrance, and they put it together in different formulas and different quantities, and so the quality just isn't quite the same. Then they tell us how to wear it, or at least how *they* wear it, but it does not make sense for them to sentence us to make sense of the essence of the essential scent that we sent for, since that one was not the scent sent for us, and the sensitivity of the particular scent changes with the wearer.

The people who came to study with Erickson in his last few years don't even understand that they missed the beginning, so they don't recognize that they were too late to learn it all the way, all ways, because they were shortchanged by Erickson's weakness and his frailty and his illness and his age. They changed and shortened the rules of learning so that they could go out and teach what they thought they learned. But what they saw was not Erickson the therapist; they saw Erickson the teacher showing them only how to

41

begin to know what to look for. He was the teacher lecturing his class, not the therapist working in a therapist–patient relationship. Because they never saw the therapist, they can imitate and teach only that which they learned as students.

The teaching seminars late in his life were made a lot more dramatic and effective by his use of tales and word pictures. This smorgasbord of stories was to be remembered for its fascination, as the diners were spoon-fed much of the main course in an effort to avoid upsetting their digestion. They had their appetizers before they ever got to the restaurant to dine, and it really would have been difficult for the chef, at his age, to select a new menu for each person; it was much simpler to offer a variety of choices and then let the guests dine on their own. When they did that, they were impressed by the variety and the significance of what they could see in each course, and they attributed all of that to the chef and his creativity. The praise of the chef really came from each diner's interpretation of what he liked best; the meal could be totally satisfying, but it could also be digested for future growth and sustenance, and could be recalled and reinterpreted as the diner wished.

The use of word pictures was an effective teaching device, but Erickson's reliance on it in those teaching seminars perpetuated the myth that he always used permissive and indirect suggestion and that his therapy was always done by metaphor and analogy. It is important to remember that the stories were used as illustrative teaching techniques. Those people who came were fulfilling their own needs and their own expectations when they chose to hear a special message for them in the significance of each story. I'm sure that each of us has been through that particular kind of enlightening experience and has benefited from it. I think we neglect, however, the premise that was the basis of Erickson's work and his style, and that is the fact that there is no set formula for working with any one individual, let alone for working with any group of individuals. It's ironic that many of us learn in our own individual ways but then turn around and try to impose only one way, the "right" way, on our patients. When we do this, we shortchange both them and ourselves.

We also shortchange our patients when we accept other myths about Erickson's work. There is, for example, the myth that if we will only trust our unconscious, our therapy will just roll out of our brain, onto our tongue and out of our mouth, and the behavior of our patient will be quickly changed in this completely spontaneous fashion. This is nonsense of the highest order. It attempts to replace years of study, practice, learning and experience with a set of magic formulas. While it is true that some of us may have more innate talent for certain skills than others, it is equally true that talent alone cannot produce and sustain success in the therapist–patient relationship. Erickson's life is, in fact, an excellent example of how talent must be maintained and fed with constant experience and growth.

Erickson's success was based on his own innate genius used in conjunction with a large number of basically self-taught skills. One of these skills was his phenomenal ability to observe the most minute cues his patients brought to him. There are few who can begin to emulate that particular skill, because we haven't had nearly enough practice. Another important self-taught skill was his ability to "get to where the patient was", and to speak the language of the patient, be he farmer or statistician. Sometimes that led to confusion, but not on the part of the patient. To so many people who were unable to "go" to where the patient was, some of Erickson's very direct approaches seemed to be confusing and nondirective as Erickson conversed with the patient in the patient's language. The patient was not confused, but the people listening, who could not speak that language, felt that it was very confusing and therefore must be an indirect approach.

I guess we could almost say that his indirect therapy was successful principally because of his extensive work with direct therapy. Erickson worked with variety and apparent spontaneity, which anyone who had spent a lifetime practicing ought to be able to do. He worked with spontaneity, but he was not spontaneous. Because of his experience and his ability to observe, he could take things that people gave him and utilize those, and it appeared that he worked instant magic. But the instant magic was the result of long, hard years of working and learning and formulating and going back and trying various techniques over and over again. His vast repertoire permitted him to draft what would appear to be an appropriate approach to a patient and, at any given time, to modify that approach by using any of the multitude of modifications he had ready when it was apparent that they were needed. It was this smoothness in transition that I think misled so many. As people missed the transition, they settled for the idea that it had to have been a metaphor.

Erickson's technique of using word pictures has caused problems for those who would follow his techniques but do not have a lifetime of experience to draw on when doing so. We are all fascinated by the tales, and we all aspire to work the kind of magic we attribute to Erickson, but I think we must recognize that, in this instance, imitation is not the sincerest form of flattery. We can only do what Erickson did if we do it in our own way. This is difficult because it requires us to put aside the myths about how Erickson worked and replace them with hard analysis followed up by years of rigorous practice. When, instead, we fall back on the myths as the easy way out, we lead ourselves astray.

There is a myth abroad that Erickson was able to come up with a new story for every patient, and many of his more recent followers strive to imitate him in this and often become bogged down in looking for stories when they should be working with the patient. I firmly believe that there are limits to the ability to come up with a *new* story for every patient and, indeed, limits to the therapist's ability to individualize the approach to each patient. I also believe that there are no limits to the ability to individualize each story for the patient, or to the patient's ability to individualize and adapt the story to his own needs.

When we recognize this ability in our patients, we free ourselves from the constant need to individualize therapy. Since the same story can have a different meaning, a multitude of meanings or sometimes even no particular meaning, why not use the same story with appropriate modifications. Consider, if you will, that every once in a while, Erickson told a story that had no meaning of any special sort. All that the story was told for was to give the patient time for the learning that was going on. It just distracted the conscious mind so that the unconscious could do its own thinking and feeling and organizing.

One aspect of individualization that the therapist must take responsibility for is the ability to determine whether or not the direct or the indirect approach is necessary. There were many patients who came to see Erickson who certainly did not need indirect therapy. They were ready and able to enter trance, and they were probably in trance before they entered. They were ready to believe, and therefore receive, the strong help that they knew was appropriate. Sometimes they needed the excuse of being ordered to get well so that they could. Erickson was capable of complying with that need in a more authoritarian fashion than anyone I have ever known. Certainly, Erickson's manner of speaking was part of his style, his approach to people, but that was not where his expertise came in.

His expertise was his ability to read the individual and determine whether the direct or indirect approach would be more appropriate. Whatever the method that was used, however, the foundation of the change was in the directive therapy, not in the direct or indirect way in which it was presented. Telling people what to do, and having them do it, is all very well and good, but we need to recognize that the telling can be either direct or indirect, but the directive therapy is the thing that brings about the change.

Erickson recognized that some patients needed the indirect approach, but others required a more direct, often confrontational approach. Many people who try to learn from Erickson have a difficult time with direct approaches, which can be emotionally draining for the therapist. As intellectuals who are more accustomed to manipulating ideas than people, therapists often prefer to discuss resistance and hostility rather than trying to provoke them so that they can be brought into play as active participants in the therapy. These theoretical discussions satisfy the intellectual needs of the therapist in a nice, neat way but do little to help the patient who needs to have these needs met directly. Provoking patients to exhibit resistance and hostility takes more of a risk than many therapists are willing to chance.

Because the direct approach is so difficult, some therapists emphasize the effectiveness of the indirect approach. They work diligently at understanding how to be confusing, how to use metaphor, how to be nondirective. I must confess that I sometimes fall into this trap myself. I suspect that the root cause is simply that we do not believe in ourselves enough. Maybe we don't believe we have the power that we saw in Erickson to make the direct approach work. We chicken out and we justify our behavior by saying that we are utilizing his indirect approach. We state our intention to follow "Ericksonian principles", but what this really means is that we lack the belief and skills necessary to make the direct approach work.

Some therapists justify the exclusive use of the indirect approach by asserting that Erickson used only the direct approach in his younger years and abandoned it as he became more skilled in the indirect approach. To those who make that assertion, let me say this: Nonsense. I knew and worked with Erickson over a period of 30 years. He was still comparatively young when he was using both indirect and direct approaches. Furthermore, he continued using direct therapy when he was a lot older than I am now. I think that he continued using it all through his life when he worked as a therapist with patients who needed that approach.

Patients were one thing, but those people who came to observe and to learn as present or future therapists were another. For them, indirect therapy and indirect teaching were not only appropriate, they were easier. Considering the number of people he dealt with and the ways he had to deal with them, it was good that he could take the easy way for the people who were ready to accept this.

While we are on the subject of Erickson's age and how it might have changed his approach to teaching and therapy, I think it is safe to say that Milton Erickson had some strongly held convictions that he kept all of his life. One of his strongest beliefs was that all therapists must work to earn the necessary credentials of their field and must then continue to learn and to upgrade their skills and capabilities throughout their working careers. As a younger and extremely conscientious and powerful therapist, Erickson frequently objected to anyone who lacked appropriate training.

I'm sorry to say that we don't hear much about appropriate training anymore. We hear that therapists need "all kinds" of training, but the appropriateness of the training is extremely important. Those people who don't take the time to learn, to try, to make mistakes, to correct those mistakes and then go on cannot be adequate therapists. We don't cure by magic or by offhand wise pronounce-ments. As therapists, we must have a plan in mind to present to the patient and be ready to alter that plan on the basis of the data that they give us.

To do this, we need constant practice, constant assessment, constant learning. This requires mellowing and seasoning and can only come with hard work and experience over a long period. Erickson main-tained that patients need a wealth of neuropsychophysiological reorientation in order to be as good as they know they have the potential to be. I think as therapists we need a wealth of experience to be as innovative and perceptive as we would each like to be. I hope that learning is an ongoing process for each of us, and that those therapists who are beginning their explorations in hypnosis, gifted though they may be, will pay their dues in time.

Erickson believed that experience counts, no matter how smooth the words, no matter how brilliant the hypotheses learned and put forth. It's ridiculous to even suggest that we can follow our sponta-neous unconscious before the "spontaneous" unconscious has enough in it to be spontaneous. It's nice to teach about change out-side of conscious awareness, but there has to be an unconscious awareness before that can happen, so one needs, as Erickson stressed, an abundant "experiential life". Rigorously trained pro-fessionals develop their awareness of these broadened interests through a symphony of movement. Moving back and forth easily between conscious and unconscious, between trance and nontrance states, is not easy. It requires discipline and hard work, but what you get when you finally play the music is well worth the practicing.

What do I see now instead of rigorously trained professionals? I see many watered-down, nondirective, metaphor-oriented therapists, afraid to take the risk of being authoritarian and direct, and justify-ing this action, or lack of action, in terms of confusion. This all sounds very much like doublethink to me. Confusion should not accompany instructions that you want patients to compre-hend and follow unless you know that their unconscious is not con-fused. I think that we need to spend more time understanding the principles that Erickson worked with and also go a little further.

I think it's time for us to enact some standards, or guidelines, for the benefit of those unsuspecting individuals who don't have the background knowledge to be able to properly evaluate the plethora of workshops professing to teach Ericksonian hypnosis. There are many who claim in their workshop brochures to have "studied with Erickson", or "trained with Erickson". What do all these phrases mean? Did the claimant spend three hours with Erickson? Thirty hours? Three years? The brochures never say. The magic now is in the assertion that the claimant spent time with the Master, but there are many unanswered questions: What kind of time? Where? With whom? At what point in Erickson's life? Did the claimant go for therapy? Did he or she go to study? Or just to have lunch?

The questions become more important and more relevant because the people who "use" the magical Erickson name should identify the circumstances under which they are entitled to connect that name with their own teaching. Why is it important? From my bias, it is important so that Erickson, unlike Big Brother, won't be accused of being on every corner and underwriting all the therapists who have ever sat with him for a few hours. Erickson deserves credit, not discredit, and tribute, not blame. There are those who would wipe out his name, as in 1984, and claim his ideas as their own, as in newspeak. There are also those who would use his name to promote their own ideas, as in doublethink. I think we need the courage and the integrity to acknowledge him as a major contributor in our work and our lives, and then move on to build our own work. We need to be originals because that is all we can be. That is what he expected of us.

At the same time, we need to agree to this credentialing so that there can be a mutual understanding of what the doublethink language means in newspeak. Everybody who teaches pretends to know the true meaning of the language he communicates so that he can show that his way is the way to speak the new language, even if he uses doublethink to rewrite the language of newspeak. However, learning any language takes time, no matter how it is taught. Unlearning an old one and replacing it with a new one takes even more effort, and we need to be patient and recognize the inspiration of the magical successes, but keep working when the successes are not magical, as often happens. Maybe if we are fortunate enough and we work long enough, hard enough, we may come to the perceptive perspective that there is no one way; there is only the way that works, whatever that may be.

As I look back over my own years of experience and learning, I wonder what I've learned outside of trance. Among other things, I've learned to be tolerant, but sometimes to be judgmental for my patients, to evaluate their state of readiness, and to give them time when they need it. More than anything else, I've learned to respect patients as individuals who have integrity which can be utilized for themselves and their benefit. I've learned that each individual has a particular history and sensibility, and that I cannot cast him or her into a mold or apply a ready made formula and expect predictable results. In Orwell's world, there was the illusion that this molding and predicting was possible, but in the real world of 1984, we cannot deceive ourselves that it can be so.

Just talking in newspeak metaphor doesn't magically produce results. I wish it did, sometimes, but I know that more than that is needed. The therapist must take a strong position in support of change. Insight may appeal to the therapist's need for orderly thought, but it doesn't help the patient unless the patient really wants to change, and that's where the skill, rather than the words, comes in. There are times for all patients when they need to know that someone is there for them. The someone needed will vary as the need varies, and the therapist must be capable of being all the someones needed at whatever times they are needed. But each time, the growth that's going on comes closer to the satisfaction of knowing that it is becoming, and gradually that becomes enough for the moment.

Gradually, too, change becomes easier, although there is never an easy time for change or acceptance. The winds of change continue to be elusive. It's difficult from one's bulwark of being buffeted by the bluster of all these changing seasons, and reasons, and winds, to sense a very slight constancy in one direction and gradually develop a leaning in that way. When we look back, we can observe the direction of that growth and know that it grows as it should to get to where it knows that it wants to go.

In the transition phase that we are now experiencing, we must learn from the past while remaining open about our future, because

49

nostalgia may be comfortable, but it's not progressive. Nostalgia is like a grammar lesson: We find the present tense in the past perfect. We must look, however, to the past not through the rose-colored lenses of nostalgia, but through the clear, well-focused lenses of our present knowledge and experience. The past must be preserved, not slavishly, but certainly accurately. When we know how Milton Erickson worked, we can choose to accept, reject or modify his methods. What we must not do is distort, simplify or reconstruct them in the image we would like them to have.

As we look back and see the sparkle of the diamond I have always considered Erickson to be, we must also see the sparks that come from his many facets. As we examine these facets, we must distinguish the fact and the reality from the myth. We cannot, however, look only to the past, because if we do, we are going to stumble over the unknown up ahead. What we can do is to use the memory from the past to enlighten our progress. I think we must expend the time to learn to expand our expectations and our horizons. I'd like to see us use rethink, not doublethink, and to keep newspeak from becoming our language by going back to Erickson's ideas for individual development.

Since it is now 1984, this is a good time to experience the passage of a good time, to speak anew about accepting the risks and the challenges of change, to acknowledge our debt to the past, but to move on to a future of careful work, rigorous analysis and hard-won experience. Milton Erickson lived that kind of life.

Question: When Erickson was direct, how did he help the patients bring about change in themselves?

T: The patient was the only one who ever brought about the change, whether it was direct or indirect. There are people who simply don't need indirectness. They can be told what to do, they need the excuse of being told what to do. They never thought of what to do, and when they go and pay a therapist to tell them what to do, he does it. Being direct doesn't mean that he couldn't get them into contract situations. I can't think of anything more direct than some of these rather embarrassing contracts that he had.

And as Jay Haley said this morning, the *ordeal* is what facilitates change, but that's still directive. What immediately comes to mind is the newly married bed-wetting couple. Asking those people to get up and wet the bed and then lie down and go to sleep had to be the most directive, authoritarian, abrasive thing I can think of, and yet it was what they needed to do in order to overcome the problem they were presenting. I really have difficulty answering this because it seems so obvious to me, because it does protect the autonomy of the individual.

Chapter Four
Metaphor
A Myth with a Method[7]

We want the creative faculty to imagine that which we know.
Shelley, *A Defence of Poetry*

Imagination lets us make the experience of trance real. And in doing so, therapy is enhanced through creative metaphor. Talking a myth is a method to let the truth be learned by appearing to not teach.

The use of trance in therapy, and metaphor as an accelerator of trance, facilitates brief therapy (and for that matter, any kind of therapy). But using metaphor is not as simple as it may sound. It requires acknowledging the many factors influencing words and mandates an ability to weave or create a myth appropriate for the individual patient's needs at the specific moment in time and therapy in which the intervention occurs. When this is done successfully, the myth assumes a reality for that individual at that point in time and makes that reality available to facilitate both trance and therapy. Understanding how metaphor facilitates therapy requires a distinction between theories of therapy and the specific techniques employed to expedite the chosen method of therapy.

Theories explain behavior within a specific context, but methods or facilitators can be seen as multiple paths to one end—the (normal) functioning of the individual involved. Thus, facilitators can be used across therapeutic approaches. In general, therapists now agree that radically different theories of therapy share methods that cross boundaries between theoretical disciplines. For example, metaphor and myth, like hypnosis, can be used in multiple approaches. Fortunately, such mixing is far more acceptable today

---

[7] Material from the original lecture, which had been deleted during editing of the published article with the same title.

than it was when Milton Erickson began his work, when the strictures of the field practically required one to declare oneself a specific type of therapist and to use the approach and methods sanctioned by that approach. Erickson's method was unusual for that period in that he combined and utilized all types of psychotherapeutic and hypnotic interventions in his therapy; he didn't feel bound by rules to stay within any one parameter. Perhaps that was one reason people had so much trouble with his therapy—they wanted to make it a theory. For Erickson, however, hypnosis was an adjunct to any type of therapy that was appropriate for the patient; it was not intended as a theory in and of itself.

Erickson's approach also was unorthodox in that he did not restrict himself to one type of therapy any more than he restricted himself to one way of approaching a problem. He always looked for a novel way for the individual to recognize his own capabilities for change, and he would do almost anything to effectuate that change. His goal was to help the patient; any approach, theory or therapy that achieved that goal was both permissible and welcome. This use of multiple approaches and theories, novel and misunderstood during much of Erickson's life, is now more clearly understood and accepted.

Because of this relaxing of the strict "one-theory" approach to treatment, Erickson's use of metaphor became an issue to practitioners newly interested in broadening their own foundation of knowledge about the use and possible impact of other theories and therapies.

Myth, and the multiple metaphors through which it is developed, facilitates trance, and thus therapy, by combining the layers of meaning inherent in words and metaphors with a story that allows the message to be a significant communication for the patient at the level at which it is needed. Ironically, the use of metaphor increases the power of the therapist by allowing him or her to be less precise in assigning meaning to the myth and thus freeing the patient to choose the most useful interpretation. The ambiguity and possibility of choice allow the patient to relate to what is needed by him rather than struggling to accept or reject an imposed framework.

Because of their pliability, myth and metaphor can help circumvent a problem endemic to therapeutic situations—the tendency of both therapist and patient to concentrate on building frameworks rather than addressing specific problems. Frameworks tempt and trap both therapists and patients. The therapist tends toward framework building in order to use the bits and pieces garnered from the patient to build a whole picture and decipher its meaning. In doing so, conversely he often will be temped to force the pieces into a framework, either preconceived or newly constructed for the occasion, and thus impose a preconceived structure on the problem.

The client has a similar and closely related tendency. Because he is entering a new situation, he may be inclined to listen more than speak. He may thus accept the therapist's framework or combine his own bits and pieces with those supplied by the therapist to build a framework of his own. This seems to be natural and necessary, but concentrating on the framework may interfere with listening and hearing because one may be listening for building blocks rather than dealing with the problem at hand. As a result, the client may latch onto an offered framework as a convenient, though not necessarily helpful, answer. When this occurs, neither the therapist nor the patient is well served. Instead, each should be assembling a new framework, or at least keeping an open mind for modifications in the existing framework.

The practitioner is under an especially strong obligation to avoid ready-made frameworks because he may be seen as the authority figure. Additionally, he may have less to gain from a new framework and thus have less incentive for the hard work of constructing one. In contrast, the client has more to both gain and lose because he is entering a novel situation. He probably sees his current position as a unique and poorly understood problem that requires definition and resolution. The practitioner may look at the same situation and see a problem he has encountered in many previous forms. The client then has more personal motivation and a stronger need to understand the situation as unique rather than common. The therapist, in contrast, must recognize the common elements of a situation clearly enough to choose an appropriate approach and simultaneously allow the client to see the individual aspects of the problem while avoiding the tendency to fit the situation into a preconceived mold. Learning to teach the clients to sense changes in belief and behavior that will improve their functioning need not stress the common structure of the problem.

It may help if therapists can think of themselves as automobile mechanics and clients as cars brought in for repairs. Mechanics listen to the car and then fine-tune it, not taking anything away, but working with and modifying what is there—perhaps using different lubricants for different speeds, reducing the discords, or removing the grating of metal on metal. Accepting this analogy forces therapists to take only what is there and stimulate it to greater potential—smoother running, longer life expectancy—rather than trying to create a new and better model. We adjust the existing model, helping it to run at its full potential. We also can teach the owner how to remove rust and put in softer upholstery. Sometimes we must even teach the owner of the car how to drive.

But with all of our maintenance, it is still the client who ultimately will drive the car and determine the desired destination. The mechanic may make alternate routes available and be present to offer directions and maps, to suggest a change of route when necessary and to maintain and repair the equipment. He does not, however, choose the destination or drive the car, although he may go along for the ride.

It is really important that the mechanic not get too committed to the vehicle the owner drives, thereby trying to keep it going longer than is appropriate, just as the therapist must recognize that the patient has the power, the potential in himself. It is not in the therapist, it is in the client. It is fitting for the mechanic to stimulate the driver to do more work. And if the therapist is a trustworthy mechanic, one that the owner has not seen anything like before, it frees him to respond by looking at the vehicle from a different perspective. It is not that something different is seen. But that one sees differently.

As with all trips, some will be short and others quite long, but always it is the destination that must be kept in mind. A trip may cover a lot of territory (or therapy) in a brief, but concentrated, time. As I use the term *brief*, I rely on both senses of the word: first, the reference to a shortened or curtailed period of time, and second, the sense of being concise and involving only the most pertinent facts and line of argument.

Brief is a matter of perspective and depends on the people, the problem, the circumstances, the readiness and the need. It also depends on the therapist, who must be willing to be concise and incisive but also compassionate and respectful. In addition, brevity can be expedited by the use of metaphor, which facilitates the speed with which the patient can respond. I categorize "brief" as three to six appointments, but generally these appointments are longer than an hour, and so some people might count them as more than one session. Although the period of treatment is brief, I expect the results to endure.

Most of the patients I typically see are referred principally for physical pain control. In the process of teaching them hypnosis and subsequent pain control, many nonphysical contributing factors become evident, and the teaching varies widely regarding the apparently common factor, called pain. If I believed the patient's initial characterization of the problem, dealing with the pain itself would be all I would try to do. But then neither trance nor therapy would be effective, and hypnosis probably would be blamed. Actually, the failure would arise from the fact that I was not dealing with the entire problem of which the pain is a symptom rather than a cause.

To achieve a therapeutic relationship with the kinds of innovative interventions I intend, I must first initiate trust between me and the patient. After an initial interview with the individual, we investigate the involvement of tension in the pain, and the patient institutes some self-control to reduce tension. At this point, the patient must begin to perceive the relationship between the tension and the pain, but he must also, and perhaps more important, accept my belief that he *can* change and control both pain and tension. This positive view of potential must permeate the positions the therapist proposes.

This positive view is communicated verbally and nonverbally. Language involves more than the way we communicate *in* words. We have sign language, body language, tone of language, touch, nonverbal communication. Trust, rapport and expectancy are the ingredients on which trance learning is based, and they are much easier to communicate if one relies on more than just the spoken word. At the same time, the spoken word has great power and flexibility, and its multiple dimensions should be understood and utilized.

Words, like metaphors, are more than simple references to objects, ideas or relationships. For each of us, any word, or group of words, carries a web of associations based on the contexts in which the words were learned. As children, we listened to and tried to make sense of the sound we heard because somehow we knew the people speaking the words understood something we did not yet know. Initially, language develops *after* understanding and becomes a way of labeling, referring to and accessing experience. How did we learn to talk? We knew what the words *meant* long before we knew what the words *were*, or how to say them. We could, for example, crawl on the floor long before we knew it was named *floor* or that the motion we enjoyed was called crawling. In a similar way, we knew the warmth and comfort of our mother's arms long before we knew the word *love*.

Only gradually did the connection between *things* and *words* become significant. Our curiosity to be admitted to that world of understanding through spoken communication drove us to learn the words for the images they inspire. And for that reason, communication through word play comes even before storytelling. It sets the stage, the background in which the performance will take place. Tapping into the *endless* energy and curiosity for learning that we had as children, but which becomes submerged or stifled as we grow, is an unending well of potential to be well.

How does word play serve as an instrument of therapy? One of the first things it does is provide the opportunity for safely exploring the relationship between the therapist and the client. It affords a means of learning to communicate trust and individual differences to the patient, the opportunity to test, to play and to discover that creative behavior is encouraged in this environment even though it may be absent elsewhere. All of these strengthen the desired change in learning set. Then, too, looking at "words" differently lets one look at the possible difference in meanings, for which the words are only symbols.

The ambiguity and possibilities for personal interpretation make words a difficult medium to control, but perhaps control is not necessary to the degree one might think. Perhaps, for example, what may appear to be the "wrong" word, metaphor or story for a given situation may be accepted by the client, using his own definition and associations, as entirely proper and helpful. There is always the danger, of course, of the reverse happening, and we must guard against the devastating potential of words that can be interpreted as being negative.

To some extent, we have an ally in this battle. There is the tendency recognizable in the child's chant, "Sticks and stones may break my bones, but words will never harm me," for the individual to assume an armor of self-protection. A further ally is the tendency of the individual in trance to recapture the child's ability to say the truth as it is perceived, even when this truth is ignored by adults who dismiss it rather than listening to what is being said. In trance, both the protectionist and truth-telling tendencies are enhanced, and the therapist must learn to tolerate and build on both. In particular, the therapist must resist the common adult tendency to dismiss bold truths that may be hurtful or just too plainly stated to feel comfortable.

As therapists, we must, in effect, travel along part of the journey we expect our patients to take and learn to recapture the magic and truth of words. As children we, like our patients, learned that we had to understand our strong and often negative feelings and harness them. It was permissible to *have* them until we gave them a word, then we had to learn not to demonstrate them. And so we learned to suppress and repress the words, and eventually even the feelings that went with them.

And we are still so afraid of the feelings that we cannot address them or deal with the conflict that this creates inside. Our deepest longings and needs and conflicts are so powerful that we respond to them with childlike emotions. To deal with those emotions requires using words that have true meaning, possibly many meanings. And so we must be careful in our choices, because words trigger emotions by way of memories.

Word play and metaphor can trigger both emotions and memories while avoiding the overly rigid one-on-one correspondence that strengthens negative responses. Riddles, nursery rhymes, puzzles, tongue twisters, charades, all can add to the intrigue of learning sets. Tapping into these learning sets by using familiar themes can lead to unconscious solving of other puzzles, using the puzzles presented at that time to do so. Another important type of word play that can be utilized with trance learning is "fill in the blanks" perpetuated at a later age when we take tests in school. We also can scramble letters to make words or develop codes, and that can be important in the secrecy of trance, as a means of keeping unconscious thoughts from the therapist or from ourselves.

In all these forms, word play can teach through demonstrating that one word can have more than one meaning. This lets us open our minds to a whole new word world of possible changes. Then, too, we learn that feelings can have more than one description attached to them. Anxiety, for example, may be seen as anticipation, and this type of relatively simple redefinition can sometimes change attitudes and subsequent behavior.

Words are a playful way to build in the therapist the kind of trust that we had in adults when we were children. Words also are useful ploys to distract the client from the fact that the words are also the induction and the utilization. "Pay close attention to the words used" means pay close attention to the symbolism in the words. We want the patient to do this subconsciously, but we must attend to the multiple possibilities on a more conscious level. We can, for example, work with words that appeal by sound, words that sound alike, words that repeat parts or the whole and so demand attention and discrimination, words that distinguish parts of a pattern, words that play games and thereby confuse the meanings and allow the "right" meanings to emerge, because words evoke constellations of meaning and experience. Those who study language use terms such as *antonyms* and *homonyms* for words that stimulate childlike curiosity and playfulness in the patient.

But word play does not end when we move beyond induction to another phase—storytelling or metaphor. We must continue to be alert to signals in words, and to listen for and provide multilevel messages. We incorporate the initial elements of word play to continue preparation for, and involvement in, change. Words are not just words; they are symbols for experience, and we must be respectful of that experienced message.

We can combine types of word play by using words that carry a meaningful message for the client's experience, such as: inhibitions are tied up in "nots". And often we make many things naughty, because they are knotty, and not just plain "nots". And we do not know about the things we "no" until it is too late to go back and pick up the pieces of the ribbon that got tied into the knots we did not know how to unknot. But you can pick at even the most painful knot and retie it into a beautiful bow that will bow to the need to know that it was once a knot, but know it is not a knot now.

As we move from words to metaphors, we take along the capacity for hearing the meaning in the words. Why metaphors? Because they tap or access both childhood behaviors for learning and also memory skills from the period before the memories have been imprinted with negative associations. In addition, metaphors contain encapsulated myths themselves and prepare the way for more complex and fascinating stories and myths.

What are myths, anyway? They are stories rooted in the most ancient beliefs of people, stories that tell of high ideals and healing truths. Myths hold an almost sacred place in the cultural evolution of mankind. They capture cultural beliefs in a communication of understanding that holds wondrous solutions. They are evolutions in themselves and thus can involve an individual in self-evolution.

Fairy tales are closely related to myths and might be considered the myths of childhood used to teach social relationships, yearnings, and values. The listening child does not seek a reason or a motivation for the story but just listens openly, with curiosity and wonder. The child does not wonder why a particular story was the one chosen at a given moment, or whether or not it has an application or a moral. The child simply listens attentively from the beginning through to the nice, neat, satisfying ending. Going back to the ideals of childhood, and the attitudes of learning instilled then, and still in us, is a most effective way to teach change by accessing long-stifled traits of curiosity, *wonder*, openness and trust, and thus expand the facts of a given experience. When such childlike listening can be recaptured through trance and metaphor, magical transformations can occur. A paragraph from a client illustrates:

In each of us lies sleeping beauty, wasted potential, dying dreams. We sleep and live in dormant twilight never knowing what it means to live, to love the bits of heaven that we can unearth deep in our hearts; not recognizing that our salvation is ever present in those parts we have disowned, denied, forgotten. The thorns of fear thwart faint attempt. The prince is courage, the kiss believing and then with these our life begins.

Since a metaphor is initially a myth, it is practically possible to propose a parable particularly appropriate for the parts of the person you perceive as needing to listen. We must meet the mind of the patient to determine motivation and then incorporate the method for accessing the skills necessary for change. It isn't necessary, however, to develop a new story for every client; probably it would be impossible to do so. But one should develop a repertoire of stories, which can be applied to many situations, and then vary the story to fit the idiosyncrasies of each situation. Developing of metaphors thus requires careful listening to the individual.

Erickson was fond of talking about the experiential life of his patients. He was also extremely knowledgeable in his ability to "go to where the patient is". His broad-based experience is not easy to acquire, and most practitioners do not anticipate having to overcome the personal health problems that gave Erickson so much knowledge about body movement, but we do need a variety of experiences so that we can relate as closely as possible to the situation of the patient. The skill of understanding and telling stories is convenient, but one must be able to listen to the story one tells in relation to the client. One must also be able to shift directions smoothly when the client takes a different tack. Flexible modification is mandatory.

The fundamental idea behind the use of metaphor is to allow the client to recognize that he has options. Stories can be remembrances, projections, pure fantasy. They can be based on things the individual likes or doesn't like, or they can be merely a simple statement. They can affect physiological and psychological domains; they can affect health and emotion and well-being. They can be used as induction techniques and as fundamental components of therapy.

It is useful to bear in mind that induction is a metaphor and that an indirect induction technique provides the opportunity for the metaphor to be effective on multiple levels. If one doesn't need to know one is in trance, then the story can appeal to both the conscious mind, which hears only a story, and the unconscious mind, which hears meaning at a deeper level. The involvement thus can be a symbol of magic for the client who experiences something that he did not control or make happen. Participating in this process can sometimes allow the patient to submit problems that he has been unable to control to the application of the same magic. Something *can* happen and that recognition alone can make the difference.

What are some examples of my brief short and brief long metaphors? One of my favorite devices is very brief and goes by the name of "Yes, but ..." This simple technique of redefinition allows the client to acknowledge the surface facts of a particular experience, but also to recognize how to alter those facts with new information that was not originally available (or not assimilable), when those facts were in fact facts. We are, in effect, asking the client to expand old memories with new information, and assume a new way of looking at all old concepts to elicit changes in thoughts, language and, eventually, behavior.

Metaphors need not be long and involved. They can be a word or phrase that taps into the memory bank of the mind, just as a single tap into a maple tree brings forth a slow, steady drip of liquid. But then it is necessary for the liquid to be boiled slowly, to distill it down to the essence of what we know as maple syrup. Thoughts are like that, too, and frequently we forget that we do not get good maple syrup production if we have not had a cold and snowy winter. Forgetting things brings other things closer in the past. Forgetting the hard winter makes it easier to remember the wonder of maple syrup.

The introduction of storytelling can also be a means of distracting the patient from the experience of pain. To tap into the child part of each of us, using words and meanings to play with, is a convenient way of accessing basic understandings. Children like to learn through puzzles. A child can be curious, can feel wondrous about the way of things. A child can look at things with a sense of newness and excitement for the learning involved. A child can thrill about arriving at some new bit of information and wonder how it will fit with other bits of information. A child can laugh and can play, or be hurt and cry, but in both cases still be learning. So using myth and metaphor to look at things from different dissociated perspectives can let one see other options, other ways of looking.

To be effective, however, the story must he matched to the individual. An individual who can accept the idea that mountainous stress contributes to his pain, for example, also may accept hearing that learning to climb both literal and figurative mountains requires necessary safeguards for such a risky but exhilarating task: a knowledge of the territory; sufficient warm clothing for changes in the weather; food for the day's climb and extra food in case of inclement weather; ropes for tricky climbing areas; hammers, pitons and carabineers for help in difficult pitches; and being roped to someone who can serve as a guide, someone who knows the route and the weather, and the best way to conquer that mountain and achieve the summit. All of the word images are accurate for literal mountain climbing but can easily be expanded to refer to any mountain, a physical or a psychological one.

And yet, another individual may not perceive the undercurrents of life as contributing to the pain experience. In this case, it may suffice to simply tell a relaxing tale for the patient to listen to when practicing the relaxation exercises connected with learning pain control. The method in this metaphor is to offer the unconscious the knowledge it needs without the conscious need to understand. In this flow of conversation, it might be pleasant to go sailing on a body of water that offers differing currents, tides and winds.

The master of the sailing vessel becomes master by learning to understand, by practicing until it is second nature, the vagaries of the wind and the water. And you have to learn when you are at the wheel how to respond automatically to those changes in the winds that come into the sails and batter them from side to side. And you find that when you do that you also learn that it isn't only the wind that drives the boat, that in addition, it's the water, the undercurrents. Because no matter how calm it looks on top, there are undercurrents always going from directions that you may not have anticipated.

And when the waves build and you find as that goes on, and you get to the top of the crest of the wave, and you are sailing straight, when you slide down into the trough of the wave, the boat goes sideways no matter how much you try to keep it on a straight course. And as you do that you learn a great deal about the under-currents and the cross-currents in the water, and the way you have to compensate for them when you recognize the way that the wind is hitting the sails. And you know that you do not sail straight and you don't really want a calm. Because if you are becalmed you are not going to get anywhere no matter how smooth that water may be. And so you need sometimes to have the wind and to learn how to tack, to go from one side to another. Knowing even though you go from one side to another, you are constantly keeping that safe harbor of your destination of the other side in sight.

And all this information helps you steer a relatively smooth course, no matter how rough the water may be. This type of storytelling does not demand anything of the client on the surface, but all the information is available to the unconscious and ready to be used to help the individual chart the future course through the storms and the calms, the undertow and the waves. And you need to know that you may not get any credit when change occurs. Also recognize the process and mental exertion requires tremendous energy and work, which need to be acknowledged by you as such, because the praise that comes from the teacher is a vital part of solidifying that change.

And so the method behind all this "myth-ery" mystery is, in a very complex way, to simply teach the patient how to change by tapping into the unconscious potential he had before words and before language. Myth uses words, language and forgotten memory skills to encourage learning by listening to a model and then exploiting hidden resources. Myths take one back to a time before problems were extant and tap into the wondrous curiosity for learning that is present but generally forgotten. Myth has the capacity to permit a different look at things, first by changing the patient's view of the past, and then by allowing new learning to be generalized to present and future experiences. When the patient returns to the present and combines his current maturity with his newly recovered abilities, he has the potential to see and understand anew. Myth thus provides a method, through metaphor, to manage to make therapy more brief.

Chapter Five
Motivation and the Multiple Levels of Trance

As I prepared for the Third Erickson Congress, I reviewed and rejected a number of topics before I finally realized that my last three papers have covered everything I could say *about* Erickson. I could not begin what is already completed.

My tribute to Erickson is thus to go on, always acknowledging that my work is the result of what he taught me. Therefore, today, I come to bury Erickson, not to praise him. It is time for me to go on, not go over, and over, and over Erickson's life and work in a fixed litany that I and my listeners may continue to repeat but will cease to hear or understand. Going over something that for me has so much emotion only desensitizes me to what was real about Milton H. Erickson and continues to be real about his work. There has already been too much talk about Erickson, too much trading on his name and reputation, and too little actual continuation of the work he started.

As Carlos Amantea (1986) said, in Part III of *The Lourdes of Arizona*:

> A whole Industry has risen about visiting the Prophet of Phoenix. One comes for a day or two, and then advertises that one has "studied under Milton Erickson." This means you can charge $1000 a day for seminars. Few pay attention to the fact that the master himself charges only $25 a day for visitors ... he doesn't care about making money, getting rich, making it in the American Dream Factory. He gives away information, knowledge, insights gives them to all comers for so little. (Page 42.)

As I see it, Amantea is speaking of all the self-proclaimed authorities on Erickson who came during those waning years, when he held "audiences", as Amantea so aptly titled them, and told stories. They came and they listened, but many did not hear and most did not learn. It is interesting to note that those who did learn from

Erickson in his "teaching" days have not chosen to, and have chosen not to, profess to understand or teach Ericksonian hypnosis—people such as Rossi and Haley and Weitzenhofer teach themselves.

Erickson taught thousands of therapists during the 1950s and 1960s in his seminars on hypnosis. He accepted the responsibility of the teaching, knowing he was teaching, and doing it deliberately, masterfully, diligently, sometimes in a Machiavellian manner, but always effectively! He taught direct and indirect, basic and advanced, but always, he taught of trance!

And he did this in a way that allowed people to open their eyes, ears and minds so that they could see, hear and understand what was being given to them and then have the knowledge and the courage to use what they had learned to continue their work, not his. He did not leave it to his students to explain his approach, nor did he expect them to interpret his work. He expected them to learn in their own way and to present their own work, not his.

Erickson was a successful teacher who had both the arrogance to believe that what he had to say should be listened to, and the humility to understand that each would ultimately hear and use what he had heard in his own individual way. Erickson would be the first to insist that his way was the one true way, but he could paradoxically insist that each "student" develop the one true way that was true for him. He had a further gift that successful teachers must have: He motivated those who came to him to want to hear what needed to be said.

My tribute to Erickson is to continue the work he taught me how to begin. As I do this, one of the things I constantly learn and relearn is that listening, and hearing, is part of the ultimate communication skill, and of course, it is an art. But there exists a still more critical skill, which is making the listener want to hear what needs to be said. Erickson possessed these skills in abundance. He knew how to present ideas gift wrapped so attractively that the intended recipient wanted to own the package. We must all learn this skill to begin to realize our own potential in communicating.

This sounds manipulative, but it is not necessarily a matter of actively doing something to change the situation so that the listener is more receptive. Often it is a matter of listening to ourselves so that we read the situation correctly and are able to go to where the person is and see the situation from the client's point of view. This putting oneself in the place of another creates a very different dynamic than is created when the practitioner is completely in charge, assumes a motivation for the client, and then imposes a schema which will fit that situation.

This is not to say that the practitioner should be passive. Listening and hearing may seem to be passive skills because on the surface they require little action by the listener. The "speaker" appears to be in control; the listener merely responds. In reality, listening must be very "active"; the listener must take in, analyze and be prepared to act on a variety of inputs. Otherwise, he is simply allowing his eardrums to vibrate to sound. The practitioner who listens must indeed be skillful. He must be able to perceive the message even when the "speaker" is not consciously trying to send it, and he must be able to understand much more than simply what is said.

Professionals in all health fields must know how to see and hear things that clients do not even know they are communicating. As we listen, however, we must be constantly aware of our own assumptions and expectations regarding what we will hear. Listening and hearing may be blocked by assumptions, even valid ones. In the best instance, the assumptions may cause us to "hear" only what we already know to be "true". In the worst case, our assumptions distort sensory information into a preconceived notion of what it should be. Such assumptions can be limiting and dangerous if they are accepted as "truth".

I suspect that assumptions about the nature of listening, coupled with the practitioner's desire to control any given situation and common assumptions about trance, have had a crippling effect on research into the nature of trance. Such assumptions have led to projects in which the practitioner has an obviously active role as both the originator of the trance and its ultimate interpreter. In this type of "experiment", the practitioner induces trance using a prerecorded tape and then observes the outwardly measurable behavior of the subject. Because the method of induction is held constant, any variation in the subject's observable behavior is assumed to be a result of the action and intervention of the practitioner during the trance. The motivation of the subject and the level of his involvement in the trance are never even considered.

Professionals can sometimes lose sight of the fact that the primary moving force behind their work should be a positive therapeutic outcome and that the outcome must necessarily be defined in terms of the patient's motivation and needs in the situation. Our experimental goals, or even our own quest for knowledge, must be secondary. Paradoxically, when we put the concerns of the patient first and do so in a way that allows us to really listen and hear, we learn much more than we would by imposing a preset scheme. Both we and our clients benefit, and the state of knowledge is advanced.

In any clinical situation, there is always the matter of mixed motivations—ours, the client's and those of the organizations for which we work. In effect, we and our patients enter into a marriage of convenience in which each hopes to gain by cooperating with the other.

This matter and manner of mutual motivational manipulation is manageable but mandates mastery of many methods. I believe that exploring trance more openly will open access to listening and hearing. In order to understand trance more thoroughly, we must begin to explore it with more liberal and inquisitive minds. I would like to propose that more research is needed and that the beginning point for the research is observation and listening. In that spirit, I would like to offer some of my observations about trance with a tentative schema for differentiating among the types of trance based on those observations.

All types of trance have the potential to be therapeutic. There is always the recognition of a learning skill acknowledged by the unconscious. We can enhance this by learning of ourselves as we observe the types of trance.

As a starting point, I would like to examine some widely held assumptions. First, trance is generally defined as an altered state of awareness. Second, generally, such states are not discrete but exist on a continuum. And third, trance behavior, even of the same person, may vary from trance to trance. A general acceptance of these assumptions is an interesting example of the ability to readily and intuitively accept ideas without hearing or thinking through their implications.

Despite the general acceptance of the continuum concept, for example, many practitioners have postulated that hypnosis and the hypnotic trance state are one state, always the same. They propose that all trances are "located" in the same state, and that observable differences in behavior or outcome result from differences in the way people respond to the situation based on the suggestions given. Thus, the observable differences between trances are explained only by the behavior suggested by the practitioner and carried out by the client, not by possible differences in the states themselves. This would indicate that the power of the practitioner is the principal influence on the individual in trance.

These assumptions probably have their basis in two phenomena of human behavior: (1) our tendency to want to control whatever situation we find ourselves in; and (2) our tendency to prefer phenomena that can be measured to those that can be analyzed and understood but possibly never measured and therefore never "proved". Faith scares us. We work with the unconscious mind all of the time but are afraid to draw conclusions from anything but observable, measurable outward behavior.

If trance is an altered state on the continuum of awareness, should there not then be the possibility of different states of trance? Since theorists generally accept multiple states of awareness, why is trance designated as only one of those states, when it can represent a number of degrees on the scale of awareness? I propose that the term *trance* can be used to characterize a subset of states along that continuum of altered states of awareness and that the differences in these states may be accounted for by differences in the motivation of the subject.

The acceptance of the common concept of hypnosis as a single, simple state is fascinating. Consider just the outer appearance of the person in trance. Consider that some trances, when observed from the outside, look perfectly "natural" or normal; that there are others in which the person "looks" trancelike or even "zombielike"; and, that there is a range of other possible appearances. These outward differences are real, but they do not necessarily indicate the depth or type of trance involved. To get at this, we have to look at the aspects of trance that may not be clearly observable. I propose that we have to look at the purpose of the trance and the motivations of the practitioner and patient before we can begin to understand these differences.

When we examine the concept of purpose of trance, we realize that there are numerous possibilities. There are, for example, trances that have a hidden agenda, those that defend from other trances, trances for relaxation, trances for fun, trances for exploration, for physiological uses, for habit control and so on. Is it reasonable to assume that trances that have such different motivational beginnings can be all the same?

I believe there are differences. I base this belief on clinical responses from patients who have experienced different types of trance; on subjective responses from patients and "subjects"; and on my own clinical, experimental, forensic and demonstration experiences. Because of those many years of differing experiences, I have done some thinking about what I have actually seen and heard and what it might imply about *how* and *why* trances differ. The basic difference I see is *motivation*.

Differences in motivation, rather than differences in instructions, may account for differences in the aware states of consciousness observed in trance. In essence, the degree of attention the unconscious needs to focus on achieving and maintaining the trance will vary depending upon the use to be made of the trance.

This is easy to understand but difficult to measure for a number of reasons. For one thing, a motivating factor can have multiple origins. For another, there can be more than one motivating factor. It is also common for types of trance to be combined, which can make distinctions difficult. A further difficulty is that much of what occurs takes place in the unconscious and therefore is not highly accessible to either the practitioner or the client. The one constant is that the trance is determined by movement toward the result desired, or, in other words, by the motivation of the client.

Erickson understood and used these differences in his work. He was a master at determining how to skillfully monitor motivation so that the unconscious would maintain the many benefits manifest in the trance. He rarely decided to deliberately delineate the types of trances nor the nuances of nudges needed, and he could and would slip back and forth unnoticed using his multitudes of maneuvers. He would also combine and confuse the meaning in the messages with other communicative tools. His purpose, of course, was to produce therapeutic results rather than a taxonomy of trance. It was enough for him to understand and be able to use the variations himself, but it may be that we need a taxonomy to allow us to understand these variations before we can effectively use them.

Perhaps Erickson's mistrust of words, especially when they are arranged into systems and constructs that we accept (often uncritically) as truths, accounts for his willingness to use the differences in motivation without classifying or systematizing them. Words are, after all, merely symbols for experience, as Erickson's frequent use of the term *experiential life* reminds us.

Erickson stressed that words alone are poor and inadequate messengers. Tonal value and body/facial expression add to (which multiplies) or subtract from (which divides) the reliability of the message. It is interesting that Erickson, in his venture to use words accurately and meaningfully, used to write out his inductions. He did not, however, use these written inductions as formulas to be repeated verbatim, but as material to be learned and practiced until the pieces were so well known that they could be combined and used to improvise an appropriate script for a given situation. And, more than words were always used. The words finally selected were varied by expressions, intonation and gestures. The written verbalizations were the starting point, not the end point, and the use to which the script was put depended very much on the audience and the needed purpose of the trance. Perhaps Erickson constantly varied the performance to be as certain as possible that the messages he gave held the meanings the person before him at that moment needed to receive. The words were simply a starting point for the communication.

Still, there are those researchers who mandate an analysis of the hypnotic trance as induced only by the spoken word via tape recorder. They are missing an indispensable component of communication that is essential for understanding what is expected and for achieving the goal of the trance. Reading, like trance, is a learned skill, mastered and used in different ways by each person who learns it. "Some persons learn slowly, then become proficient. Others take to it rapidly, and continue enthusiastically. Many learn just enough to satisfy their own selfish purposes, which often involve passing the necessary tests. Some persons read extensively for a while, then lose interest and proficiency. Of course, some people learn but never really use the knowledge." (Pearson, Thompson and Edmonston, 1970, page 3.)

People who learn trance may do it similarly: They may learn rapidly and well, or they may learn slowly but thoroughly. They might learn superficially. They can learn from good, bad and neutral teachers. They may learn but choose not to use the knowledge. They may learn but be afraid to use the knowledge. Some graduate with a degree and go on to professional practice. Many, unfortunately, never progress beyond the kindergarten stage—they never understand the portentous potential of what they have learned.

Most neophytes are preoccupied with learning about how hypnosis affects them and what they can do with it. Their responses are influenced by their degree of learning, just as a beginning reader may not be able to make sense of fourth-grade books. At the other end of the spectrum, advanced learners develop their own internal cue systems so that when trance is appropriate, the mechanisms are activated through the autonomic nervous system. They have learned trance thoroughly enough that they can use it as a means to whatever end is appropriate at the moment.

The view that there is only one trance state may be correct in the sense that a given individual might enter trance consistently in the same way, and the observable behaviors that indicate that trance is present might be equivalent. Nevertheless, an individual might obtain different results from trance, and there must be some way to account for that. I think that the behavior in trance and the results of trance have not been thoroughly or systematically studied because of a preoccupation with studying trance induction. We are focusing on the vehicle, while the important aspect is the journey and, even more important, the destination. We may take many routes to the same destination, or conversely, we may take the same vehicle to many destinations. The destination and what we do when we get there is of ultimate importance.

When we first adopt a particular mode of travel, by car or plane, we can be understandably obsessed with the details of it, but later the mode becomes so familiar that we see it for what it really is: a means to an end. We miss something very important if we continue to focus on the vehicle long after it has become routine and second nature.

As I go on, I want to emphasize that the types of trance I propose are a function of the sophisticated trance only. Sophisticated individuals are in a position to evaluate what is needed *by* them and *from* them both *for* this trance and *from* this trance. Sometimes an intense involvement is indicated, but at other times superficial participation will suffice. Patients ponder price, and once they buy the cost, they then weigh whether the work is worth the fee and the reward.

It seems reasonable for sophisticated individuals to establish their own internal cue systems, accessed through their autonomic nervous system. It also seems natural that once trance is learned, it becomes owned, to use (or not to use) according to choice. It becomes the goal of the practitioner to speak a language that will permit intrusion upon the hypnotic state with appropriate guidance and suggestions. The person entering trance determines both the mode of transportation and the destination. Examining trances from the point of view of the client's motivation leads to a proposal of six distinct types of trance:

1. *Clinical*, in which the chief motivation is self-control or self-help;
2. *Experimental*, in which the motivation is money, mankind and self-learning;
3. *Demonstration*, in which the motivation is learning and/or teaching;
4. *Entertainment*, in which the motivation is the desire to entertain;
5. *Forensic*, in which the motivation is recall of past events; and
6. *Spontaneous*, in which the motivation is self-control and self-help.

The distinguishing characteristic in all cases is the motivation of the person entering trance, and the variations in motivation determine the variations in the quality and type of trance. Each of these types of trance can contain within its subgroup light, medium and deep trances. Each of them can include all or none of the phenomena of trance, depending on need. Each of them can be obvious or covert, based again on the sophistication and motivation of the person entering trance. All six types, and all types of trance, are defined by the significant behavioral, physiological and emotional changes, which are, in turn, influenced by the motivational structures involved.

Let us first consider the *clinical trance*. In the clinical trance, the individual is motivated by a desire to increase his personal learning so that he can increase self-help or self-control. The learning and self-control may involve physiological, physical or exploratory—emotional needs.

In clinical trance, the individual's only concern is himself; no outside element enters into consideration. For instance, the person about to utilize hypnoanesthesia and control of bleeding for surgery is only focused on that objective. Similarly, a woman who decides to use trance for labor and delivery in obstetrics focuses only on that. If a dental patient's bruxing (grinding his teeth) damages the temporomandibular joint, and he enters trance with the goal of controlling the bruxing, nothing else matters. If a psychotherapy patient wants to recover some traumatic memories that interfere with life adjustments, that is the purpose of that trance. There may be multiple factors responsible for the development of the problem, but the need is specific.

In each of these situations, the motivation is self-control and self-help. The importance of using trance for purely personal learning is paramount; nothing else matters! If the practitioner views this situation purely from the outside and as a product of how the trance was induced, he will miss most of what is actually happening.

An *experimental trance* may be induced in the same way as a clinical trance and may, in fact, look the same from the outside, but it is in reality different because the motivation is quite different. In the case of experimental trance, the motivation factors include money and mankind.

The individual goes into the experimental situation with full knowledge of the following facts: He has volunteered to participate in an experiment. He is informed about the experiment. He has been assured that the experiment cannot do him any harm, and further, that, if at any time he wants out, he can leave the experiment. He has also been assured that the experiment will be of benefit to mankind, that the results will help society in some way. In addition, he knows that he will receive some type of remuneration for his participation—if not financial, then some other reward.

So, this person goes into the experiment, which will be of a specific duration, knowing that he has nothing to lose. He can do anything asked of him, he cannot be harmed, he may learn something that will be of value, and he will be rewarded. He may walk out anytime he doesn't like it. His motivation, then, is *money, mankind* and maybe some *personal learning*.

Contrast that with the individual lying on the operating table with a surgeon about to cut open his abdomen. Such a person cannot easily hold up his hand and say, "Stop, I've changed my mind." The differences in motivation probably lead to differences in the depth and nature of the trance.

The third distinct type is the *demonstration trance*. In this type of trance, the individual has a narrow range of requirements. The person volunteers to participate in a demonstration, knowing that the situation will be a fairly neutral one. Trance phenomena, and sometimes just "trance", will be demonstrated, either to him alone, as a learning procedure, or to a group, in a teaching situation. He may, in fact, be learning trance so that he can use it in a future clinical situation, but the learning is separate from the use of it; the trance is only a demonstration.

Demonstration trances are used routinely in classes teaching hypnosis, as the best way for practitioners to learn how to work with trance. Usually, the volunteers are from within the group learning it, and the person who volunteers can both teach others by the demonstration and learn from the trance experience itself. In the demonstration trance, then, the motivation is either *teaching or learning*, or both. The clinical, experimental and demonstration trances are all recognizable as types that occur in therapeutic and teaching situations.

The fourth type—the *entertainment trance*—is quite different. Understanding the motivation and use of this type of trance may help us to understand where our difficulties in utilizing clinical hypnosis first arose. Years ago, stage and lay hypnotists were popular and were commonly used for stage performances, after prom parties and so on. Even today we have popular, nationally known hypnotists such as Damon and Kreskin, and many lay hypnotists entertain for groups and private parties. Because these early entertainer-hypnotists were the only source of knowledge about trance, they became involved in teaching hypnosis to medical practitioners who sought this knowledge for its possible therapeutic value. As the doctors then began teaching hypnosis to other health practitioners, they taught it in the way they had learned it from the hypnotists. It thus retained its aura of magic and control. Trances were created so that subjects demonstrated "zombielike" behavior. It was not until the emergence of serious professionals like Erickson that we began to shed the "mystique" of hypnosis.

What about the people who make fools of themselves by following the commands of the lay hypnotist? Does this not demonstrate that the hypnotist (and *his* motivation) are in control? This situation does indeed demonstrate the skill of the hypnotist, but it is his skill in choosing subjects, not his skill in manipulating motivation, that we witness. He cleverly conceals the antecedent variables in the stage show, but they are there, and they influence events.

Consider this situation. The hypnotist gazes out on a crowd. When he asks for volunteers, he gets two types: He gets the extrovert, the ham, who really wants the opportunity to show off. And he gets the introvert, who is elbowed up by friends and is too intimidated to refuse. After a few suggestibility tests, the unsusceptible individuals are escorted off the stage by the assistant, and the audience promptly forgets about them. From the 16 to 20 people who volunteer, the hypnotist selects the best four or five and "uses" them.

But, they do stupid things! Doesn't this show that the hypnotist is in control? Yes, they go into a trance at the hypnotist's urging as part of the contract they made when they came on stage, and they crow like a rooster, or they run through the audience selling newspapers. They may even eat an onion and make it taste like an apple, knowing all the while that they are playing an enormous trick on the audience, since they do know what they are doing. It is a great opportunity for the subjects, the extrovert and introvert alike, to have the chance to show off. They can have a marvelous time!

But then the hypnotist says, "In a minute I am going to wake you up," and in their newly acquired sense of time distortion, the subjects immediately think, "I made a fool of myself, how am I going to go back and tell my friends I knew all these stupid things I did!" But then, the wily hypnotist finishes the sentence with, "And when I do, you will not remember a thing." The subject, of course, acquires a valid, instant amnesia, which solves his problem of going back to his seat with vivid memories of what he has just done. He can respond to the jibes of the audience with, "I didn't do a thing, he made me do it all," pointing to the hypnotist, who is quite willing to take the glory (or the blame) and look like the "magician" who controls people's minds. But the contract and *motivation for the entertainment trance* is fulfilled to *entertain*.

The next type of trance to consider is the *forensic trance*, a type which has aroused considerable controversy in both the courts and therapeutic circles. There are those who claim that hypnotically enhanced memory is valid, and others who claim that it is unreliable. An examination of the subject's motivation for entering this type of trance may help our understanding of the situation.

The *motivation* for the only valid forensic use of hypnosis is to *enhance recall*. Individuals in trance can still think, can still lie (often better with the aid of trance, since they are better able to control their responses), can still misremember, and can still enhance their memory with unconscious remembering. Enhanced recall can only be used as a guide or clue. Corroborating evidence must be the conclusive material used to make decisions or judgments.

Although courts are not ready to concede that hypnotic memories are as valid as memories recalled through "normal" means, we should begin to think about the nature and application of memory in forensic situations. We recognize that regular memory, especially of traumatic or long-past events, can be faulty. Yet those memories are routinely permitted in evidence with the understanding that they may not be complete or fully accurate but nevertheless present one type of evidence about the events in question. If we treat hypnotic memories the same way, hypnotically enhanced recall should be as valid as any other type of recall.

A further interesting point to consider is the distinct probability that individuals, particularly when they are under oath, can go into a self-induced trance caused by the stress of the situation. This type of trance is generally not recognized because it is not externally induced, and there may be no externally observable phenomena that can be identified as evidence of trance. This illustrates the urgency of understanding trance more thoroughly. Until we can measure trance, we cannot accurately predict who is in a hypnotic trance at any designated time.

The possibility of self-hypnosis under stress illustrates the next type of trance, a catch-all category that we do not know how to investigate or even acknowledge: the *spontaneous trance*. This is the trance that individuals go into when the need to achieve or the need to survive automatically accesses unconscious resources not usually available to that person. The motivation for the spontaneous trance is the same as the motivation of the clinical type of trance, *self-control* and *self-help*, and so we come full circle.

What then is the difference between the clinical and the spontaneous trance? The difference is that the spontaneous trance requires no outside person to induce it. It is a trance that is entered as a result of an immediate, urgent need. Because none of the person's usual responses will meet the recognized need, the reserve potential of the unconscious is activated, and trance results. The "miracle feats of physiological control" that exist in the literature—the mother who lifts the 250-pound refrigerator off of her 3-year-old boy, or the farmer whose arm is severed in a tractor accident who walks miles to the doctor's office without bleeding—may be instances of this phenomenon. Looking back on these events suggests that trance made the feats possible.

The possibility of spontaneous trance may have far-reaching implications. As we begin to explore and learn more about the immune system, and about the chemical components of thought, we should also examine the abilities that hypnotically skilled individuals possess in an attempt to determine the relationship between accessing altered states of consciousness and controlling bodily processes, organs, glands and the immune system. Consider, for example, whether spontaneous remission is any less possible than superhuman feats of strength if we consider that trance and the access to the immune system may enhance physical capacity and capability.

All six types of trance I have described are patient or individual motivated. There is one further type of trance, however, that must be mentioned, the *involuntary trance*, which is *operator motivated*. I know very little about this type of trance but have talked with some practitioners who have encountered it, and I do know that it exists. I first heard rumors of it back in the 1950s from an attorney member of the American Society of Clinical Hypnosis. Only now are some of the things that have been done with drugs and mind-controlling techniques involving hypnosis starting to become known.

At one time, I believed that nobody would do anything in trance that was against his will or beliefs. Since then I have encountered situations that lead me to believe there are trances that are induced utilizing other psychological techniques and/or drugs, and that these techniques result in undesirable consequences. Hypnosis is not the primary controlling factor, but is a technique used to create and to absolutely control the behavior. The drug-induced trance is involuntary and therefore dangerous. I do not know enough about it to discuss it in any detail, but it is a subject that we should all be aware of and one that certainly warrants further investigation. It exists; I know about it. I don't know enough about it, but there is a myth to be dispelled.

As health professionals, of course, we are primarily concerned with understanding the healing trance, and more research is also needed in this area. More research might be stimulated if motivation were considered as the basis for defining trance, categorizing it, and identifying the kinds of trance that individuals will go into based on their personal motivation. There could be parameters connected with each of the types of trance that people will understand.

I am proposing a research methodology for the study of the *utilization* of trance, rather than, as so often happens, the induction of trance. That method would involve using sophisticated individuals who already know how to go into trance, or even unsophisticated individuals who can learn how to go into trance. Criteria would have to be established for testing for the presence of a trance state that all individuals must attain, *any way and with any method of induction that will work for those individuals*. Once the individuals meet the criteria and after the trance-entering behavior is documented, standardized approaches can be used to test for the defined experimental criteria. The preliminary requirement would be that the person entering trance must be permitted to reach trance any way that is best for him. Then the experimental standardization can be established after the trance is achieved!

As we go on in our search both to enhance our understanding of the relationship of word to knowledge and behavior, and our understanding of the altered states of *awareness* of trance, we consciously and unconsciously pay tribute to Milton Erickson, who was forever curious about the ways of the how and why and what. Today, Erickson's influence on therapy is being acknowledged in a broader sense because of the sense, not the non-sense, of his techniques.

As we are motivated to look to the future with the knowledge gained from the past, we expect that more answers will lead to more questions, and the language of trance and motivation will continue to speak for itself.

References

Amantea, C. (1986). "The Lourdes of Arizona, Part III", *The Fessenden Review*, 11 (3), 42.

Pearson, R. E., Thompson, K. F. and Edmonston, W. E. (1970). "Clinical and experimental trance: What's the difference?", *American Journal of Clinical Hypnosis*, 13 (3), 1–7.

Part II
The Language of Hypnosis

This section opens with an exploration by Camillo Loriedo and Dan Kohen of Kay Thompson's critical influence on the development of the language of hypnosis.

In "The Languages and Metaphors of Kay Thompson", Camillo Loriedo evokes a musical metaphor to explore the remarkable harmony of Kay Thompson's masterful therapeutic communications and describes several fascinating examples of Thompson's complex nonverbal communications. In "Teaching the Language of Hypnosis", Dan Kohen defines what he believes are Kay Thompson's most important contributions.

"Language to Effect Change" (Chapter Six) was Kay Thompson's last major teaching workshop and is a treasure chest of her teachings. Many of her favorite inductions, metaphors and clinical vignettes are included, besides a wide variety of demonstrations about how language can elicit and effect change. She closes the chapter with an inspiring discussion about the development of her butterfly metaphor.

Chapter Seven, "Metaphor, Analogy, and Word Play Development", explores the very important processes of both developing metaphors and tailoring them to meet the unique needs of clients. Several important therapeutic themes are demonstrated, including substitution.

The Languages and Metaphors of Kay Thompson

Camillo Loriedo

When I first met Kay Thompson, she was giving a presentation during a hypnosis congress. Her ability to use so many different forms and levels of communication, or "languages" at the same time immediately gave me the sensation of being deeply immersed in listening to a symphony.

Each language reminded me of the sound of a musical instrument. Her voice's tone variations appeared as intense as the exquisite notes of a violin, and through playing with words she produced melodies reminiscent of great piano virtuosos.

The flow of her stories and metaphors was as intriguing and absorbing as the music of a magic flute, and the nonverbal language she used to express a meaning was elegant and as pleasing as the sound produced by the touch of gentle fingers moving on the harp. The harmony of the ensemble was so masterful that one could hardly distinguish the many levels of communication that she was able to convey. And in fact, only later, after having attended a number of her "live concerts", I realized how the absorption in the music facilitated the acceptance of the content by the listener.

The Conversation

Kay's language usage was very complex, but it never appeared to be complicated. She used easy and simple words that developed special meanings through their varied combinations, not because of their individual sense. These additional meanings created the effect of spreading the sound in different directions, applying the persistence of echo to the original melody.

In therapeutic conversation she played with words, as if she were performing a symphony, guiding the audience in a fantastic voyage around a meaning to explore emotions of different intensities. Although orchestra musicians follow a score, she adapted her performance to the unique needs of each audience, following the track given by her listeners. For example, when a client exhibited exaggerated tension because of her fears, Kay transformed "tension" into a peaceful and relaxing experience, as in the following example:

Pay Attention to the Tension

And it demands a risk of confronting your fear and saying its okay to be afraid and don't let it stop you, and it seems that people are like that. They deal with tension and you can pay attention to the tension that you need to attend you, which may be one of the reasons that you know that you don't have to have that (symptom), because you have a different kind of attention. And when you tend to those items one at a time you discover that kind of attention to the tension doesn't get rid of the tension. And you need to learn to tune out the tension by tuning in to it before it becomes a tension and to tone up the peaceful, calm, gentle experiences you have explored before in the passage of time, those minutes, days, weeks and months of comfort and happiness.

The Metaphors

Sometimes, instead of expanding the meaning of the word and playing with all its possible connotations, Kay preferred to use the same word as the core element of a brilliant metaphor. In a similar case, for example, the fearful tension of a patient could be gradually transformed into the usable tension of guitar strings. Once the metaphor was accepted, then tightening the strings a little bit more was described to the client as a necessary step in order to make the instrument perfectly tuned. And once the proper tension of the strings was reached and the instrument was tuned, she explained, no additional tension was needed, and the instrument was finally ready to use the strings' tension to produce harmony and consonance. As in the case of the guitar strings, many of Kay's metaphors transformed a difficult situation or problem into a resource or an advantage.

Initially, she outlined the canvas, very carefully preparing the words and concepts that she wanted to emphasize for a specific situation. Then she delivered her messages within a concert of vocal tone variations and by the poetic phrases that gave the reverberating effect of rhyme.

One of Kay's favorite metaphors was entitled *Electric Potential*. She used this metaphor very frequently, maintaining the initial structure, but slightly altering the content in order to adjust to the listener or to indicate a special direction to her thoughts, as in the following example:

Electric Potential

If you think about teaching people hypnosis and teaching them to tap their potential, it's kind of like learning about electricity when you took physics classes. You learn which switch activates which voltage. And you used the switches only when it was appropriate to use the voltage. All I know about switches is you push one of those and something happens to the lights up here. But the switch can be left on or it can be turned off, depending on what it is you want to do. During the conditioning pulses in physics classes, you get a lot of short circuits, which you get when you overuse the power that you have or overload the circuits you have. They are supposed to happen, because then you are supposed to understand the mechanism. When something goes wrong with that kind of circuitry or that kind of voltage, you learn to do something about it.

I see the electric potential in each person, not just each patient, for learning to really understand the message, the language of hypnosis, because that's where the meaning is. I wonder whether we really listen to the messages that people give? Whether we can develop some pattern in the patter that we provide which potentially portrays the perfect patient that each of us would like to see. I wonder whether there are those here who truly hear what it is that I am saying or what we are talking about. Or if your unconscious feels that that is kind of a disturbing sort of knowledge.

Nonverbal Language

One of Kay's most extraordinary abilities was her use of very expressive nonverbal language. The mobility of her eyes was absolutely unique. She could express her opposition or her strongest support to the other's ideas by changing the direction of her glance very rapidly. While the rest of her body appeared relatively immobile, she would initiate a little gesture, and a new language was immediately activated. Kay could, better than any other person I know, use gestures to represent very complex metaphors. Some concepts that are difficult to put in words even for a sophisticated speaker, as well as some phenomena that are hard to elicit even for an experienced therapist, were elegantly sculpted in the air by a few little movements.

Although her use of verbal language was poetic and as effective as a surgeon's knife, she could also elicit every possible behavior without uttering a word. Every form of pain and suffering was very rapidly softened, removed or cancelled, just with a few well-designed gestures. She often used verbal communication to obtain a specific goal, while nonverbally either enforcing the words' effects or working in another completely different direction.

She could easily induce trance in her clients without speaking, and I've seen her suggest even anesthesia, in otherwise "impossible" clients, using only the force of gestures. While the few other hypnotists who know how to perform in a similar way are usually ready to emphasize their "special" ability, consider it as a personal power they possess and are not keen to teach others, Kay always considered her repertoire as simple and offered to teach what she knew. She was a very generous teacher and liked to explain very clearly, step by step, rendering accessible even the more complicated interventions.

Generosity and Sensitivity

Her generosity and sensitivity were recognized and appreciated by both students and clients; she loved to give to everyone. During all the times she visited my Institute in Rome, she never forgot to bring a little gift for every teacher and supervisor (there are about 20!), and for the secretaries. She also generously offered personal help. She immediately recognized when others were suffering and didn't wait for a verbal request to offer her discreet but effective support. On several occasions she sensed my frustrations before I was even aware of them, and promptly provided advice and suggestions.

It may be hard for people, who didn't have the chance of meeting her personally, to believe that she could do all these things. It is equally amazing that she always had a gentle smile and was very natural and at ease, and thus, her actions seemed almost effortless to the observer.

Teaching the Language of Hypnosis
Dan Kohen

I believe that the most important aspect of Kay Thompson's teaching was her use of language or what she called the language of hypnosis. Kay was the consummate teacher. She was confident, matter-of-fact and, ultimately, an ongoing, ever-present model of everything she taught, requested, urged, challenged and expected of those of us fortunate enough to be her students.

That said, the most important example of her modeling was in her use of language, and the way she wore her awareness of it. Kay taught about the essential and integral role of language, and more importantly, our thoughtful, respectful and careful use thereof, and believed this to be the most appropriate and effective utilization and application of clinical hypnosis. Kay's unique emphasis on the multiple meanings of words and phrases, and the multiple layers of understanding and growth, has become an essential underpinning of effective clinical hypnosis.

Learning to hear and carefully construct our own language teaches people how to listen carefully to others' language, to really hear here what people were and are saying, *now*. And it teaches us how to listen much more carefully in all modes, to watch carefully so as to not miss subtle nonverbal cues clients/patients may communicate. Kay's focused sensitivity to subtleties of communication is the essence of the pacing and leading we know to be the functionally mandatory ingredients of effective clinical hypnosis. And effective clinical hypnosis is fundamentally therapeutic communication.

Kay's teaching about language and its appropriate, subtle, refined communication at various levels of consciousness, represents the ultimate and defining gift she gave to clinical hypnosis. As Kay taught, it is through language that hypnosis (and therapy in general) has its most powerful and enduring effectiveness.

Chapter Six
Language to Effect Change

There is at the bottom of all of us a similar kind of linguistic inclination and I think laughter is one of the best indications that we all come from a common base. I'd like you to read the phrase, "Richard and Robert purchased a retriever" without pronouncing the "r's". The way you do it is to think differently and say, "Dick and Bob bought a dog," which gives some indication of the way I hope you are going to be thinking at the end of this morning. Words are symbols for experience.

You can think like a child, which is one of the best ways to think!

I think what we are into with words, is the increasing recognition of the significant impact of verbal and nonverbal communication on the outcome of patient treatment. The language utilized can influence the physiological as well as the psychological progress of the patient. Holistic medicine, which is simply the acknowledgment that the mind and body are one unit working together, must play an important role in the psychodynamics of an effective doctor–patient relationship. I got into this business from the physiological viewpoint and got into dealing with the psychological aspects of it. You need to realize that's where I come from in most of what I am saying here.

As far as I am concerned, the utilization of hypnotic techniques in your practice has a great deal to do with the intensity of the interaction and the impact of the response.

I think it's the obligation of the therapist-doctor to stimulate the imagination and demand recognition, by the individual that you are working with, of his or her own potential. And consciously that can be a rather disturbing knowledge, but on an unconscious level, I think it is really much more appropriate. It's not a matter of actively doing something to change the situation so much as it is listening to ourselves. Because we get signals from the patients all the time. And we need to learn to do what Erickson was so famous for, and that was to go to where the patient is and see the situation from the client's point of view. And that is a very different perspective and one that too few of us are able to pay attention to. The idea that we can accomplish this through words is a major responsibility.

Responsibility is not a duty but a voluntary act in response to the needs of another human being, according to Erich Fromm (the well-known psychotherapist). So that responsable action has a personal expression.

I think that when we are working with hypnosis, it is important to decide, not on the depth of trance, because the client is going to determine the depth he needs, but on the goals of the trance. Once we teach people to relearn this skill of hypnosis, which many of them have forgotten that they ever knew, they will decide on what depth is necessary to reach their goals, as long as we stand out of their way.

The acceptance of the symbolism of words acknowledges the integration of metaphor and analogy just to develop options, and of word play to convey multiple meaning messages. The language of hypnosis, then is going to turn out to be the therapeutic tool for change.

I'm fascinated by the fact that neuroscientists tell us that the brain doesn't seem wired for logical thought. Why do we have receptors that bind to PCP and angel dust? Is maybe their purpose possibly to force us to play? Otherwise, why would the brain have receptors for crazy-making drugs? Maybe, to imagine, to envision, to experience either through the breakdown or breakup of our normal structured channels of thought. To encourage a return to an earlier age, when words were symbols for experience and meaning.

I've talked a lot about the way that language develops and the way children develop. I think that vulnerability is one of the issues that we need to pay attention to. When the client comes in to you, they are vulnerable. And when that happens, it's like storytelling with children. When you tell a child a story, the child doesn't think about the moral, and wonder, "What am I supposed to be learning?" The child feels how good the words are and that makes them more vulnerable. You can slide the message in without them being suspicious about what you are doing. And it provides a background, a stage on which the later performance of that client is going to take place because the client in that vulnerable state taps into the endless energy and curiosity of a child. And isn't that what we want?

If that client wasn't stuck, they wouldn't be coming to you. If they could do it themselves, they wouldn't need you. So we need to tap into a resource that they have not been able to reach: and that's the curiosity and the energy of a 3-year-old. I wish I had it! This idea of being able to tap that unending well of potential to be well. Even in playing with those two words, it makes your mind think differently. That's how word play works. Word play works. Is it play or is it work? If it is work but you can make it play, isn't it going to play out so that the work, in itself is going to be more beneficial for the person who was listening to it? That was brand new. When I started thinking about work and play, it seemed very natural to use the words that way.

That's what you do when you open your mind to the options, to hear the possible other interpretations of the words that you say all the time. You talk to yourself all the time. You have learned how not to listen. Hypnosis is a means of making you able to listen again with the ears of a child and with the truth of a child. It makes you look at words differently. It isn't that you see something different, it is that something different is seen. What you are seeing is the same thing but the way you look at it, the possible differences and the meanings of the words, opens a whole new world.

We go to lecture after lecture after lecture that promises to give us the answer. The title of every one of those lectures is always the same. The title is: Why you should think like I do! If it isn't the title, then I shouldn't be up here talking about it. If I don't believe it, I shouldn't be talking about it. But I believe the real puzzle is not to find the answer, the real puzzle is to define the question. Is communication important in mind-body healing? Can I have an impact on the patient's physiology through my words and my actions? Is there any scientific basis for the belief in the relationship between emotion and physiology? Thank God for Candace Pert (research scientist and author of *The Molecules of Emotion*), because I now have this scientific basis for the beliefs I have always had.

How can I help my patient to achieve that goal and arrive at the desired destination? That's the real question. There is no answer, no single answer, because it depends entirely upon the patient. I once read in *New Age* magazine something that I will paraphrase: We empower patients by encouraging them to develop their own strategies for managing illness. It assumes that the unconscious mind comprehends the nature of disease processes and how to resolve them, an assumption consistent with the healing system's diagnostic capability.

Whether or not we make that information accessible to waking consciousness and then encourage patients to act on it is the question. The body knows what it needs. There is no effort to answer, just to state the question.

And we are giving permission, I hope, in the child's way, because children speak truth and that's what you really want. We want people to be able to understand and express their feelings freely, after a lifetime of having learned to suppress words. If words are symbols for meaning and experience, when you learn to suppress the words, do you not also learn to suppress the strong feelings that go with them? If you get back to the learning sets of word play, then you're going to get unconscious play with other kinds of puzzles, puzzles like riddles, nursery rhymes and homonyms. Reframing words, which have feelings associated with them, can change the attitude about the feelings.

How many of you can describe the physiological responses that go with the word anxiety? Everybody says, sure I can. Palms get sweaty and your heartbeat goes faster, and you get either warm or cold depending on the way you respond to stress, and you breathe faster, and you worry. That's anxiety. Would you also define for me the physiological responses that go with the word anticipation? You are anticipating going out on a date or to a conference you have been looking forward to. Your palms get a little sweaty, your heart beats faster, and your mouth gets a little dry, and you get a little cold or warm, depending on the way you do it. Isn't that what I just said about anxiety?

Anticipation is a very different kind of feeling, isn't it, than anxiety? By reframing the physiological response to anxiety into anticipation, all you are really doing is getting the individual to recognize that they have more control over their physiology, and that they can begin to look forward to something with much more anticipation that they previously would have looked at with anxiety. There are so many of those instances that we just don't listen to. Working with trance accesses listening behaviors that are not readily recognized or more appropriately utilized. This is what metaphor and analogy enable you to do.

What happens inside your head, when you are listening to the radio for the weather report, that makes you miss the weather, and still get hung up on a melody or worse yet, a commercial you didn't want to hear? And the commercial goes round and round and round and you can't get it out of your head. Where does your mind go when you don't hear those things that you said you wanted to *hear*?

Hypnosis in the unconscious state can offer confusion of the conscious mind to produce breakdown of the normal channels of thought with the transactions, "trance-actions", which result, causing positive permutations. Trance-actions versus transactions are one and the same but are really different. All that means is that the acceptance of the symbolism of words acknowledges the integration of metaphor and analogy to develop options and word play to convey multiple messages. I said this before. I hope that you heard it differently this time. Because the language of hypnosis can be the therapeutic tool for this trance-action.

A metaphor is a story. Children learn to listen to stories. Therapists learn to listen for metaphor, ideas to be given in a word, a feeling or phrase by the client and then to elaborate or build a story around that significant word. What that says is that developing metaphors demands really close attention by the therapist. It isn't necessary, practical or possible to develop a new story for each client. You don't need to. They don't know that you used them before. I think that's very important. You need a repertoire of stories to build on and then they can be spontaneously adapted to many situations.

One of the criticisms I have heard of Erickson's writings concerns the story of Robert when he got his leg cut.[8] When you read this story in different versions, you get different "visions" of this story. Were you really listening to that word play? That was appropriate. In poetry we call it poetic license. But when Erickson did it, he was not telling the literal story of Robert, he was telling a metaphor to the client to be used by the client in the most appropriate way. The variations that he gave the story had nothing to do with the actual fact of Robert's slice on his leg. It had to do with what it was that that particular client needed to hear. The idea behind a metaphor is not to be literal; it is to open the options.

Metaphors don't need to be long and involved. I'm notorious for opening my mouth and closing it 90 minutes later! I can give a metaphor that will be as short as one that is kind of like, the tap of a tube into a maple tree that starts the slow steady drip of syrup. But that syrup has to be boiled down and distilled for a very long time before it actually becomes the maple syrup that we know and love. But it starts with that first tap into the maple tree. The need to have the courage to simply make that short sentence metaphor, and then back off and wait for the client to do what they need to do, is the important part of it. And sometimes, that takes guts.

One of the other things that I really get upset about is I will hear someone do a magnificent metaphor, absolutely magnificent, and when they finish it, they say to the client, "Now, what that means is …" Whose confidence is low at that point? Yeah! It's the therapist. Don't waste your time telling a metaphor if you are then going to turn around and explain why you told it, because that really doesn't help. One of my favorite ways of getting into a metaphor and reframing at the same time is to say, "Yes, but." It permits acknowledgment of the actuality, but then reframes it with new information that was not accessible at the time.

I think that profound messages can be given very simply. Contract words are little words that we use all the time and we don't pay attention to—*when, then, not, before, until, after*. When you say,

---

[8] Erickson's story involves acknowledging the serious cut on his son's leg and then engaging Robert's interest in his healthy blood and whether he will get more stitches than his sister got when she hurt herself etc.

"When this happens, this is going to happen but not *before* you are ready," has it happened yet? These little words are important, that we stick in the middle of, or on the end of sentences, that people don't hear consciously but hear on an unconscious level. With the verbal and nonverbal communication that you are using, you can get really, really fascinated by them.

For someone with migraines, the statement, "You don't need to have those headaches anymore" gives permission to look at the headaches from a different perspective. The conscious mind tends to hear "need" but the unconscious mind hears "anymore". Apparently simple words like anymore are deceiving in their simplicity. Because what they do is validate that individual. It says, you may have had a very legitimate reason and need for those headaches at that time, back where you came from, and that was okay. But based on my permissive encouragement, I didn't say, "Do you need?" I said, "You don't *need* to have those headaches anymore." Whether the headaches still serve a useful purpose will be the unconscious evaluation and looking at their future destination and whether or not it's time to explore a different route. That's very different from saying, "You don't need to have those headaches." Or the more common questions, "Why do you want or need those headaches?"

Are you ready to give up those headaches *yet*? That isn't a yes or no answer. Because, with yet said, there will be a time when you *are* willing to give up those headaches. That is the important part, opening the possibility of change. Opening up new memories by giving them old information and getting the individual to think about it differently. When you say, "You know, if you think back to when you had dinner last night, and you think about who sat across from you at dinner, or you think about what you had for dinner," you are doing a regression. All I asked you was six words, "You know, if you think back."

Regression doesn't have to be running a movie camera backwards. Regression doesn't have to be going into a very profound trance and working your way back. Sometimes that's appropriate because there's a lot of intervening material. In order to think back, they have to regress. It's the only way they can do it. Are you aware of the impact of your words? Pay attention! [Thompson tells one of her favorite metaphors about looking back at one's childhood and changing perspectives: see Chapter Ten.]

You are expanding old memories with new information in a way that they can look at them differently. Simply giving new information is not enough. It has to be reframed so they can make use of it, so they can utilize it. The induction itself *is* a metaphor. If it is indirect, then the conscious mind can hear the story, while the unconscious hears the multiple layers of messages. Making a metaphor, from something the client said which jumps out at you, is confusing to the conscious mind and refreshing to the unconscious mind, because it gives it the freedom to follow.

Are you all familiar with the sand bucket induction? It simply involves asking the client to hold both arms out in front of him, and asking him to let his unconscious choose an arm that the bucket is going to hang on and to put the sand in the bucket. How many of you could talk sand bucket for 45 minutes and be comfortable doing it? On the other hand, how many of you could talk sand bucket as utilization of a metaphor for 45 minutes and be comfortable doing it? I have a couple of examples.

One was a lady who was stuck at not being able to lose weight. And the therapist brought her into the group as a potential hypnosis volunteer to show her hypnosis. That was all we were going to do, and sometime down the line, she could use it for her particular weight problem. And she put her arms out and proceeded to hold her hands there for 45 minutes. As we talked, what she heard were multiple meanings in words, because practically every word that came out of my mouth had a multiple meaning.

She was finding the way to weigh the weight that she was waiting to weigh—the weight in that bucket. What does bucket represent in slang? It represents the derriere. So every time that we put sand in that bucket she was paying attention to the weight in her bucket. And talking about not being able to overlook the weight of the sand in that bucket: I would throw the word sand in regularly, so that she wouldn't get too clearly the discrimination between the weight she was waiting to learn to weigh and the weight in the sand bucket. And when you are dramatically overweight, it's hard to overlook that overweight, because you can't look down without looking over the weight that you wished that you didn't weigh.

The more we talked about the sand in the bucket, the easier it became for her unconscious to hear the multiple messages about this weight she was learning to weigh. And as we talked a lot about her getting a handle on this, because after all, we had a handle on the bucket, she could reach out a hand to the therapist who was working with her. She came out of the trance and her hand did eventually go down, and she was very comfortable with having learned about hypnosis, which was a *very* interesting experience. And she was seriously going to consider whether she was going to use it with her therapist for weight control. And she never quite figured out why between that appointment and the next one she dropped 14 pounds. And if you are going to use the induction as the utilization as the metaphor, then you'd better be prepared to talk a very long time about whatever that particular induction technique is.

The other one was a biophysicist at one of my universities and he needed to have some dental work done. His dentist couldn't do his dental work because he gagged. We spent a very long time working; it was 12 visits, it was not brief therapy. On the other hand, he hadn't been able to go to the dentist for 40 years. If you divide those 12 visits into those 40 years, that isn't your twice a year tooth cleaning kind of routine. But the sand bucket routine became again a very important induction technique-metaphor for him, because we got nowhere pouring the sand in the bucket, until the phrase changed just a little bit to "and the weight of that bucket is kind of like the weight of that burden you have been carrying on your shoulders for such a long time". And then the arm moved.

And I thought, okay, let's follow that path. Combining the weight of that burden and looking forward to letting that weight on his arm go down, the unconscious heard many multiple messages that it was able to accept. When we were finished, he left with tears in his eyes and said, "This is the first time in 40 years that I believe I may be able to do something about this." Twelve visits later, I took him by the hand back to his dentist, so that I could teach the dentist how to talk to him, so he wouldn't negate everything that had been done, which is a very important part of what I do.

Therapists have to keep in mind that the outcome of the trance, this altered state of awareness, has to be defined in terms of the patient's motivation and needs. And this matter and manner of mutual motivational manipulation is manageable but it mandates mastery of many methods. Were you listening to what my words said? Were you listening to M, M, M's? Does it matter what you were listening to? No. Because the part of you that needed to hear the one, heard the one, and the part that needed to hear the other, heard the other. Trance is going to vary depending on the use that is going to be made of it. It certainly can be influenced by the doctor. A good therapist can help a patient. But boy, a bad one can sure keep that person from being able to go into trance.

Erickson's frequent use of the term *experiential life* reminds us that words are simply symbols for experience and meaning, and that we started out knowing more about symbols than we knew about words, which by themselves, are really poor messengers. That's one of the reasons I reject experimental trance. Experimental trance demands that you use the same wording, the same inflections, in the same way, on a tape recording and doesn't take into account individual differences. No wonder it fails. I don't think it's valid for clinical kinds of transitions. I have my particular philosophy about types of trance based on motivation. I believe that experimental trance serves a useful purpose, but not one that's very much help for me because I am a clinician.

When you are going to use an indirect induction, it can be used early on. You kind of have to recognize that you can push the start button on that marvelous mind machine that each of us owns and starts us driving down memory road. The question is whether it's going to be a rough and rocky road or a smooth and lovely lane. I took my mother to Scotland a few years ago. Their back roads are a lane and a half wide and there is no protection on either side. And I came to a sign that said ROAD WORK AHEAD. And then came to another sign that said, "You have been warned!" Are we warned?

Let's take a trip and see the relationship to the linguistic vehicle that we are driving, because we want to have as much of an impact on the patient's response as we can. I think that Candace Pert made it clear that we are having an explosion of knowledge and understanding of the biochemical basis of emotion and the body-mind connection. She demonstrates that we can, through hypnosis, imaging and suggestion influence the immune system. There's a lot of us who have been saying this for 40 years but nobody has ever given us scientific proof. Now we have scientific proof and PET scans and we have all these things we rely on, to say, "See, I told you this works." The same chemicals that are released in various emotional states are found in the immune cells. And the receptors for these chemicals, including PCP and angel dust, are found in the brain and in the immune system.

Neuropeptides and their receptors are a road map of how the mind and body are interconnected and of the pathways of the three systems. Back in the dark ages, when I went to school, we were told that there were three systems and they didn't talk to one another. And I kept thinking, they are all in the same body, how could they not talk to one another? Now we've decided that it's okay that they talk to one another and influence us. These receptors are interconnected through the internal information highway, so emotions can be manifested throughout any of the three systems of the body. We have an interstate and an intrastate highway map and it's under construction right now. As we drive these new main highways, are we going to be able to learn the short cuts that are going to take us to our destination, by asking directions and learning to understand the words we get from the answers?

The largest number of message vehicles coming from the brain are kept on this straight road, not by juxtaposition of nerve cells and close intersections, but by the specificity of the guidepost receptors in a very complex wide ranging pattern, almost like gas stations, distribution stations. The receptors serve as the mechanism that sorts out the neuropeptides and the information exchange in the body, the same way a traffic policeman dictates which traffic has to keep going and which traffic is allowed to park. And you've got to have a special sign to be able to park in those places. This leads to the conclusion that the receptors for the neuropeptides are the road map to the biochemistry of emotion which is the parking place for these responses. But there are *lots* of wonderful parking places, receptors other than in the limbic system, which for many years, we thought was the only parking place around.

We are talking about the brain, the glands, the hormones, the spleen, the bone marrow, the lymphatic and the circulating cells. This is where the information carriers are coming in. This is our information theory that we are working with. The mind is composed of information. It has a physical substrate which is the body and brain. But I am concerned about this immaterial substrate that carries the information constantly flowing through these parts.

How is this mapping important? It's very important to you. Because you, as a healer, constantly do things which have the potential to alter the biochemistry of the body, the physiological–psychological homeostasis or balance of the body. This is what we are trying to do and this is what we *do* all the time.

What we are doing is taking our words to tap into the physiological substrate so the individual can control, not only his mind, but his body, his responses and his behaviors. There are a great many people who have worked with hypnosis for many years who thought that they knew what it was that they were doing. Years ago, I said that I keep finding things out that I did not yet know that I knew. But the things that have made my life so much easier have been things like surgery, auto accidents, and knee replacements and things like that.

It's a little bit unusual for somebody of my generation to quote Malcolm X, but I happen to think that this is a particularly good statement from him. "Only those who have experienced a revolution within themselves can truly reach out to help others."

I think learning to think in a different way, being open to the options that hypnotic language can give you will let *you* have that revolution within yourself to be able to reach out and help others. To listen differently and to be able to work with those people to get them to the place that they would like to be. Why is this important to you? Because you are a healer. Because you constantly have the potential to influence other people. This is what you *want* to do. This is what you *chose* to do.

You need to understand that we recognize that roads are intended to be smooth, balanced, and well-traveled ways to a destination. But then sometimes a contractor decides to do some road construction, which interferes with the time it takes you and possibly the direction that it is going to take you, to get that individual to travel to their destination. You may find one of those road work signs ahead, and if you do, then you'd better be warned. In that case, travel may be accomplished best by just kind of slowing up and choosing an alternative route. Sometimes the best way to travel may be in an altered state vehicle. When you are in that altered state vehicle and you reach a major detour/construction, it is convenient to have a car that functions on automatic, so your mind does not have to constantly worry with shifting gears. You can let you mind cover other routes, while the vehicle crawls slowly along the traditional route.

Of course, there are those times that your attention wanders too far; you decide to stay awake by deliberately putting the car in a lower gear, which demands what? It demands that you pay more attention to the driving. And there are a lot of people who like the satisfaction of being able to shift gears and to have more control over that vehicle that they are in. They like it that way. They want to do it when they want to do it, not when the vehicle says so.

I think it is important to decide, not on depth of trance, but on destination. I think that it is fascinating to me that words are so powerful, but they are so often ignored. It's kind of like after you have driven through a red light or a stop sign and the policeman can issue a ticket or issue a warning, so you know how to interpret the importance of that red light or that stop sign. But you also know that it depends on the mood that the policeman is in, whether you get a ticket or warning.

In the context of driving, you also have to know how to operate the car. And teaching people to drive can be done in a great many ways. There are always those people whose parents taught them how to drive. What did they do? They learned all their parents' wrong habits and they just carried them on forever. There are other people who take driver training. I know one woman who has taken driver training seven times and still has not passed her test. Some people are so anxious, and she falls into that category and hasn't begun to look at it as anticipation, so she won't even take it any more. Other people fail the test because they are arrogantly overconfident that they can do anything. And what we are hoping for are the lucky ones who really understand how to drive a car, how to gauge distance and closeness, and how to avoid accidents, so they are competent and they pass the test.

But after all this teaching, what happens? You get your driver's license. Do you remember when you first got your driver's license? If your mother wanted a loaf of bread from the store that was half a block down the street, you'd go get the bread if you could drive the car, right? But now there aren't too many of you who still have that overeagerness and overenthusiasm for driving because it has become routine. Unless you come across a very different kind of road or there's a pothole ahead of you and you have to suddenly become alert, driving becomes very ordinary. You need to shake up that ordinary in order to really understand the *best* way to get to your destination.

We had friends who took trips east coast to west coast, and they changed drivers every 50 miles. If they were in the middle of a city and the 50-mile mark came up, they stopped and changed drivers. It took them a long time to get across the country. But this was the way they did it. Other people started refusing to take trips with them, because they couldn't stand that. There was no way they were going to do it any other way. They couldn't *hear* any other suggestion. Other people need to be distracted to endure the journey. But man, they focused on those 50 miles. I'm not sure that they ever drove enough that their skill would improve with practice, because they were too busy watching the odometer.

I think that trance is kind of the same thing. Correct semantics, good operating technique, considered approach, that's all that most people require. But how does the mechanic explain the principles of the car? One of the things that happens to us is that we think that we know best.

By the nature of my profession I am forced to do difficult and sometimes potentially painful procedures to repair the heap the patient drives up in. It is necessary that I do this carefully. I have to explain about the necessary repairs on the basis of how the car had been taken care of in the past, what is necessary now to get it in good running order, the maintenance that is going to be necessary to keep it in that condition, and how much it would cost to get it repaired, so it will hold up for many years.

About that time, the owner has heavy concerns about my working on the car. I believe that the explanation for that concern lies in the area in which I as the mechanic am going to be working. This vehicle is *his*. And they have traveled down the road together for a good many years and they expect to be together for a lot more. If I understand that trip, I can respect and refine the work that needs to be done without getting them too upset and angry with me.

I hope that I can teach the driver how to better drive the car. But in the ideal world in my office, there are 8,760 hours in a year and I'm going to see that person, maybe for three or four. What chance do I have? I'd better reach the unconscious, because the conscious resistance has been there for a long time. One of the things I have to acknowledge is that no matter how much I teach, no matter how hard I work on that vehicle, no matter how bright and shiny it is, it is still the owner of the vehicle who is going to take it away and drive off into the sunset with it. There comes a time when I have to be able to enable them to do precisely that.

The driver wants to depend on my integrity and my knowledge. You, as the doctor-healer have to serve as the authority figure. And you are going to get vehicles who are going to be frightened, fearful, antagonistic, sullen and hostile, all based on previous experience on the roads that they have been traveling along, not necessarily to you. Your first job is to earn trust and understand about the development of these attitudes and then proceed to change their perspective to a present day reality. How do we do that? How we earn that trust is a really important part of the things that we do.

It's time for a participation exercise. I would like you all to stand up and pair off and face one another. One person take one step closer to your partner. The other person take one step closer to your partner. UH HUHHH! The first person take another step closer. You're running out of room yet? Are you listening to the increased noise level yet? The first person, take your right hand and put it on your partner's left shoulder. The second person, do the same. What happens when you do that? It grounds you. The aloofness and the strangeness in that distance between you settles down and isn't that strange. That's all, but I would like to talk about it.

Because we are the authority figure, you have no problem invading your client's personal space. Dentists invade their patient's personal space about as much as you can. Most of the time they do it without so much as a by-your-leave. The respect and the trust we need from that individual is also something we have to give. It can be given in a verbal or a nonverbal way and we need to pay attention to that.

Now, obviously personal space varies based on your background, based on where you live. There are lots of studies that have been done that show that people in Scandinavian countries like three feet of personal space. And in Mediterranean countries, you exchange breath if you are really friends. In the United States, ours is about 18 inches. When you get within that space, you start backing off. When you go to a party and watch people, you notice that there are people who like to elbow you and touch you and the people who resist that are constantly backing away.

Those kinds of nonverbal communications are in effect in your office. Because you are in charge, you are not generally so aware of when you are getting inside that person's personal space. It helps if you ground yourself and your client. When you did the exercise, as you got closer and the noise level went up, when you put your hand on their shoulder, it stopped. There was implicit permission that this was something you were allowed to do. When you are working with people, you may come out and ask them how comfortable they are.

Nonverbal communication is very important. When you go in to take someone's blood pressure, and you are here, and they turn around to give you their arm, and make it a big deal that they are doing it. I work with a reasonably large number of agoraphobics. I remember being in the middle of extracting a molar. I was making a valiant effort to be gentle, but the tooth wasn't cooperating. I was elevating the tooth and the root fractured and I thought, "Oh, dear!" Later the patient said she was looking at my face and my face was so calm and composed that she knew everything was in control. I think dentists play a different kind of poker.

Therapists need to practice the expressions they put on their faces. It is important that you be able to be an actor, not that you be

106

insincere. Simply that you do not have this aloof kind of distance, that says that you don't care. This was one of the qualities that I was most taken by with Erickson. I know that you are supposed to remain objective and not get involved in the patient's problems. But remaining objective doesn't mean that you are not compassionate. There are some people who can do both, and Erickson was one of those. But Erickson, in addition to writing out his work and practicing his verbal presentation, practiced what the expressions were that he would put on his face, that he wanted the client to think that he thought.

I think that this is very, very important. I think that each of us needs to be able put the expression on our face that is the symbol for the words and experience that is going on for that client at that particular time. I say that I am putting on my wide-eyed sincere look. And when I put on that wide-eyed sincere look, it says that what I am saying is eminently reasonable. As the authority figure. I expect that my patient is going to do it. When I do that, it usually involves telling my patient to stop bleeding or to turn off pain. For me that is eminently reasonable. I know they can do it, I expect them to do it. My expression says that they will do it. I suspect that if I had a video camera, I put that expression on my face when I was saying that. Those words go with that expression so far as that individual is concerned. That request is one that is enhanced by the expression that I put on my face.

The expression enables me to teach that individual self-regulation via metaphor. What I say, how I say it and the way I look when I say it, are all important. Because in that patient's vulnerability, especially with somebody standing over him about to cut him open with a knife, there is a regression to a simpler time, when words were more eloquent and went straight to the meaning. Patients can tell you things about themselves at times like that, which they might not tell you at other times. Early on I said that my orientation to hypnosis comes precisely from the fact that I can get used to talking with patients, but just about the time I get comfortable talking with them, somebody comes in and wants surgery. And they don't want anesthesia or bleeding, and most of the time I am the one doing the surgery.

It demands a more intense level of commitment on my part. I can't get away with just words. They are going to prove to me whether or not my words were effective. It's simple enough to say the words that you want to say. You need *feedback* in order to know whether what you said was interpreted and acted upon. I think that not all of you are going to have the opportunity to do surgical procedures. You need to get a different kind of feedback from your client and it needs to be both verbal and nonverbal.

When I talked about what I really do, it related to a different kind of situation for each of you, by stimulating memories of past events. Each of you had some kind of memory of having been to a physician or dentist who did more than just talk with you. They did some actual work. And so I was asking you to remember a regression experience. When you do that, you can become so entranced with really knowing all there is that you need to know about how to make the memory of that experience change into something that it wasn't when it began, only because you had not thought about it as being what you didn't think it was.

What did I say? Does it matter? It makes sense. I don't know whether I can diagram it. It speaks to the conscious mind because I say it so seriously and so thoughtfully, you *know* that I must be saying something important. But you can't follow it. You also know that your unconscious mind is hearing and making perfectly good sense of what appears to be nonsense, by getting the essence of the sense of what it is, that gives you the sensation that there is something essential in what I said.

Everybody in this room needs to learn to do some of that. You can't preplan it. It is a spontaneous, childlike ability to see words as symbols and say that they can be other things and to change that perspective of the individual to get them to look at things differently. The wide-eyed, sincere look opens the options of the patient.

In the world, people are used to seeing images on television that are symbols for experiences that the advertisers want us to adopt and recognize. As responsible individuals we are aware of the significance of the words we use and need to talk to more people about it. We have a revolution exchange. We have all kinds of information flowing back and forth. Maybe one of the things we can do is teach people how to resist the game playing that goes on in words, to teach people to look at the words that the games are being played with and analyze what is behind the words. Of course, I don't think they are going to be able to analyze all the unconscious kinds of things I am talking about. I do think educating people about the importance of words is going to be a very important part of the future of what we do.

It's so important that we pay attention to the kinds of things we do, the things that we are talking about, and the kinds of things we want that individual to do. This long and involved trip that we were taking is really an important trip, in the kind of driving you learn to do with your clients, and the ability you have to permit them to do things that you didn't know that they knew how to do. One of the fun word play games is a takeoff on K,N,O,W.

You really don't know everything that you know that you know, but it's all right if you don't know everything that you know that you know, as long as you know that you don't know everything that you know that you know, and if you know that you don't know everything that you know, but you know that if you need to know it you'll be able to use it, then you can go right ahead knowing that you don't know everything that you know that you need to know.

The only way I can get through the confusion of words is by being in trance. That's the only place that it makes good sense. And that's the place where I expect that the unconscious is going to be able to hear it.

This is a little aside. I have never been able to not know which of my fingers lifts for ideomotor signaling. That's my problem. When I'm working with somebody else and I ask for finger movements, if I would prefer that they not know which finger lifts, I have this doubt in my head. Because I can't do it, I don't have the confidence. I'm an advocate of the Chevreul pendulum, because I think it's far harder for the client to tell which direction the pendulum is moving. I don't have them sitting there and staring at it. I have something between it and them. How many of you are familiar with the Chevreul pendulum? The pendulum has four directions in which it can move, other than standing still: clockwise and counter-clockwise circle, vertical and horizontal straight lines. There are four answers for any question: yes, no, I don't know and I don't choose to answer, otherwise known as, it's none of your cotton pickin' business!

But when I talk with the patient, I will get them to set up the signals they are going to use for that day. Frequently, they will change signals. The next time they are not going to use the same signals. I ask, "Which direction is the pendulum going to move if the answer to the question is going to be yes?" I have a very well-trained pendulum. "And which direction will it move if the answer is no?" I'm obviously not watching it. "Which direction if the answer is I don't know?" Then the pendulum slows down. "If you want to hurry it you can stop it and start it again." What did I say? If you want to hurry it, you can stop and start it. Hurry and start and stop are very conflictual words so the client has to think through those. And we are left with I don't want to answer, which is the last direction. It's much more difficult for the individual to cheat. There are those people who will cheat if they are using finger signals. It's much harder for them to tell which direction the pendulum is moving. I think the pendulums are so much fun and I have a major collection of them. The one I really like is when all else fails, you get this one out and hit them on the head with it.

How many of you still do structured formal induction techniques? *Not enough hands.* Every time that you do one, you learn something new. Every time you do one, you get good physiological feedback from the person you are working with. I'm a real advocate of them and I still do formal induction techniques, and so did Milton Erickson. In later years, when he was much more incapacitated, it was much more difficult to do them. It was a lot easier to tell stories because the people who came to see him wanted to hear him tell stories anyway. Recognize that you need to sharpen your skills to keep them refined. Formal structured induction techniques will help you to do that.

Also, when you have a client who is cynical, scared, resistant, difficult or desperate, it can be very useful. When they hold their arm out and the arm goes down or when they do a levitation and a hand goes up, or stare at a spot on the ceiling, and their eyes close, *something happened*, something outside of their conscious control. Their problem is outside their conscious control. They have tried to deal with it and they couldn't. If by using hypnosis, this can happen outside of their conscious control, maybe, just maybe they can deal with their problem outside of their conscious control. That is a very reassuring and a very helpful kind of feedback for that individual to have.

I like working with people who have been told that they are resistant. I think that resistance is kind of fun. I see it as a challenge to me. I think that the person who demonstrates resistance is very smart because they are getting a second opinion. If someone comes in and I look at them and say, "Boo!" or "Rumpelstiltskin" and they go GULK into a trance, they are pretty gullible! They don't know me. Why should they trust me at that point? But if they come in and give me a hard time, then I am impressed with how smart they are to do that. If I am able and willing to deal with them with hypnosis and an induction and we succeed with that, then they have the validation that it's probably all right to trust me with their "real problem". That's one of the fun ways I look at that.

The other one is to say, "Uh, well, uh, I don't, uh, I'm not, uh. I'm not real sure that hypnosis and trance are appropriate for you to use with your weight loss or your cigarette smoking or whatever your problem may be. Uh, I'll tell you what. Today we'll teach you about hypnosis and when you come back next time, we'll decide whether you want to use it for your problem or not." What did I just do? I took away their need for resistance. Let's face it. Everybody thinks that hypnosis is kind of fun, once they find out that it isn't control by another person, that is.

They come to you with the belief that, "If I go into trance, I am going to have to lose weight. If I go into trance I will have to stop smoking. What did I do? I just said, "Oh, No! Uh uh, that ain't the way it works, folks! We will teach you about hypnosis today. When you come back the next time, you and I will decide whether ..." It gives them the freedom to have the fun of learning about trance and hypnosis without having the obligation of having to use it for their problem. Once they learn about it, of course, they will probably want to use it for their problem. But that has nothing to do with me. It's fun to choose to look at resistance that way. It's simply getting the person to understand that hypnosis isn't what they thought it was, which is what I think that hypnosis is anyway.

If you think about teaching people hypnosis and teaching them to tap their potential, it's kind of like learning about electricity when you took physics classes (see electric potential: Chapter Eleven).

And if you think about ideas in the four corners of the quarters of your brain, the things that come forth from these let you go forward pretty well. Three-fourths of what we think is not truly intellectual in the hemispheric sense, because it's only this front left quarter that is truly intellectual. If you think about the right hemisphere, the abstract side, as having a front of the brain as well as a back of the brain, you have one quarter in the front and one quarter in the back. And then you have the left side, which is the side which is left, and you take the one quarter in the front and the one in the back and you add that and you get two, and when you add those up you get four. And you can look forward to an additional gain from this kind of addition.

When you add things up in this way, one is when you win and when you win, it means you gain. But sometimes the only way that you can gain is by losing, because when you lose, then, are you really gaining? If you win only what you gain by losing, you understand that some losses can be very positive gains, especially if you don't need to have it all add up. Because if it does, and you think you know what you are really listening to and have heard, then possibly what you do know, is not what you are consciously willing to know that you know. Because if you do and then you discover that comparing that to what you do not know, the three quarters that I mentioned earlier in adding up the gains and losses, is reflected in the kinds of things you see when you look into a window pane. And a mirror can truly be a pane. And I wonder when you look into that pane, I wonder whether it's very painful to see what you see in that sea of wavy scenes that you see? And do you see the scene that you see or the one you want to see? And can you see where you were and when you were there and where you were when you were where you are?

Because looking through a very clean clear pane to the other side lets you understand where you can go, as you merge the mirage of wavy lines in your lives into a marriage of past events which have shaped us, present events which surround us, and a future that adds up. Just by knowing that one on one side and one on the other side is a gain, so it's okay to finally win by understanding that you can learn to gain by losing, and still know that you know everything that you need to know. Because by doing that, you can be what you want to be, which is the sum total of those four corners of the quarters of the brain. But if you chose that, recognize that it involves a risk. It demands expansion of those very comfortable walls behind which you hide and through which we refuse to see or be seen, even though it may be a pane. And if you confront that fear and recognize that it's okay to go ahead anyway, then the good feelings that make it all worth while are the kinds of additional things and positive responses that you generate from a recharging of enthusiasm and a renewed look at the current language of metaphor and word play.

Is anybody in trance? I didn't ask you to go in one. All I did was start talking. And what I talked about made sense. My nonverbal communication said that this is just a report. I can listen to this. And then the unconscious gets sucked into it, when the conscious mind is still struggling to make sense of it. This is probably the one [induction/metaphor] that I have done the most, which is why I tried to follow the structure which I have used. So many natural, everyday kinds of things are really very trance enhancing. Trances start a trend of transferring the tendency to trance out temporarily by tempering the tenor and the tempo of the time, tempting us to theoretically take this trip together. And you seem to be seen to transcend the mundane into the magic of a mosaic of many memories. When you store that mosaic of memories in your mind you discover that it's there to be pulled out, whenever it's appropriate for you and whenever it's something that you believe is going to help your client. One of the metaphors I'm having a lot of fun with is about a butterfly. (In the following discussion, quotation marks are used to distinguish the metaphor from Thompson's discussion about the metaphor. All of the text is by Kay Thompson.)

"I'm always truly fascinated when I watch a caterpillar because change has a beginning, a middle and an end. The end for the caterpillar is the beginning for the butterfly. And I watch a caterpillar, kind of all fuzzy and tenuous creeping along, determined on its journey, and it has some pretty long, hard and lonely times to go through. And then I see it bound by a tight cocoon held very rigidly by the fine ropes that made the shell. And the cords that bind it may be silken, but they smother. And there's a struggle to leave that prison."

And this is the point at which if I am telling it to a client, I change my pronoun. Up until this time, I have been using "the" and then I say, "I hear the beating of 'your' wings" and at that point, the client becomes that butterfly. Up until that time, I have just been telling a story about "the" caterpillar and "the" cocoon. It doesn't sound like much. But when you are doing indirect work, be very aware. In the one which I just did with the hemispheres, when and how did I change from "the" to "you" and "your"? What difference did it make? It makes a lot of difference!

"And I hear the beating of your wings, little caterpillar, butterfly fighting to be free, because always deep inside is a vision of what you are meant to be. A lepidoptera, even the name is magnetic!"

Now utilizing things like lepidoptra, is one of the things I have a lot of fun with. If you insert something like that in the middle of a discussion, it peaks that childlike curiosity and interest. One of the ones I use a lot is *"levator labialis superioris ala que nasae"* the longest name of the shortest muscle in the body. It is a muscle that lets you wiggle your nose. I would challenge each of you the next time you wiggle your nose, try not to think about *levator labialis superioris ala que nasae.* When you are working with someone, and you attach or you ground or anchor them with something that's fun and something that they can use and laugh about, then it's a lot more effective for them. And *Lepidoptra,* for many people is that kind of a word, magnetic.

"And finally the cords that hold the shell begin to split. And you creep out and you balance tentatively on your new legs. And then as your wings dry, you begin to spread them and the air catches them and startle. When they flutter, you fly away. As you look back at those dried up left behind parts, which *stay there,* as you know you will never forget, they once happened to be a part of you. That jail is never more. Because what people don't really know is the reputation of the butterfly as a fierce fighter beneath that fragile exterior, defending home and family."

You'd better go home and read about the butterfly, if you don't know these are all true statements.

"And so you are a survivor of that sort. Even more now, you can appreciate the beauty inside, as well as what shows outside that you have become."

And then you talk about the sunny days when you fly around and have a great time everywhere, but then you talk about the rainy days when you take refuge under a leaf and hide, knowing that the sun will come out and dry you, warm you and comfort you.

"And you've got these magnificent colors that shine for everybody to see. And the rhythm of the poetry of your being is reflected in the beating of your wings, and its sensitivity, the truth of the vision in you. So having been touched by the promise of that loveliness, and the elegance and grace of those gloriously colored wings, we wait, we wait, sure and secure in that special way for the rest of your journey into light."

It doesn't take long. You can tell the story however you like and it can have so many multiple meanings for so many, many people, that it's a good one to have in your repertoire.

I said there are short metaphors. Isn't it convenient that nature gives us all a kind of pressure cooker safety valve, in tears? If you think about all the storms we endure and the heavy thunder and lightening and we get swept up in the damage and the torrents of the floods that rain down. But our enthusiasm is never washed away. And we know the floods will create our refuge in quiet pools. And those who survive the storm are the ones who get to see the rainbow. It doesn't take long. You play with it however you like. They all don't have to be two pages.

When we come to the edge of all the life we have and must take a step into the darkness of the unknown, we must believe one of two things. Either we will find something firm to stand on or we will be taught to fly. You all are about to fly.

One of the things you ought to know about me is that when I first went to these seminars, the way that you found me was to feel along the wall for the bump in the wall, and you would peel the wallpaper off, and I would be hiding behind it. I was not born vaccinated with a Victrola needle. If I can do it, so can everyone in this

115

room. You have to work hard to be loose enough. Remember, I am a dentist, so that means I am compulsive, conformist, lacking in leadership, lacking in responsibility, an individualist whose ethics go down while I was in dental school. If I can break that rigid frame, those silken cords that bind me, and turn into a butterfly, then everybody in this room can do the same thing. And that's important. You just have to practice.

One of the things I do is plagiarize freely, otherwise known as research. How many of you are familiar with comedy groups? People can get a whole audience caught up into being childlike. Metaphors do not have to be long. How many of you are familiar with the song "The Rose"? (see footnote on page 134.) Every single line in that is a metaphor.

Some say love, it is a river that drowns a tender reed. Metaphor!

Some say love, it is a razor that leads us all to bleed. Metaphor!

Some say love, it is a hunger, an endless aching need. Metaphor!

We don't have a corner on the market. That's why I plagiarize. I have a folder marked poetry, because other people say things so much better than I can. One of the sayings by Thoreau has saved my life more often than I choose to admit, because I have difficulty writing to someone who has lost someone they love. I just quote Thoreau, "The pain of loneliness and loss is but a measure of the love we know." That is one that has gotten me out of some very difficult situations. I say to my patients who come in grieving, "Wouldn't you feel bad if you didn't feel bad?" It makes them look at feeling bad in a different way. It gives us the opportunity to start to talk.

But the idea is to get you to begin to open your own options, not just the options of your patients. And in the paradigm of change, we spark the energy that oscillates within us. We link in series the transformers that recharge our storage batteries with direct rather than alternating current. This conduction of positive polarity discharges the negative current and the resistance is impeded. We are galvanized as we remember to ground the voltage charge so the meters register only commutation values and we are safe.

René Daumal wrote a metaphor in *Mount Analogue* (1959). It has become of my favorites and is relatively short and talks a lot about what we are doing here and about what we take home with us.

> You cannot stay on the summit forever. You have to come down again. So why bother in the first place? Just this. What is above, knows what is below. What is below, does not know what is above. One climbs, one sees, one descends, one sees no longer, but one has seen. There is an art of conducting oneself in the lower regions by the memory of what one saw higher up. When one can no longer see, one can at least still know. (Page 103.)

My patients do wonderful things besides using hypnosis. We are taught that we have to get everybody in touch with reality. But sometimes it doesn't take very much to turn reality upside down and make it fantasy. And sometimes it is hard to tell which is which. But as long as the person can function in their own reality or their own fantasy, what difference does it really make?

References

Daumel, R. (1959). *Mount Analogue* (R. Shattuck, trans.), London: Vincent Stuart.

Chapter Seven
Metaphor, Analogy and Word Play Development

There is a line in a popular song about how to turn down the noise in your mind. I think that's what hypnosis lets us do. It lets us turn down the noise in our mind so that we can listen to the music that's there. Sometimes it's pretty hard to distinguish between the noise and the music when there are other things like pain or discomfort or people interfering. Really, the ability to distill and clarify, based on previous experience the individual has had, is very important.

I think about Milton Erickson as someone very fond of trees. I use trees as symbolism for a lot of the things that I do. If you think about a tree, you also have to think about the way the root system works. I come from Pittsburgh where maple trees are very popular and they have a taproot that is very long and if you cut that taproot, the tree dies. So if I get transplanted from Pittsburgh, and that cuts my taproot, then I will have trouble surviving. I wonder if you heard "trance-planted" from Pittsburgh or transplanted from Pittsburgh? And how often have you heard me say, trance-lates early? And *trance-mutes* and *trance-forms*? And I wonder why we call it trance, when we have so many permutations of the word trance, all of which have a relevance to the hypnotic phenomena and to the hypnotic state and to the language we utilize when we are talking about hypnosis?

A lot of Erickson's foundation and those roots, the things that he did, were processed through his trunk and went out into the branches. What you had on this tree were first generation branches and second generation branches, and the seeds that fell out of the first generation branches making a smaller circle, and the seeds falling from the second generation branches making a wider circle. From that seed is a little bit of the original. Everyone is individual and is growing in a different way and everyone has to wonder about what it is going to grow to be.

Are you going to graft anything on that branch? Are you going to take learnings from other systems and graft it on that trunk or foundation or on the branches? The yin and yang and the meditation and elements of that can be grafted on that branch.

We have to learn to prune the dead wood. We are not very good with that when it comes to Erickson. Everything that has the Erickson ambience connected to it has to be sanctified and purified and put up there. I don't think that's true. There are people who came to visit Erickson and didn't partake of any of the branches of the tree and went away explaining the need for explaining the change in themselves by explaining him, so they write books. There are people who *do* have the knowledge and the understanding to have been grafted onto that tree.

You need to be selective and decide how much is the real trunk of the tree, how much has been grafted on and how much is bad wood that has not been pruned away, and how much is pure, and how much is blended fruit. I have a tree in my yard that has five different kinds of apples and yet they are all apples. You have to sort out which apple it is you want. You find that a tree never fruits directly from the trunk, does it? It always grows out of the branches and has to change and be modified. If it doesn't have the trunk's solid base, it never has the chance for the fruit to grow and it never has the strength that it needs.

What we are doing with learning hypnosis is that kind of growing process. You have to be smart enough to decide which kind of apple you want from that tree and recognize when you need to prune the dead wood. And you have to be discriminating in your choice of utilization of what you learn from the trunk of that tree as well as from the branches. It's really difficult today with the proliferation of the ability to graft. Every time I use that word, I hear it in a number of permutations. It's important to read and learn and to begin to have knowledge about all the people who spent time with Erickson and with hypnosis and make your own decisions based on knowledge about hypnosis. Don't accept what I say, but you decide how it is going to graft onto the knowledge you already have in your own trunk and in your own solid foundation. You decide and make the choice about what it is you want to do.

You want to talk about metaphor and analogy? We just *did*! Isn't that what we always do, when you give an example? That was a fairly long one; metaphors can be a single tap into a maple tree that starts the liquid dripping out. What you have to recognize is how long it takes for the maple syrup to be boiled and how much steam is given off before you finally get that pure amber liquid. And how many grades there are of amber liquid. Some are darker and not quite as good and some have some sediment and some have a gorgeous color, texture and odor—what we think of in our memory as real syrup.

Anything that you say can turn into a story that has a lesson. Those are the lessons people learned to listen to with pleasure and satisfaction when they were young. Some therapists pile story onto story onto story. If the stories don't have relevance to the person and they are not personal, they aren't going to get into the memory process, into that information cell that creates the change we want. You need to have information about the person, you need to know what they like, what they want, what their interests are. The neat thing about that is, finding that out gives you the opportunity in the interviewing process to initially establish the relationship with the person.

I mentioned a lady with a migraine. I had never seen her before and I am *fishing*. I said, "Where did you come from?" She mentioned a university on the East coast. "Where did you come from originally?" She said, "Where did I grow up? Oh, well, ___ , a small town." *I thought, I'd rather be lucky than good.* Because I knew someone who lived in that town, and there was the connection. There was *no* chance she wouldn't know that name. I knew they were well respected and it was going to give me credibility and that's what I needed. That's what launched the relationship we had. That gave me the information that I needed to be able to start working on the three metaphors I utilized when we were talking.

It's not nonsense kind of talk and it's very important that every word that comes out of your mouth be focused on this goal you want. The words that happen before hypnosis happens are just as important, because they are giving you the information you need to connect with that patient. How do I know what to say? Sometimes, I don't know how I know, it just comes out. It comes from this store of stories that I have, that I have a feeling for that person. There's no way, absolutely no way, that I can deny that sometimes it's a connection with that person that I don't understand, but I just have to go with it. You all *do that*. You have that. When you do, listen to it!

When a patient talks, sometimes a word they say will light up in neon and it charges out at you. And you think, there's my metaphor and my story. "It's really driving me," or "I'm overwhelmed." There are so many driving stories you have. What do you have? I get on the road and move onto the interstate and kind of settle down, and as I settle down, I see that my gaze eliminates all the distractions on the side and focuses about 500 yards down the road. That's how far ahead I want to be looking for things that are happening. As I drive along, I pay no attention to the other cars, except the ones on either side of me that could impact on my driving. (see also Chapter Twenty-two).

I know that if I get back on the highway, because I have to get to this particular destination, that sometime in the future I always have the option to get off onto that side road and enjoy the benefits it gives me. Erickson would tell a story like that and at the end of the session, 20 people would come up to him and say, "Dr. Erickson, how did you know? You told that story exactly for me!" And all 20 reasons were different. The people heard what they needed to hear in the story. There were enough elements of reality for them to be able to identify with that particular problem.

I have a metaphor with a flower and the seed gets planted and it has a tough time growing (see Chapter Twenty-two) and eventually it grows this bud and this gorgeous flower. You can think about a lot of reasons for that. (Kay tells a story about creating a story for dental students about to take their boards, see Chapter Fourteen). But I'm certain that everybody in this room can think of a different kind of utilization for the flower metaphor other than passing dental boards. You understand that stories can have multiple applications.

People accuse Erickson of not telling the truth about stories, like the one about when Robert cut his leg. I have heard at least four versions of that story. I think its called poetic license. If it is a patient interested in healing, we are going to focus on the healing aspect. If it's a patient who has a problem with blood, we are going to talk about the bleeding part of the leg. If it is somebody who is going to have a lot of sutures, we are going to talk about the question of whether Robert could have more sutures in his leg than his sister had when she had her sutures. You are going to give it the slant that it needs, not for accuracy, not for truthfulness, because that isn't important. What is important is the impact and the message that patients can apply to themselves. It doesn't make a bit of difference whether it is a true story about Robert in every detail because that's not part of the project or goal.

If I say to some of my patients that "your tooth is periodontally involved and unless you take care of it, you are going to lose that tooth," there are some who become defensive and say, "I take perfect care of my teeth, how dare you say that to me and I'm going to tune you out!" And they do. If I am working with that kind of patient, I might talk to my assistant. "I'm really concerned about the periodontal involvement on that patient we saw yesterday. I recognize she really thinks she's doing everything she can for that tooth. But we are going to have to persuade her that she needs to do x, y and z if she is going to plan on keeping that tooth. I think we should get her in and talk to her about that."

We have this gossip listening and the information is dripping down on my patient and there's no denial because we are talking about somebody else and she can listen with this sense of curiosity and wonder. When we're done, she says, "Gee, Doctor, do you think that same thing might be happening to this tooth down here?" I can put on my wide-eyed surprised look and say, "Gee, Mrs. Jones, I hadn't thought about it. But now that *you* mention it, yes, I guess it could be very similar." Then I launch into what she needs to do. When she asks *me*, she is going to listen, she's going to pay attention. It's about weaving these stories in ways that people don't put up their defenses. That's why you tell stories. When you confront some people head on, they can't hear you, they don't want to hear you, and so they are not going to hear you.

You get a number of stories that can be useful for all sorts of different things and then you modify that story for each patient. You can modify whatever story it is to tell it so it will be appropriate and relevant for that particular person. Metaphor and analogy is a comfortable kind of communication but it needs to be relevant. With the woman with the migraine, she had a little butterfly pin on. I thought, Hey! she has a butterfly pin on, she chose that butterfly pin, she picked it out and she decided to wear it today. Who am I to fight this?

I said, "You know I understand that you have been really restricted by these headaches and have been held down and haven't been able to get free of them. It's kind of like a caterpillar that I am so fascinated by watching." And I take the caterpillar into the cocoon and here we are into the restriction and I talk about the cocoon and the silken threads that wind it up and how very difficult it is and I can hear the beating of the wings inside trying to break free. And I talk about the beginnings of the breaking down of the cocoon, and the butterfly coming out and standing on the limb tentatively and these wet wings beginning to expand and then I start on the beautiful colors of the wings. As the wings dry out, the butterfly discovers suddenly, kind of accidentally that it can fly. We do this gorgeous flight and these nice things that happen. We put in this rain so the butterfly has to hide but it knows that the sun will come out again.

Who knows why she wore the butterfly? Maybe it was pure coincidence. Who knows why I chose to go with the butterfly? It was very appropriate for her because of the things that it represented. The symbols behind the words made it easier for her to understand that maybe it was time for her to break free of that cocoon and try her beautifully colored wings and she did. You look at different kinds of things. You look at people who always come in wearing drab kinds of colors. You wonder whether their life is that kind of brown.

I was on a color kick one time. I was doing this palette of colors in my talking: red, orange, yellow, green, indigo and violet. I'm telling this patient about red and passion and orange and fire, and yellow and sunlight and life. She was sitting and getting more and more rigid and withdrawn and unhappy. I said, not what's wrong, but "What's going on?" Because if you say, "What's wrong?" they automatically assume that something's wrong. If you ask, "What's happening?" that gives them permission to talk to you without assuming that it's negative. She said, "I don't like your colors." I said, "Those are *my* colors! You can see any colors you *like*!" I give you the affect so you understand that my hypnosis is *not always quiet and peaceful*. She got a grin on her face and promptly went into this nice trance.

I found out later that she was an artist and was seeing monochromatic browns. Never in my world would there be monochromatic browns. I was imposing my trance on her and that ain't fair. Luckily, she told me what I was doing wrong. I could say, what was true, "It's my trance, you do your own." I changed my verbalization because she was the one who was important. It's those kinds of little things that sometimes we miss that can really help. When we are talking about a beach and they don't like a beach, they go off on their own trip and that's fine. If we sense that the patient isn't where we'd like them to be, we should be smart enough to recognize that and maybe next time not use a beach.

Think about a beach. How many of you have a hot, sunny, warm, sandy beach? How many have a rugged coast of New England rocky beach? How many have a beach in the night with the moon and waves breaking on it? How many have a stormy beach with the waves really crashing? Look at all the variety. If you are going to talk about a beach, you and the patient need to agree what kind of a beach it is. Cart before horse is not a good thing to do, whether you are telling stories or just doing a hypnotic induction. Beach images conjure up different stories for patients. If you want to use your metaphor, you need to accept the fact that the patient needs to understand where you are going to be, before you tell that story. It's appropriate when you are choosing metaphors.

If you take something away from a patient, you leave this *huge* void. What are they going to fill it in with? Taking something away is only half the story. The idea of hypnosis is that it needs to be replaced with something good. What do I do with a habit pattern, such as thumb sucking, that is established? I need to have something in its place. If I am dealing with a child, I start with the obvious, "Which thumb do you suck? The right one? Well, why? You are right-handed. If you sucked your left one, you could get a lot more thumb sucking done because since you're right-handed, you have to take your thumb out of your mouth to do things, but if you sucked your left thumb, you could do a lot more thumb sucking." Who just went into trance?

What I am saying is very logical, very truthful, and very matter of fact and the kids recognize that. I say, "Why do you suck your right thumb? I have patients who come in and suck these two fingers," and I show them. And I say, "Why did you pick on your right thumb?" They say, "It tastes better." Gotcha! I say, "How do you know?" They say, "It just does." I say, "Well, have you every tried your other thumb, have you ever tried any of your other fingers?" They look at me as if I am really weird. I say, "I will get your parents to lay off nagging on the thumb sucking—" That's just the way I say it, "if you will help me with an experiment. I'm doing some research and trying to figure out why people pick the fingers they do. Is it a deal?" They say, "Yeah, it's a deal."

I take a sheet of paper and outline their hands and label it Monday, Tuesday etc., and you have 10 days and 10 fingers and on that day that's the finger they are supposed to suck. And they agree with it. And I tell their parents to lay off nagging them about the thumb sucking. That's an attention getter and negative attention is better than no attention and I know that! And so on Thursday, when they are supposed to be sucking their middle finger, they hear from their siblings and their parents, "Get your finger in your mouth, what finger are you supposed to have in your mouth, you don't have your finger in your mouth, come on." They are not nagging about getting their thumb out of their mouth. They are simply reminding them about the finger they are supposed to have in their mouth. And, generally, I don't think 10 days is enough of a trial. That's not fair. We have to do another 10 days.

By the time they come back after the second 10 days, they are so sick and tired of having to remember and being reminded of keeping their finger in their mouth, that they can't wait for me to thank them profusely for helping to find out whether that thumb really does taste better and it doesn't and to give up having to go through the tedium of sucking their fingers. It gives them something to have in their mouth when they go to sleep at night and gives them something to fill in this void of no longer sucking their thumb. It makes very good sense in terms of the presentation I give to the child. It is very reasonable. Why do they suck their thumb? Why don't they suck those two fingers? I don't know. Maybe they can help me find out. If that's what I am really after, it comes across as being just as sincere as I think it is.

Substitution in a positive way can be a very positive response, instead of just expecting someone to eliminate something. It gives them something else to do. We have a lot of pressure and stress and are frenzied. We need to understand that people need to know how to deal with that and how to do something with that. I use a metaphor that talks about winemaking and the fermentation process for that.

If you have an audience that does not drink alcohol, bread making is something you can talk about. One of the things I think can be very useful, is to recognize how much emphasis there is today on natural foods and on cooking and baking, and baking your own bread. I'm not very good at baking bread but I am having fun trying. The first time I had yeast which was out of date and so couldn't use that and had to get some new yeast and bread flour. Bread flour is different from regular flour because it has more gluten in it than regular flour. That's really important. That one ingredient, that one little item makes a difference in the success of the bread you are going to make. Are you listening to it with the ears of the patient?

So, you mix the flour and the water and the yeast. You have to make sure that the water is just the right temperature. If it isn't, it's going to kill that yeast and you are going to be down the tube. You are not going to have anything but a rock for bread. The first time I made bread, it was so bad and so heavy, we took it mountain climbing because it was the only bread you could sit on and not hurt it. I have gotten a little better at that. When I set the bread aside in its pan, I love to watch it and I wait and I wait. Then it gets to the time when I can really have fun because I need to knead that bread so much. When I knead that bread, man, I push it down here, and the bubbles pop up here, and I go after the bubbles. I can knead that bread as long as the patient needs me to knead it. Then we put it aside and let it rise again. If we've done what we needed to do in kneading it correctly, then what we have is an even distribution of all those little bubbles of pressure, of air throughout the bread. Then we talk about baking it and having enough moisture in it, and you can drag this out as long as you want to.

If you have a patient who occasionally has outbursts, you will have a loaf of bread with an occasional bubble that is bigger than some of the others. When you slice it, it has an occasional hole in it, but it doesn't affect the taste of the bread. You see how easily you slide into it. All of the silly little details you put into it make a difference in terms of the unconscious interpretation of how to deal with the pressures of life. This is what it is really talking about.

I had a patient who was having trouble with family and transplants and things like that. With the follow-up, I talked about telephone communication and the old-fashioned party line. I knew she would remember party lines and I talked about how sometimes the line was busy but every time the line rang, everyone would get on the line. You had nothing that was private. A student asked, "What was that with the party line?" I said, "Her family." She had a family that was like that and fit the party line image. It made sense to relegate her family to the old-fashioned party line which we no longer use and no longer need. They did all this stuff to her and now she is in the newer age. It made perfectly good sense to her, although some of the people listening were confused but it wasn't a confusion technique.

Where does this come from? I wasn't born with this repertoire of stories. I talk about them, I listen to them, and I make lists and notes. Every time I tell a story I think about the additional ways to use it. I cheat. I use poetry. Poets say things better than I ever can and would. I spend a lot of time in airports and look at cards. Some have the best metaphors I have ever heard.

Everybody who came up today for clinical demonstrations closed their eyes. Not all your patients are going to do that. You need to be comfortable with them sitting there, staring at you. You need to have an outline in your head, so if they are going to be staring at you, you aren't going to be able to sit down and read.

When you are going to terminate trance, I'd like to hear a little more contrast in your voice at the end of it. You are not using your voices as the instrument they are. I would like to hear *lighter and lighter* and *heavier and heavier*. When you are asking them to terminate trance, bring your voice back to its "natural", to its louder register because that will clarify for the patient that this really is to be the termination of trance. If that's all you do, they'll still get the message. One of the other things I'm challenged about is that I'll say, "Thank you very much for your cooperation." People say, "Therapists don't thank clients for having done this work." You are not thanking them for having worked with you; you are thanking them for cooperating in the trance state.

I say, "May I borrow that manuscript on your lap? Thank you." Take it back. "Thank you." What did it mean when I said, "Thank you?" It was the end of that interaction. When you say "thank you" to a patient, what does it mean? It means the completion of something. It's a real clear message of termination when you say thank you. That's the end. There ain't no mo'. You don't have to really, really elaborate with termination of trance. You say, "Thank you very much." It sounds so easy and so simple. It's almost as easy as saying, "and how was that?" When you change from the present tense to the past tense, that also means that it is over.

Everyone makes a thing out of starting the trance. We all need to get into that mode. My signal to myself is to say, "Okay, I'm ready to go." The other thing is when I look at the client and say, "You know, it's kind of like ..." When I hear myself saying that, I know I'm going to tell a metaphor. Start hearing what you say. You have your own internal cues. You'll say, "oops," that means I'm going to do x or y. It is fun to pay attention to the cues you give to yourself. We sometimes spend a lot of time getting ready, because we just don't want to take the plunge into starting the hypnosis. If you get yourself some words or cues, it is easier to start into it.

Part III
The Nature of Trance

In his commentary, "And Her Words Will Go On", Akira Otani shares fascinating teaching vignettes about the nature of trance.

Chapter Eight, "The Case Against Relaxation", opens this section with an interesting deconstruction of the experience and meaning of relaxation in a hypnotherapeutic context. In addition to exploring multiple perspectives on relaxation, Thompson suggests that a more active physiological trance may be more conducive for many of the objectives of trance, including managing pain and gaining control.

Chapter Nine explores "facilitating trance as a relationship" through an imaginative metaphor of keys, locks and combinations. Both simple and straightforward, this chapter is a careful and studied examination of tailoring a variety of approaches and techniques to the unique needs of clients.

In Chapter Ten, Thompson presents her important thesis that all hypnosis is autohypnosis, teaches a simple self-hypnotic technique, and demonstrates a dual induction (see Chapter Twelve).

Thompson introduces Chapter Eleven with an animated story about the presentation of her first conversational induction in public. The following historic lecture gives readers an opportunity to study the evolution of the conversational induction and some of Thompson's favorite inductions, by viewing them in their earliest stage of development.

James Auld and Kay Thompson copresent Chapter Twelve on the dual induction. In Auld's chapter introduction, he discusses important aspects of the dual induction and some of Thompson's unique contributions as a teacher of hypnosis. Following Thompson's intriguing story about the spontaneous creation of the dual induction, is a wonderful example of the "jazz" ensemble that Auld and Thompson create in the two dual inductions they weave together.

And Her Words Will Go On

Akira Otani

Milton Erickson is said to have told his patients and trainees, "And my words will go with you ..." when giving hypnotic suggestions (Rosen, 1982). Among those of us who trained with Dr. Kay Thompson, her words continue to reverberate in our hearts and minds. While many of her suggestions and stories were clear to us immediately, others were unclear at the time when we heard them. Like hidden messages planted deep in our unconscious mind, they blossomed only later when we were ready to accept them. This is how Kay trained us. To help the reader appreciate how powerful and elegant she was as a supervisor and mentor, let me share two of my favorite vignettes.

My first contact with Kay was during the annual clinical hypnosis workshop at West Virginia University (WVU). After one of her presentations on hypnotic language, I mustered the courage to ask her some questions about trance induction. She smiled at me and said, "You must have been studying my writings!" She then invited me to the faculty lunch on the last day of the workshop "as her special guest". I felt flattered and accepted the invitation. At the faculty lunch, she had me sit directly across the long table from her. When the lunch was about to be over, Kay began thanking each faculty member for his or her contribution to the workshop and hoped each person would come back next year. While these greetings continued, I kept wondering what she would say to me? After all, I was her guest, a nonfaculty member, to be greeted last. When she finally completed expressing her gratitude to all faculty members, Kay looked me in the eye without saying a word. I could feel all faculty members turning to me at the same time. Then she said very slowly, "Well, Akira ..." Another pause. I found myself going right into trance on the spot. As I did so, I heard myself telling her spontaneously:

"Dr. Thompson, it was wonderful to be here with you. I hope to come back next year!" No sooner did I make this unexpected commitment to the workshop than she replied with a smile, "All right, Akira. I look forward to seeing you, too, next year!" I have since then gone back to the hypnosis workshop every year! It all started with this sophisticated invitation 15 years ago. The intrigued reader may study what hypnotic technique Kay used with me in this encounter.

Kay always expected her trainees to master hypnotic language as a means of communicating genuine caring to the patient and thereby to enable empowerment and healing. "Write down suggestions," she would tell us, and, "Practice, practice, practice!" The latter became a motto among the WVU hypnosis study group members. Believe it or not, some of us devised and swapped our treasured hypnotic suggestions with each other, like kids do with baseball cards! Some were very fancy, particularly those with twisted metaphors and confusing word plays. Kay was a master at them herself. Yet, she frequently reminded us to go back to the basics. Observe the client very carefully and pace him or her with appropriate suggestions. She showed us that hypnosis was interpersonal communication in which the hypnotist would utilize the client's own resources to promote behavior change. This definition of hypnosis is straightforward and clarifies how hypnosis differs from guided imagery or progressive muscle relaxation, both of which require the patient to follow the therapist's predetermined scripts. For this reason, mastering the language of hypnosis is quite demanding and requires constant, diligent practice on the part of the therapist.

Kay demonstrated her artistry in hypnotic communication on many occasions. One of my favorite recollections is her supervision on trance work with a rather noncompliant volunteer subject. I was giving him suggestions to "notice the heaviness in your hand as it gets pulled down to your lap". Despite my desperate effort, unfortunately, his hand stayed still. Kay came over after a while, picked up my hand quietly, and began pushing it down toward my lap. As she did this, the client's hand started responding and moving downward as well. I immediately noticed a sense of ease in my verbalizations and could feel the trance deepening in the subject. After this fascinating session was over, I could not wait to ask Kay what she did to help me. She replied, "Akira, you kept suggesting the heaviness in his hand without conveying to him the sense of heaviness. So I applied pressure on your hand each time you said 'heavy.' Put weight on that word. Your unconscious mind picked up the message quickly and took over the rest." I had no conscious recollection of heaviness in my hand. Yet, I vividly remember her intervention making a noticeable difference.

As the reader can imagine, this episode still fascinates me. It is undoubtedly one of the most memorable clinical supervisions I have received in my entire training as a psychologist. She taught me in this simple yet powerful firsthand demonstration what hypnotic communication was and how subtle cues could carry so much weight in our communication, even without our awareness of it. Her teaching is still fresh in my mind.

The lyrics of "The Rose", Kay's favorite song, ends with the verse, "Just remember in the winter, far beneath the bitter snows, lies the seed, that with the sun's love, in the spring becomes the rose."[9] This captures the spirit of Kay. As a gifted and caring supervisor, she gave many of us a chance to blossom into roses when spring came into our lives. No wonder she loved this song dearly and shared it with us.

Reference

Rosen, S. (1982). *My Voice Will Go With You: The teaching tales of Milton H. Erickson*, MD, New York: Norton.

---

[9] Lyrics from "The Rose" by Amanda McBroom. Copyright Warner-Tamerland Publishing Corp. and Third Story Music Inc. All Rights Reserved. Used by Permission of Warner Brothers Publications. U.S. Inc., Miami, Florida 33014.

Chapter Eight
The Case Against Relaxation

Ancient and modern teachings in the literature concerning hypnosis present one or another model of relaxation as the primary means of teaching hypnosis to individuals. Relaxation is a practical, useful tool for many people, such as the apprehensive medical or dental patient, or the patient in therapy who can use relaxation to stimulate recall and reduce anxiety. Relaxation provides enough adjunctive benefit to the patient to enable the doctor to treat him. What it is critically important to recognize is that, for many people, hypnosis is not synonymous with relaxation, and that complete dependence on relaxation will often retard the individual who is learning the technique.

Relaxation techniques teach the patient to expect the doctor to "do" the hypnosis, since the patient is required to participate only by sitting and listening and relaxing physically and mentally. Further, relaxation techniques demand that the patient "go into a recognizable trance", which means that he should *look* relaxed, with his eyes closed, his body loose, and semislumped in a chair, and relatively unresponsive to stimuli. The nature of relaxation encourages the doctor to use the "I want you to ..." approach to the patient; to expect compliance at least, and possibly complete subservience. Before a patient can progress beyond relaxation, he must learn that this stereotypic response is not a necessary component of trance, nor a true indicator of hypnosis. Perhaps one reason so many people find it difficult to acknowledge the spontaneous trance is that it does not require relaxation. It is easy to demonstrate that closed eyes do not imply relaxation: think of the many regular dental patients who keep their eyes closed, but who most definitely are not relaxed. Many a patient who wishes to use hypnosis during surgery, childbirth or some other traumatic procedure is apprehensive because the doctor continues telling him to "relax ... relax ... relax ...". The patient knows he is not what he perceives as relaxed, at least on the physiological and emotional levels; though he may be quite capable of undergoing surgery and controlling pain and bleeding, the process requires such hard work and concentration on his part that relaxation is the last thing on his mind. The patient does not need to relax; he needs confidence in his ability to control his autonomic nervous system.

For 25 years I have taught individuals hypnosis. I have increasingly turned away from the relaxation-sleep model and have demanded more from the patient than that he sit there and listen to me drone on and on, until he becomes so lulled that relaxation is the natural consequence of boredom. In the more active physiological approach, the patient is taught and expected to rely on his own unconscious and to learn that his unconscious can initiate behavior which his conscious mind is not controlling, nor even expecting. When he understands this type of trance, he is more willing to accept active responsibility in the cooperative venture of getting him well.

He recognizes that at no time is he "under the control" of the doctor teaching him hypnosis (although he may be restricted in what he can learn if the doctor's teaching is inhibited). The patient learns that he can—and must—talk, walk, react, think and, in general, interact and participate in the procedure. One of the most important aspects of the nonrelaxed trance is that the patient is more immediately aware of his own control. When he is encouraged to move around, talk and do whatever he needs to do spontaneously, he realizes it is *his own trance*. He also learns to take responsibility for himself.

The confusion which surrounds the doctor–patient relationship in a situation involving hypnosis may be partly explained using the terms *to, for* and *with*. The earliest concept of hypnosis required an authoritarian doctor-hypnotist who did something "to" the subject-patient. This evolved into a relationship in which the doctor-hypnotist did something "for" the subject-patient. The modern approach is one in which the doctor-facilitator does something "with" the patient in a cooperative teaching-learning situation. Patients with whom I work understand that once they have learned to achieve trance, "You have your job and I have mine." I assume that the patient will do his part, which may or may not include relaxation.

There are real semantic difficulties in interpreting the word *relaxation*. What does the doctor mean, and what does the patient understand, when the doctor continually emphasizes "relax, relax, your whole body is getting heavy, loose, limp and relaxed?" To the doctor it may imply being comfortable and it may certainly include the ideas of dissociation, cognitive control or the letting go of anxiety; sometimes it means safety. For the patient these same words must imply a change from anticipating the worst and dreading the unknown, to feeling secure in the knowledge that everything is under control. Relaxation is convenience and the freedom to concentrate on the task at hand, and the realization that the patient is in control of himself. How difficult it is for the doctor and the patient to understand one another if all that is communicated in words is the need to relax, which may well be interpreted by the patient as mere muscle looseness, lethargy and a disinclination to function or think.

What are we really communicating to our patients? Are we saying what we think we are saying? Do we permit the patient to transcend our words or do we restrict him to a narrow, literal view of trance and its associated behaviors? A doctor asks a patient in trance to "control" his bleeding; does the doctor mean "control", or does he really mean "stop"? Do we pay enough attention to the meaning our words have for the patient? One way to improve communication, which I have been encouraging for years, involves tape recording our sessions with our patients, and later studying the recording to determine all possible meanings of what we have said. This may oversimplify the problems, but at least it is a start toward understanding our own interpretation of "relaxing", and patients' understanding as well. This exercise can help us to clarify the meaning of our words.

One wonders why facilitators continue to talk about and insist on relaxation as a precondition for hypnosis. Do we need to see this relaxation to believe our patients are truly in a hypnotic state? Would it shake our confidence in ourselves if the patient did not "look" as if he were in trance? Surely, if we can learn confidence in our ability to work with a patient under any circumstances, we need not demand that he "prove" to us he is in trance. Erickson says, "My learning over the years was that I tried to direct the patient too much. It took me a long time to let things develop and make use of things as they developed" (Erickson, Rossi and Rossi, 1976, pages 266–7). Perhaps the cultural and professional educations we have received make us unable to trust the patient to control himself. Possibly our own experience of trance, or our lack of experience, inhibits our willingness to trust the patient's unconscious.

Attitudes toward clinical hypnosis seem to divide facilitators reliably into two categories: those who have experienced hypnosis for themselves, and those who have not. It is difficult for me to accept anyone's interpretation of trance in anyone else, if he has not experienced usable trance in himself. Clinical trance is so often indicted as a nonmeasurable, subjective, interpersonal response that we must recognize how greatly our understanding and interpretation of the experience is influenced by what *we* have undergone. For too long practitioners have assumed that an external, "objective" view of the state of clinical trance is more valuable in helping patients than an internal, "subjective" view. I do not accept this. Valid descriptors can be obtained using, for instance, the Gracely, McGrath and Dubner (1974) verbalization technique, and this should be done.

We should ask those most directly concerned—the patients and the doctors who have experienced trance themselves—how *they* define relaxation, and whether or not it is a necessary condition of trance. (We might also ask these doctors who have worked with hypnosis before and after having themselves experienced clinical trance, whether that experience changed their understanding of hypnosis or their approach to their patients.) In my own very small sample, both patients and doctors who work without relaxation maintain that the trance is the patient's own; that relaxation is not necessarily a part of it, and may in fact detract from it; but that until a state of close communication has been established, the patient will necessarily rely on a literal interpretation of the doctor's instructions.

It is understandable that the manipulative, practitioner-centered approach to hypnosis has prevailed in the practice of medicine in the United States: until recently, most of the doctors who used hypnosis had been taught it by stage hypnotists. The stage hypnotist could not discard the concept that he was indeed doing something "to" his subjects. In fact, the same authoritarianism extended to most aspects of the practitioner–patient relationship. Recently, however, the humanizing of the health professions in general has resulted in the widespread notion that the patient has both the right and the obligation to involve himself in his treatment—particularly when that treatment includes hypnosis.

Too few clinical patients and too many experimental subjects have been involved in the study of relaxation. In the laboratory situation, in which the urgent motive of pain-control does not really obtain, experimenters may well view the hypnosis as a surrendering of self-control by the subject. Even in the clinic, some doctors rely on tests to determine whether a patient will be a good "subject"; if the patient "fails" the test, the doctor relieves himself of the responsibility for working with him and the patient accepts the judgment that he will fail at hypnosis. (The role of the healer is exchanged for the impersonal demands of the instructor, and the self-fulfilling prophecy is completed; Rosenthal, 1966). Those patients who remain are taught to "relax", and, in general, they will do well; the rest are not counted, and the score for "relaxation" remains high.

It is important to remember, also, that even when the doctor provides the patient with a legitimate opportunity to learn hypnosis, the patient may—for a variety of reasons which are not immediately apparent—either refuse to go into trance, or prove unwilling to use trance in working with his particular problem. Erickson, as far back as 1952, emphasized that the induction of trance is not the same as the utilization of trance (Erickson, 1952, pages 78, 83).

In my opinion, when the patient is learning to induce hypnosis, the doctor should explain to him that hypnosis is a normal, natural, human capacity, that learning it is a process that is curious and interesting, and can even be fun, so that while an individual is in trance he can do all the things he normally does, but that he *gains* certain controls over himself. The patient's active participation must be acknowledged, and he and the doctor must recognize that his conscious and his unconscious minds may have different expectations of appropriate procedures.

The patient's physical appearance has little to do with the situation; he will achieve a trance profound enough to accomplish whatever it is that his unconscious recognizes as necessary, whether or not he *looks* as though he is relaxed. He will certainly concentrate fixedly on the demanding task at hand, and, as a result, will appear to ignore outside interference, but that does not mean he is relaxed. Indeed, it may mean just the opposite: he is relaxed only when he is *not* required to call upon *profound* trance, or to control his autonomic nervous system.

The advantages of eliminating relaxation as a precondition for trance include the elimination of the need to relearn the nonrelaxed state, the admission of more natural responses to the therapeutic situation, the recognition of spontaneous trance, and a freer communication between the doctor and patient, which should result in a more comfortable use of hypnosis and its more wide-spread acceptance in medicine.

References

Erickson, M. H. (1952). "Deep hypnosis and its induction", in L. M. LeCron, (ed.), *Experimental Hypnosis* (pp. 70–114), New York: Macmillan.

Erickson, M. H., Ernest L. Rossi and Rossi, S. I. (1976), *Hypnotic Realities*. New York: Irvington.

Gracely, R. H., McGrath, P. and Dubner, R. (1978). "New methods of pain measurement and their contro", *International Dental Journal*, 28, 52–65.

Rosenthal, R. (1966). *Experimenter Effects in Behavioral Research*, New York: Appleton-Century-Crofts.

Chapter Nine
Whose Story is This, Anyway?
A History of His-Story

This is a story about an exceptional man and his impact on an extended, self-selected family. But it is also a story about all those people in that self-selected family who want to be like him. But the end, yet the beginning, of the story is about the people who will benefit from his teaching as it filters down and is filtered down through all the ones who follow him.

His story is like a cascading waterfall on a powerful river. There is the main torrent of water, which, after it falls, continues to flow on as the river. But there are also drops and little streams and fallout from the waterfall that spray/stray far away, while others fall close to the mainstream, and others dry up before they ever land. Then there are others that start their own stream instead of rejoining the existing river.

But this particular story can only be my story of how I perceived his-story. So it is a story of how I use what I think I learned from Erickson to help those who have special needs that must be met before they are able to learn trance. It will also speak to my two primary beliefs, those of motivation and the need for inexhaustible and unending practice of basic skills with hypnosis! I will address basic techniques in utilizing hypnosis and trance.

The essence of these stories is the distillate: the result of straining the original product repeatedly until it is reduced to a potent potion, a portion of which can be applied sparingly as we learn how to mix it with our own ingredients to produce a product that is particularly personal and pleasing. In this way, each of us takes the essence of what we saw in the substance of Erickson and each of us strains it through the sieve of our own perspective, thereby creating a new product. But in our insecure, needy, greedy way, we prefer for a while to interpret it as the original, and so the essence takes on many different extractions or configurations, none of which is the original, each continuing a filtered distillate of the original, until we forget that it is not the same as the original.

I wonder what it is that is in the molecular distillate that I absorbed from Erickson. I reflected on how I use what I think I learned. I am sure that my view is influenced by my clinical utilization, which requires a reorientation of the patient's physiology, not just psychology. And I don't always have a lot of time to accomplish this change "within their heads" before I go in to change some physical thing in their heads.

The intensity of my physical intervention utilizing trance requires development of a belief in the physiological alterations that can be activated and achieved during the hypnotic trance. We physicians and dentists do not have much time to work through the bonding and transference that occur with the use of hypnosis directly, but they need to occur, indirectly, with the guidance of the doctor. About the time I get comfortable with just having to talk to people, I get a patient who is scheduled for surgery, and often I am also doing the surgery, so there is a different level of need and urgency and a deeper sense of commitment on my part.

There are a number of general opportunities I utilize to help this particular population with their special needs. Most of these patients have tried hypnosis before without success. I believe that the work I do with hypnosis is grounded in: (1) my learned focus on the foundation of motivation for change within the patient; (2) my learned willingness and perceived obligation to employ every means to enhance and restructure, reinforce, and build on that motivation; and (3) the conviction that there is the potential for change. In looking for commonalities in what takes place, I find a consistency in my acknowledgment and appreciation of individual differences. I cannot utilize others' predetermined approaches like frozen entrées, or even canned recipes, although I may start with the same cookbook. Nor must I rely on theories in those cookbooks. I must work with the ingredients on hand and I must have a taste for what is simmering with this one patient, different from any other I have seen, demanding a new adaptation of any recipe.

I find a constancy, in that all patients have within them the power to change, given the appropriate motivation and relearning. The change must fit their belief systems. We, as therapists, cannot do it for them. Accepting the patients' potential and the multiple variations in that potential, makes it possible to work with those needs and motivations. The more the therapist can speak the true language of the patient, the better the patient is able to understand.

It is difficult to determine the "across-situations" incidence of consistency. It is the mixing and shifting back and forth from one approach to another, as required, that makes Ericksonian trance so difficult to analyze. He had the skill to be able to do the complex, simply.

But always, enhancement of motivation is the key I use to open the options the patient has locked out. Erickson understood and used these motivational differences. He was exceptionally smooth at slipping back and forth unnoticed, using his master keys on any locked door that presented itself. He would also combine and confuse what was behind the doors by using additional communicative tools. Neither the burglar nor the locksmith cares what combination of tools gets him into the valuables. I am not concerned about where that lock came from in the past. I am concerned only that the patient is ready to change the future.

Motivation can come from different motivating factors, and a motivating factor can have multiple origins. One door can be opened with many keys, and one key can open many doors. Since much of what occurs takes place in the unconscious, it is difficult to track. One constant is that trance is tracked by movement toward the future, as determined by the key motivation of the client.

Set One

How do I determine which key to use for the door that I am to help open? My first task is to determine the type of door and lock. The initial meeting is an inventory of the problem doors, so the patient is encouraged to talk, while I take scrupulous notes. Much can be learned without asking. I do ask what is being asked of me. The objective is to listen actively and observe carefully for the nonverbal communication as well as for the words. Then it is time to make a judgment, based on the perceived motivation.

The first personal skill, then, is in deciding what approach the patient needs, so that you can affect the effect by a change in your behavior and an offering of trance. The offering must vary, so you must know how your key fits each door, and this requires practice.

Each of us must practice to acquire the skills and techniques to express the appropriate aspect of our personality for that person in the personal way it is needed. One of the things that always was impressed on me in Erickson his-story was to note his rigorous practice and self-discipline. He wrote out verbalizations and monitored his own behavior, ready to shift immediately as he observed minute changes in the patient. Because of his care and compassion for each person who came to him, he did all this to enrich his ability to reach the patient. He would listen intently for the tumbler to fall and act quickly when it did.

Practice, patience, creativity and commitment—and always to work hard—these provide the rosin that smoothes the key for teaching trance. After you master basic direct, indirect, permissive, authoritarian and confusion approaches—only then focus on storytelling and metaphor.

There are still those who say they just open their mouths and let their unconscious speak. It is okay to trust in and rely on the spontaneous unconscious, but only after there is an abundance of knowledge and experience in the spontaneous unconscious to rely on. If you are contemplating using a combination keyless lock, make sure you can remember the combination.

Set Two

Once you know the many master keys you have available, how do you decide which key to begin with? Formal, informal, direct, indirect?

If hypnosis is the last hope for the client, formal trance is essential. I cannot just talk to that patient, because he has tried that and everything else. He talks to himself all the time and has learned how not to listen. My job is to teach him to listen again.

Two A

With formal trance I am rigid and I am structured, but I am also very permissive about things that don't matter, such as feet flat on the floor or eyes closed. I do not want to overload and distract the patient with things that are irrelevant to the trance.

The traditional approach sometimes involves asking the patient to do things that may seem a little silly. The key here is to identify them first as ridiculous, before asking that they be done, which takes away the excuse and embarrassment. I may say, "Look, I'm going to ask you to do something silly, but that's okay, do it anyway. Hold both arms out in front of you, like this ..." The safe, traditional approach provides you with invaluable feedback and lets the patient know that something is happening outside of his conscious control. This is reassuring. You both know the combination has the potential to be effective on that lock.

Two B

Indirectly approaching the formal technique reduces the stage hypnosis attitude. One way I might do this is to put on my sincerely curious attitude and get the patient involved in questions and factual observations that lead gently into trance. By pointing out the obvious, one defuses the defenses and resistances and lets the key work more easily.

The "Have you ever ...?" and "Did you notice ...?" questions narrow from generalities to specifics and utilize the specifics of different physiological attentions, abilities and inabilities. This gentle, slow development of logical attention to facts mixed with memories lends itself to an awareness of the different state that is developed.

Gently turning the key can slowly bring it around. Sometimes locks that won't open can be oiled more easily than forced. When you acknowledge facts in a way that demands looking at the facts differently, it also demands looking at the faces differently.

Set Three

"You can't make that key work. It can't be done. It isn't the proper way." That challenge becomes the induction technique.

"See if you can" is a very effective system for defusing resistance, as well as removing the belief that the therapist-doctor must be in control. "See if you can balance your fingers exactly evenly on your knees. Of course, you know you can't, but try anyway." The published Erickson case of "See If You Can Pace a Little More Slowly" includes that type of challenge (1967).

If the challenge is an acceptable one, the individual not only goes into trance, but learns that it was pure personal skill that provided that opportunity.

Set Four

Teach hypnosis separately from the problem and from utilization of trance. There are at least two doors into different parts of that house, and we will go in using a key for a different door in a different way.

Patients may perceive a threat to their symptom inherent in going into trance. It is almost as if there were a contract stating, "If I go into trance, then I am obligated to use hypnosis for my problem." If the patient is not yet certain that is her goal, then the easiest way to address it is simply to resist going into trance. The therapist, therefore, not approaching the issue directly but approaching it nevertheless, says, "All right, today we are going to teach you about hypnosis. That is all. Next time you come in we can discuss whether or not you want to use it to help you with your problem." In that way the patient is free to learn trance. Once it has been learned, it probably will become an appealing system for unlocking the possibilities within the problem.

Set Five

Another belief in my locksmith system is that I am glad if the door doesn't open easily, as if it were already unlocked. It takes an intelligent person to want a second opinion, and to get it by testing me. It makes sense for the referred patient to be skeptical. I express my admiration for the person who comes in critical and suspicious, asking many appropriate questions. The patient who gives me a difficult time during the initial appointment is reassured that I respect his hesitation and recognize that he is not "gullible". As the patient continues to challenge me during the induction, he demonstrates his wisdom. After all, once I pass the test the patient is then free to trust me to be responsible in dealing with the real reason for which he was referred. This acceptance on my part permits me to see through the more abrasive patient to the scared yet hopeful person within, the person I want to help.

Set Six

"This key used to work. I'm sure it still will."

With all patients I maintain a "Yes, but" philosophy. It follows the principles of reframing and is an important part of defusing the importance of the symptom for the patient. "Yes, but" can be portrayed in a number of ways, all of which indicate that you agree with patients, but then by adding consequences or getting them to look at things from a different perspective, you get them to see the advantage of change.

Set Seven

"It may be important that you keep this key, even though it doesn't fit very well anymore" is the next step beyond "Yes, but".

No matter what patients say in a negative fashion about the symptom, I can defend the symptom. This validates their integrity in having the symptom, removing the need for them to feel guilty for not giving it up, and unconsciously supports their own esteem. In this interaction I permit patients to point out to me all the bad, negative things about their symptom, while I emphasize all the positive things about it.

I also express my serious concern about what can ever take the place of the symptom, and I must be convinced by patients that they can live quite nicely without that impediment. I may voice my concern about having them give up the symptom, and I become quite resistant to the idea of change. They become committed to convincing me that they can, should and must give up the symptom and change! Reluctantly, I can then agree to continue to work with them to get the new key.

Set Eight

One key technique I have used for years involves pointing out to the patient how the symptom might have actually been needed and useful at the time it was acquired. Then I become curious about how it got "sidetracked". Somehow, the training never progressed beyond that sidetrack. We wonder about how to get that sidetracked train car out onto the main line so we can change the destination to a positive one. I remain very respectful of the patient's right to have and have had the symptom.

I wonder aloud about the mechanism, determination and persistence that let the symptom continue to sidetrack the patient and what it was that blocked the tracks. Did no one bother to let him know the schedule had changed, so he could make arrangements to hook up with a new train? This lets the rest of the world go by every day, riding in shiny new trains, looking disdainfully at that old car off on the side, getting ever more dusty and rusty and out of date.

But then a train aficionado comes along who recognizes value in that old car. It had a good strong structural foundation, with a frame constructed of top-quality metal and wood, better than many builders of today use. First, it is necessary to clean and restore the inside, and that is quite a job. We have to throw away the moth-eaten upholstery and get rid of the mildew smell. Eliminate the musty, mold-infected velvet and change to smooth, fresh leather. Clean the dirt and soot off the windows so one can see through the panes again. Clean the darkened interior until the light wood paneling glows richly. Scrub and wax those hardwood floors until they shine, too.

Once the inside is clean and resilient, it's time to renew the function of the car. The electrical system must be sandblasted and wires checked to eliminate short circuits, and the power of the generators increased. The mechanical system must be overhauled and lubricated and any necessary parts replaced. Then the shell of the train car can be cleaned and dents removed. Finally, it is painted, waxed and polished. There is no resemblance to that rusty, dirty, old car that sat stalled on that sidetrack for so long. Now, with small, gentle moves at first, it can begin to approach the main track. Its function has been restored, and it is ready to be attached to the newer, faster cars that come by.

It selects the train and track with the destination that pleases it, and goes on its way, leaving behind the residue of the renovation, ready to rejoin the main line. It can look back on what it once was, proud to know it learned to know what it needed to do to become what it is going to be.

Set Nine

"This key just doesn't work."

Acknowledging the patient's strong willpower by formally and directly trying to hypnotize him and succeeding in failing will satisfy the patient's need to resist and to know that he retains control. He can also take pride in countering my best efforts, and that pride permits him to feel sorry for me and conciliatory toward me. That allows us to go on and just be curious about the problem, asking a few questions about it and wondering about the facts of it related to life. An indirect trance induction can be utilized. Since he has already demonstrated that I cannot hypnotize him, there is no longer any need to resist, which he knows he could always do if he chose to.

Set Ten

"Let's give up on this key."

After you have worked diligently and unsuccessfully with patients who succeed in failing to go into trance, what else can you do? You explain that in a minute you are going to ask them to complete this experience. As you say that, you can see the clients take a deep breath and heave a sigh of relief at having successfully resisted all your efforts. Right then they drop their guard and their resistance, and you have about 15 seconds to make one or two powerfully worded suggestions about the next visit, including the enhanced trance-ability they may discover.

Set Eleven

What of the door that appears locked, but is ready to go to pieces when touched in the right place?

Once I have made my paradigm shift and set aside my assumption that I knew anything at all about how the world worked, I have broadened my options. Now I can demonstrate to patients that the usual way is not my way, which encourages them to respond more spontaneously.

Each meeting is a unique encounter. As we tailor the therapy to each person's patterns, we must be ready with quick on-site alterations when the unexpected fit presents itself.

Sometimes, the therapist introduces the concept of confusion in order to help the patient be receptive to change by disrupting the normal impulse pattern of the thinking channel and opening new lines of communication. Trying a newer, more suitable lock may lead to the discovery that the fit is much more secure than the old way that seemed so safe.

Make quantum leaps in diagnosis and pull the rigid rug out from under patients. This requires risk. Go further than strict theory might, but leave the interpretation open to patients to resolve.

Little words can be contract words: Hook the unconscious, which hears them in ways the conscious mind does not. When you think back, remember that you were asked to do regression, to go into trance at other times, in other places. Regression is what I asked you to do with the remark, "When you think back, you remember when." It was done so simply that you did not need to realize it was a request for a regression. When you pay attention to the little contract words, then you begin to understand their power, and you can try them out. Have you done that *yet*? We must pay attention to the word's power, since words do possess power. Be possessive about the power of words, those symbols for experience and power for change. In summary, language and motivation are the combination of keys I work with to open these doors long rusted shut.

The language of trance can be the therapeutic tool for change. Language reflects back on all the things Erickson taught me to learn. The intricacy of the simple words provides the opportunity for multilevel messages and manages to manipulate the mood of the moment to maintain the method by which we mean to maneuver the change.

All of these methods cross barriers from one theory to another, just as Erickson combined and utilized all types of intervention, not bound by anyone's rules to stay within any one parameter. Today, this is an acceptable and desirable approach. Just as times change, so can people change.

This basic piece of my story as unlocked from his story can add to your repertoire for health and growth, a synonym for change, the essence of Erickson's life and his-story.

References

Erickson, M. H. (1967). "Further techniques of hypnosis-utilization techniques", in J. Haley (ed.), *Advanced Techniques of Hypnosis and Therapy: Selected papers of Milton H. Erickson, M. D.* (pp. 34–5), New York: Grune & Stratton.

Chapter Ten
Autohypnosis

Autohypnosis must be practical. It must be useful in order for it to work. It isn't fair to use hypnosis only for yourself without giving your patients the opportunity to learn it also. Autohypnosis can be spontaneous. But the easiest way to learn autohypnosis is to have someone else teach you how to go into trance, and when you are in that trance, give you a signal or a system that you can follow in order to achieve hypnosis yourself after that—heterohypnosis for autosuggestion.

If all hypnosis is not autohypnosis, if we really do something to our patients and we control the trance, why are we so careful about it? Why do we have to worry about what we say? If we're the ones in charge, all we have to do if we misspeak is back up or say to the patient, "Hey, don't do that because after all I am hypnotizing you." If they are in charge, and they control the "stop and the go", then it stands to reason that it has to be autohypnosis.

If it is then autohypnosis, what do you need to know? You need to understand that autohypnosis can be and should be structured with an outside standing awareness. When you are teaching a patient to go into trance, you have to reassure them that if someone sticks their head in the door behind us and yells fire and they are in trance, then they won't sit there and burn. My reaction to that is to explain to them that I have two responses. I can come out of trance and run out of the room or I can stay in trance and get out of the room. If I stay in trance, I will probably beat everyone else out of the room because I function better in trance. And they kind of giggle and that explains that without making a big deal of it.

When you are using autohypnosis, the patient needs to understand that they *will not* ignore appropriate signals. With the mother who has the new baby at home, the baby is sleeping and the mother decides to takes a nap and the baby starts to cry. If Aunt Mary is there to tend to the baby, the mother doesn't need to wake up. If Aunt Mary isn't there, the mother wakes up. Autohypnosis is the same thing. If we are around to take care of the patient, they do not have to pay attention to outside noises and sounds. This nonsense about "You will not hear any other sounds but my voice," is exactly that. It is nonsense! On the other hand, "you need not *pay attention* to anything except the sound of my voice", is what you are really saying to the person. In this relationship, you can scan and decide if these fringe things need your attention, and if they don't, then you just continue to listen to the person who is doing the talking.

When you structure autohypnosis, what happens if the patient doesn't come out of trance? Will they go in trance at home and stay in it forever? Certainly not! The person goes into trance for a specific purpose, even when they are at home. When the need is fulfilled, there is no longer any reason for them to stay in that trance. When you teach autohypnosis, you can do it in a spectacular way or you can simply say, once they have been in trance, "The next time that you come back in my office and you put your head back in my chair, that will be a signal to remind you of how to reach this very comfortable state." And they come back and put their head in the chair and, "*Whew*, there I go again."

I had a patient who did this and one day came in and was sort of giggly. She said, "I had the funniest experience. I went to the opthalmologist and sat down in his chair and couldn't stay out of trance," because it was so much like my chair. So that is the whole part of the conditioned response that the patient has. As far as I am really concerned, autohypnosis is no big deal, once the patient realizes that it is in fact his trance. A friend of mine finally realized this after using and working with hypnosis for four years. Bob Pearson and I were doing a dual induction and she finally got this absolutely magnificent grin on her face. And I said, "Are you willing to share what your grin is about?" She kind of hugged herself and said, "Mmmyyyyyyytrance." And everybody in the audience sort of went *wow*! Because, if they ever had any question, that took it away. It was in fact, *her* trance and nobody else's.

I used to think that I was doing something to someone and had this head that was getting bigger and bigger because these people were doing all these things that I told them to do. And then I started having patients spitting in my eye, figuratively speaking. And I discovered that if I gave them appropriate suggestions, they wouldn't do them; they would ignore me. And I learned a lesson from that. Now I try to gauge suggestions based on the fact that I can go into trance too. I can tune into the patient, be alert, be functioning on all my levels and have a patient say to me, "You were really inside my head. How did you know?" And I say, "It just felt right." They don't have to know I'm in trance. There is nothing wrong with functioning in trance as long as you remember that the reason you are in that trance is to help the patient, and that your own autohypnosis needs to go on for yourself outside the office.

What do I do in terms of teaching autohypnosis? When I was doing monthly workshops for the American Society for Clinical Hypnosis (ASCH), we had a standard procedure to teach people how to go into trance. What it demonstrates is how easy it can be and that rehearsal is a good thing. All it includes or involves is you take your thumb and index finger of your hand and pinch them tightly together. Then you take a deep breath in a minute and hold it until I count to five, and at the count of five you let go of your breath and finger, and just kind of float with each additional breath. I'll give a couple of instructions and we'll practice.

The other thing you recognize is that I tend to be rather straightforward and kind of offhand and casual and just expect that people are going be able to do these things. I *believe* that hypnosis is a normal natural capacity. I think that there are tricks to helping people find out that they have that capacity. I don't think I need to be really quiet or that I have to have any extraordinary situation. It's just a matter of communication. That's all. Some people communicate better than others in every situation. And you can learn, by practicing, by paying attention, and by caring about your patient.

Thumb and index finger tightly together. Take a deep breath. Hold it. 1, 2, 3, 4, 5. Let go and take three more deep breaths, and with each breath pay attention to your body and its comfort and its relaxation. Almost as though you were going down steps into this more profound kind of comfortable state. And when you get to that third deep breath, you are at the level where you can talk to yourself when you are at home or at any other appropriate place.

At that point you can say to yourself, I have gone into trance to give myself these suggestions and I am going to listen to them. And an appropriate suggestion that you can give yourself now, is that any time in the future that you pinch your thumb and index finger together, and take that deep breath and let it out, that will be a signal to your unconscious to pay attention to its ability to go into trance and listen. And after you do that and your unconscious knows that it knows all that it needs to know, you take another couple of deep breaths and terminate that particular experience so you can practice it again.

And when you do this, it's really interesting because the room gets really quiet, much quieter than the average quiet room in a normal situation.

Okay, let's do this again. Index finger and thumb together. Take a really deep breath and hold it. 1, 2, 3, 4, 5. Let it out. Take those three more deep breaths. And do your thing. Because it's kind of like a recipe, where everybody gets the same ingredients. But it's the way you cut up the vegetables, the way you cook them and mix them up, and finally the way that you apply your own special flair that makes any recipe particularly yours. And so when you know that you know everything that you need to know, even though some of it you didn't really know you knew; but now that you know that you don't really need to know whether you knew it, you can let yourself know everything that you need to know in order to do this, any time you know you need it. And when that one gets processed at the level at which it's understood, that's really what it's all about.

Now, always, rehearsal is important. When you first learned how to walk, it took a lot of practice and you fell a lot. And when I first learned this, it took me a lot of time. The reason I like this way, is the autohypnosis signal that I was taught was to hold out my arm and stare at my thumb, which would be irresistibly drawn toward my face like a magnet and my hand would drop into my lap. And frankly I find that a little embarrassing to do at a party. It's much easier when I have a glass in my hand to stand there, when I have been cornered by the biggest boor at the party. I can say, "Yes, oh really, you don't say," and respond appropriately to this person here, and listen to the conversation there that is more interesting there and the conversation over there, and send help signals to my husband who is on the far side ignoring me.

Hypnosis and autohypnosis, particularly, has to be *practical* in order for you to use it and that's what it's all about. If it's unobtrusive, it doesn't mean it's ineffective. And that's the secret in terms of what I consider to be the bright-eyed bushy-tailed trance. It's an ordinary everyday thing that I just rely on to happen.

I had my automobile accident and there was the hypnosis, and if I ever questioned it before, I don't question it anymore. I am conditioned to utilize it for survival, because I shouldn't have survived and I did. And I don't think there was any other reason.

Question: About working with someone who has difficulty finding time to practice hypnosis because of their family responsibilities.

T: If they say, "I really can't," then I tend to say to myself, the person is a martyr to the family or something of this nature. And I say, "You know, I really think you owe this to your family." And I think if you explain this to the family, how much better Mommy is going to be able to cook, and to wash, and to clean if she had this 15 minutes, that they will set aside the time. And it's like doing homework. And you set aside the time for Mommy to do the homework. And I find that the family frequently insists that the patient practice. And I agree with Erickson's philosophy and so does Jay Haley, that if the person isn't really committed, you deliberately add an inconvenience to it, so that the inconvenience involved in the contract makes them want to commit. It's kind of like with a screaming child, you are pulling the rug out from under the patient.

We have an experiential session and in order to do that we need two microphones.[10]

They need to experience the experiential session. What kind of experience do you think they should have in it? Does that put us in the position of having to teach something? It means it's up to them to do the learning even if we don't do the teaching, and it depends on how many blanks we leave. So, if you fill in the blank, then it's no longer a blank, and what you fill it in with determines how you

---

[10] Note: This will contain Thompson's part of the alternate dual induction and then her part of the simultaneous induction. Ed.

feel about having filled in the blank. And if old learning is going to end, but every ending is a new beginning? And you end where you begin only if you begin that particular ending at the beginning of the last beginning. I prefer thinking about beginnings more than endings because endings imply leaving. And if we go on, how we go on doesn't really make any difference as long as people attend to what they didn't know. (End of alternate part of double induction.)

But does it really matter? When you pay attention to people and when the two people you are paying attention to are two people, as long as you have two ears, you can hear different things. The same as with two eyes, you can see different things. And you are down to the very grain of truth and you grind them but only if you need them. And, as long as your body needs them, it doesn't make any difference what you think about, what you talk about or hear as long as you go on listening, and not really paying attention, but training your unconscious mind to do the things it needs to do.

As you listen, the kind of trip your mind takes, is the one of finding out that you can expand your horizons beyond the limits of normal culturally induced trance. And that the trance that you reach as you learn the kinds of things that you already know that you know, lets you free yourself to expand into a different atmosphere and a different culture, moving out always into a more evenly understood and more readily recognized significant sort of thing. As you listen to him, as he offers his feelings about this and as you don't listen to me while you listen to him, and you listen to him while you are not listening to me and vice versa; it doesn't really matter what you *hear*, what really matters is the message that we give.

The ability to be in your own trance is as important as the ability to help your patient be in hers. To expand into the experience of moving out and up and learning that you can function with your eyes wide open communicating with your patient, working, being bright eyed and bushy tailed. Letting yourself move wherever you need to go while you are doing this, whatever location you need to focus on, and go back to kneading bread or needing stimulation or excitement, because those are the kinds of things that make us aware of the universality of man. And the ability that he has to reach out to other people and to help them with that particular expectancy that dentistry so often misses. And as dentistry becomes a more aware and sensitive kind of experience, you find that the things that were missing from your life in the dental school and in the practice, you can fill in by virtue of working and listening, and hearing the things that you really need to hear.

And that you don't really have to be quiet, that you don't really have to be "out of it", that you can hear and respond and function at a higher level with trance than you can function in your normal tense, distracted state, and that's important and appropriate. And as you learn that and as you do that, playing with it becomes more fun and you kind of wait around for all the right things to happen As you go on sorting out the sort of things you need to order your priorities, in order to get them in order of wants, wishes, and needs. And when you get that done, you find that the cooking that you do is really in order that you don't lose track, that you stay on top of things. Because there is nothing more boring than a dentist who is boring. I couldn't stand being that.

The mind is an amazing machine. It really is! It has over 10 billion neurons and there is a lot of room up in there for us to do other things than those things that we have learned to do. I really don't think that we work enough with those. I don't think that we understand or go far enough or push ourselves enough. And that the reason that so many physicians, dentists and psychologists are afraid to push those boundaries is because they are afraid they are going to look foolish. As I said when I talked about the screaming child, I'm not afraid of looking foolish because that's not something that threatens me. And that may be one of the reasons I'm willing to make all these crazy kinds of remarks and responses and efforts. And I think that being willing to try, and to test, and to move out is important. I'm firmly convinced that the worst that can happen is that nothing happens, but it's very rare that nothing happens.

When you find out that you can really tune in to two people and listen to two people at once, and that you can process everything that both people are saying, it opens up for you some better understanding of the multiple levels of hypnosis that Erickson talked about all the time. I don't know how to *tell* anyone how to function in the bright-eyed bushy-tailed trance except to model it. And I think that kind of modeling may make some people say, "Hey, wow! I'm at least as bright as she is. If she can do it, I'm going to do it too." And that's in many instances why I do use so many "I" statements. I never say "You can do this" without letting the patient know I really believe that they really can. I think that's very very important.

Question: About how often does Dr. Thompson function in bright-eyed bushy-tailed trance?

T: I am eternally not in trance. Because trance is hard work! For those people who have only used trance for relaxation and Whoopee! it isn't. But, when you are using hypnosis in the clinical sense, when you are using it to control pain, to stop bleeding, to do therapy, whatever, to increase the speed of healing, you are expending a great deal of energy. It's much easier for me to be in my normal, tense distracted state.

When I come home from one of my four-day workshops, my husband would pick me up at the airport. I would get in the car and he would say, "Have you had dinner yet?" I would say, *"Grump."* He would say, "Would you like to stop and eat on the way home?" I would say, *"Rrump!"* And he would say, "Okay." And I would collapse. Maybe the next night I would be willing to talk with him.

Because I am extending much energy to scan, remembering what's done and what needs to be done, and people who have asked different questions. I couldn't do that without hypnosis. I honestly believe that I couldn't do that. Using the portions that are appropriate when they are appropriate is right. There is no way that I'm aware that anybody could stay in trance all the time.

I was in an auto accident. I had two broken legs, three broken ribs and a depressed sternum. I tried biting my tongue in half and almost succeeded, clobbered six teeth, and had a TMJ problem, 60 sutures in my forehead. I had a brain concussion, I was unconscious for 30 minutes, and my eyes didn't focus for two days. I never hurt and I didn't bleed.

I had a very bad time in the hospital because I went in as Mrs. instead of Doctor. Because I didn't hurt, there couldn't be anything wrong with me, and so they let me walk on my two broken legs. They didn't believe for a long time that I actually had broken ribs and I had to let them hurt on the third day until they would take me down and re-X-ray my ribs to see that I did have three broken ribs. I was in the position where I know my body well enough, that I could play that silly game. Most patients are not sophisticated enough that they can do this. In that instance, I stayed in trance in parts of me for 7 weeks at least. I was working on increasing the speed of healing. They said it would be 12 weeks before I could walk again. I was walking and lecturing in Vermont in 7 weeks without a cane.

Now something was going on. When I thought about it, different times during the day, there would be this kind of blush that would just kind of take over my body. I was scanning to see what I needed to do in order send the necessary kinds of cells to the parts of me that were healing. I know that. And, gradually, they just spread out further and further apart until I no longer needed it. But I'm an 18-hour-a-day person. Except at that time, after about 10 hours I needed a couple of hours sleep, because I was spending so much energy on that. Patients tell me the same kind of things. When they do this, it does take work and they are tired. And I think that's perfectly reasonable. Because that's why patients don't stay in trance all the time. We have to acknowledge the fact that it is a lot of work.

We're going into the psychological significance of the oral cavity, which is one of my soapboxes because I get concerned that for one thing, physicians and psychologists don't recognize the impact that dentistry has on the body. And they don't recognize how important it is. Every dentist knows more about medicine than any physician knows about dentistry.

I don't care whether you believe in Freud and the oral, anal, and genital phases of development therapeutically. You cannot deny that this is the way the body develops (see Chapter Nineteen), that the oral portion of this body that we own is the first and most important part of the body. What happens? The child goes to the dentist. We invade that highly significant area. We take away his ability to communicate except by crying, and we do things to this mouth that is so important to him, frequently before he can even understand this. For these reasons I firmly believe that the hypersensitive mouth is in fact a normal mouth.

There is another angle. We have this philosophy that guilt is always punished. If you sin, you deserve to be punished. How many people in this room have never eaten a candy bar, or drunk a coke, or had dessert? How many of you always brush your teeth after every time you put anything in your mouth or floss every time you put any food in your mouth? Do you have any liars in the group? We understand and reconcile that.

If you get a patient who has a poor oral adjustment and they don't do everything they should do for their mouth, they come to the dentist, knowing they have sinned and they deserve to be punished. Who do they elect as their primary executioner, but the dentist? When they have a cavity, they deserve it, they deserve to be punished. We punish them and fulfill their need for this particular retribution. Then they can go out and hate us and feel absolutely great for themselves, because they have done the right kind of penance. And sure that may be an extreme, but there are people who fit that category.

Now there are people who say to me that you can only do hypnosis within your field of competence. Now Milton Erickson said, and I firmly believe, that dentists who limit their practice to dentistry, are doing psychological therapy limited to the field of dentistry for all the reasons that I have just mentioned. We need an awareness of the kinds of things that go into this particular situation or we are not going to be able to do the dentistry with comfort within ourselves, as well as with our patients. I don't think that the average patient is going to a therapist to have these dental problems handled. We can handle them by ego strengthening and by support via hypnosis, and by helping them understand that change is possible. Hey, people are ambivalent about change and it requires effort, and people do not like to change and they are going to resist it, unless we can give them the understanding that where they go with this change can be to their benefit.

I did this metaphor, "If you think back to when you were a kid ..." (see Chapter Fourteen), at a workshop and a group of people were going on a tour that afternoon. One woman came back and said, "We went back to the house I grew up in and everything you said was true and I didn't believe it." Most people realize that. That kind of metaphor works for them. You have changed in other ways.

Anytime that you can change, there is the potential that you will change more. And that is what we are dealing with.

Another thing is that I don't do archaeological kinds of research. I'm not interested in why the patient has the problem. If the patient wants to know and needs to know, I will refer them to a therapist who can deal with that situation. I don't know why the problem started, I don't care why the problem started, all I care about is that you want to get over it. That's the important thing. They can have 87 kinds of excuses. Whether they are the real things doesn't matter.

I remember a demonstration. One patient, the wife of a doctor, had a problem with gagging. We were taught to get the patient to go into a trance and regress. And then you would say, "Did the problem occur before the age of 20?" Yes, with their finger. (Ideomotor signaling.) "Did it occur before the age of 10?" Yes. "Did it occur before the age of 5?" No. "Did it occur between the ages of 5 and 10?" Yes. "Did it occur when you were 7?" No. "Did it occur when you were 8?" Yes. "Tell me about it." And the patient then said, "Well I went into the hospital and had my tonsils removed and it was really terrible." And the doctor said, "Well you are no longer 8 years old and that was done when you were a little girl, and it doesn't need to bother you any more, and now that you know why you did it, you have insight and you don't have to gag anymore."

And so the patient came out of trance, and low and behold she didn't gag, and she could take a tongue blade and stick it way down in her mouth and had no retching at all. She is declaring, how wonderful it is, how marvelous it is that she doesn't gag anymore. And her husband was sitting in the front row and looking rather puzzled and said, "But, Honey, you never had a TNA."

Remember when I said that hypnosis did not need to be truth serum. The most interesting part of that is that even though she never had a tonsillectomy, she still had her tonsils; in fact she did not have to get back the gag reflex. Having once learned that she could get over it, for whatever reason, she didn't have to get it back again. If the patient is willing to accept something as having been the reason, sometimes that can be as helpful as knowing the real reason. I'm not saying that patients don't have problems that need a therapist. The way in which their dentist deals with a lot of their problems gives them enough support to be able to handle them, because we don't have enough therapists to handle all the patients who have dental problems.

Question: About working with people who have neurological problems

T: We've done some work with some physiological problems which respond to direct symptom removal. I think that patients can learn to deal with neurological problems and that hypnosis can definitely help them. I remember when Erickson was confined in a wheelchair, somebody in one of the audiences said, "If you are so damn good, why don't you help yourself?" I remember very distinctly. He took his left hand and elevated the right arm very slowly. He used silence very effectively, never said a word. He waited until it was up in the air and proceeded to give an anatomy lesson on the musculature, the enervation, and the blood supply and to name all of the doctors who had examined him and told him, that at no time, in any circumstances, ever in the future would he be able to move that arm. Then he very quietly lowered the arm, he had been holding up in the air for 10 minutes. And then he said, "Does that answer your question, Doctor?"

For that reason I believe that it is worth trying to help patients. The worse thing that happens is that nothing happens. We've gotten into some fairly interesting kinds of things. Why not? Because frequently, the mental distress that the patient is under increases the tension, thereby increasing the neurological response and making the deficit worse. If all you do, for instance, with a cerebral palsy patient, is teach them how to relax and be more comfortable, they will have better control with that kind of comfort. If all you ever do is teach your patients how to relax, which I think is only the beginning of hypnosis and not always necessarily the beginning, rather than the ending, they are going to benefit from that and so are you! Let's face it, working on a nice, easy comfortable patient who is not having spasms and sitting like that and making it difficult to get into their mouth, makes your life a lot easier. And that's part of the reason for using hypnosis, isn't it?

Question: How do I cope with a patient who abreacts?

T: The facetious answer is very carefully. My feeling about the person who abreacts is that they need to do that in order to get it
"out of their system". I use a lot of body language and organ language and verbalization. The first one I ever had did it spontaneously. She had a dental procedure at the age of 7, was sitting in
a dental office and looking out the window at a pawn shop ball
revolving across the way, and it put her in a spontaneous trance
and ruined her dentistry for the next 34 years.

When I have a patient who abreacts, as a general rule, I talk to
them while they are in the trance, and explain to them how nice
it is that they are able to get all this pent-up emotion out of their
system. How safe they understand they are in this situation and
how they have been longing to be able to do this. How much it is
going to help them to have that kind of understanding and relief
and release. When they have had sufficient recognition of how
much of this memory has been retained, and how really, really
painful it was, then their system can quiet down again and they
can understand what they need to do now in order to handle it.

Chapter Eleven
The Mythical Trance
The First Conversational Induction

I was challenged one time by some traditionalists that you couldn't do conversational inductions. I decided that you really could. I was doing a presentation in San Francisco at the ASCH meeting that year and I thought, "Oh! Fun!" And so I did! It's called "the mythical trance".

Right smack dab in the middle of this formal lecture, I lit into this, "I see the electric potential in each person, not just each patient." It was really fascinating to watch people. Some of them had to get up and walk out. The people who really hate my guts had to leave, because they could not stay. A lot of them, who didn't like me or what I was trying to do, went into their trance to stay out of the trance I was asking them to go into. Which was fine. What I was demonstrating was *trance*, whether it was the one I was requesting or the one they went into to stay out of the one I was requesting. It didn't really matter. It was absolutely fascinating.

Now I'm in such a bind whenever I give a presentation. People expect that I'm going to do something like this, and so I usually put in a short paragraph and they say, "Oh, Wow!" I don't have to do anything else, because they do it all anyway.

That was the very first one and I worked very hard on it. I was really making an effort to prove a point. And I think I did. And people pick up on it. When I start out, doesn't it make sense? By the time you find out that I'm doing something else too, its okay.

This one I read, because I was so afraid I would get lost.

The Mythical Trance

When Dr. Wain [Director, Veterans Hospital] first asked me to write a paper, I questioned whether to agree because I did not believe I had anything new to say about the utilization of hypnosis and I generally try to provide both useful and practical information. After some deliberation, I realized that perhaps I could do something philosophical and practical, too, since both are important elements of any paper I prepare. I then thought about how many people really had not heard what some of us have been saying for years regarding Milton Erickson's approach. There are those who teach and have used the name of Erickson's approach but they do not truly appreciate the skill, work and effort—the true genius— involved in what he does, this thing called "the mythical trance".

Why is it called "the mythical trance"? What is meant when we say we "use" hypnosis? Does it mean we are going to practice on somebody? Too often, we get involved in the induction technique and do not progress from there; once we master the technique, what then? It comes to using it and that involves the perfect trance. We teach people to go into the perfect trance. The only problem is that sometimes the perfect trance is the one we require to meet our needs rather than the one that satisfies the patient's needs. For most of us, the ideal trance patient responds appropriately to the induction technique, quickly and easily goes into a recognizable trance and becomes, which is even better, a somnambulist along the way. He will then go into trance at a prearranged signal, listen and obey all our instructions. Unfortunately, there are not too many people who meet all of these requirements.

This paper will discuss some of the results we should realistically expect trance to achieve. Basically, we should expect the patient to learn to use his own autonomic nervous system and to tap his own unconscious. At the University of Pittsburgh, we have been teaching a course in hypnosis for 21 years. During those years, there have been many changes. In place of the term *operator* or *hypnotist* (which is not consistent with our beliefs) the term *facilitator* is used to refer to the physician, dentist or psychologist who helps the patient to go into the trance. The facilitator then applies his own skills and methods as a healer, be it pills, prescriptions, surgery or psychotherapy. He is still only able to help the patient to heal himself.

Interestingly, with regard to hypnosis, a number of people have noted that the success of hypnotism seems to decrease as the facilitator gains experience. Some of us may ask: "Why are we more successful as beginners than we are after we have been using hypnosis for a while?" It might be that beginners have not yet begun to be afraid to believe; because they are still so full of enthusiasm, hypnosis has not become a habit, and they have not backed away from it. As Mark Twain said, "Nothing so needs reforming as other people's habits."

I was taught, over 25 years ago, in an apprenticeship type of program that demanded that we learn a lot by ourselves and that assumed that hypnosis was a very unusual, special kind of state. It was believed at that time that all one had to do was learn the induction technique and that everything else followed. I do not believe that any longer, but I do believe that Dr. Erickson's methods and techniques have resulted in a much wider range of current approaches to therapy and that he was very much ahead of his time. Books such as that by Watzlawick, Weakland and Fisch (1974) permit the reader to understand not only the authors' acknowledgment of Erickson's influence but the influence his early work is having on therapy today.

The early seminars satisfied an early need. They eliminated the curious and the magic seekers: they came, and when they found out that the workshops were not particularly flamboyant, they left. There were a few diehards who came back again and again, and every time they learned a little bit more.

I learned that therapeutic hypnosis is a goal that both doctor and patient must agree upon and that it only works when the patient wants it to work and agrees with the signal to be worked with. Also, I gradually learned to believe what Erickson taught about relying upon the patient's unconscious; it is the patient's trance. The patient sometimes needs the facilitator to give options and to give permission to use and learn more about hypnosis, more about himself on an unconscious level, but basically it is the patient who is going to do whatever is going to be done with the hypnosis. Erickson taught the patient to develop new and unorthodox ways of communication as well as new and unorthodox ways of looking at things, that would enable him to recognize things that he normally would not bother to look at.

I went through phases in learning hypnosis. I started out with a lot of curiosity then went into a kind of skepticism. At that point, I would attend a workshop, listen and try what was suggested there. That the suggestions worked caused me to spend a lot of time in that particular phase because the knowledge that it worked was also a little bit scary. There is no way that one can honestly believe that one is not doing something to a subject. All of our training teaches us that when someone does these kinds of impossible things, he must be doing something pretty weird; thus, the positive reaction transfers to the omnipotent reaction.

There is something similar that applies to a great many of us: At some point, I recognized that if I am doing this to the patient, then there is no way that I am going to let anybody else do this to me. I refuse to be under anyone's power or control. I have to reach the stage at which nobody can hypnotize me. If one does not get stuck at that stage, then hypnosis really starts to become useful. It took me awhile to get past that point because I was not about to let anybody else hypnotize me.

My patients came through and taught me, and they rejected me when I tried to get them to do things I wanted them to do but that they did not want to do. Finally, I realized that it might not be necessary for me to give up control in order to go into the trance. I went on to acknowledge that it was indeed the patient's trance, and, as the doctor, I could cooperate with the patient. Then I reached another scary phase, one of not really understanding the patient's behavior. I was not sure that I was going to be able to respond appropriately to whatever the patient might do. At that point, I still felt that the magic was in the induction technique. As I moved beyond that phase and into using the hypnosis, then I began to understand that it was all right not to understand and that I could, as I said earlier, begin to rely upon the patient's unconscious, realize the kinds of things that he is learning, and be flexible enough to negotiate with him. I learned that hypnosis is not one sided, and in fact it can never really be.

Where did I go from there? Erickson's ways were again influential: he would sit down and work, write and outline and practice the gestures and the words that he was going to use. I went through a period of time when I had to sit down and outline, work and plan. I think it has resulted in a great deal of benefit to my patients and some, at least, to the workshops on hypnosis.

At present, my greatest interest is in the nonrelaxed trance, otherwise known as "bright-eyed and bushy-tailed trance", though I think that relaxation can be useful too when a patient is anxious and uptight and needs to learn to relax, but I think that if you stop there, it can retard the individual's ability to use hypnosis. Unfortunately, too many doctors refuse to allow the patient to develop beyond relaxation and so they never really utilize the patient's full potential. Personally, I am not comfortable with the patient who has to be "zonked" in my or anybody else's chair. Therefore, the patient takes an active role in the treatment and in the induction. This allows the patient to maximize his own potential, rather than just withdraw.

After 26 years in hypnosis, I expect and I hope that I am the youngest of the elder statesmen involved because I do feel like an elder statesman. Much of my work in hypnosis centers on my doing much traveling and teaching both in the United States and overseas. I hope that this is going to be the means by which I can continue to grow, challenge, communicate and develop. Every once in a while, I wonder why those of us who have been in this field for so many years are still here. Why are we still teaching hypnosis when so many others have quit or only pay lip service to it?

In response to the above questions, it appears that teaching people hypnosis and teaching them to tap their potentials is like learning electric circuits in physics classes when one is studying electricity. One learns what switch activates what voltage, and then one learns to use the switches only when it is appropriate to use the voltage. The switch can be left on or it can be turned off depending upon what one would like to do. During the conditioning pulses, however, there are going to be a lot of short circuits. They are expected to happen because they provide an understanding of the mechanism. When something goes wrong with that kind of circuitry and that kind of voltage, one knows it, and one learns to do something about it.

I see the "electric" potential in each person … not just each patient … for learning to really understand the language of hypnosis, because the language is the message, and the message turns out to be in the language. How many of you really listen to the messages people give? How willing are you to let yourself listen to what people say? I wonder whether there can be developed some pattern in the patter I provide which potentially portrays the posture of this perfect patient that I talked about earlier ... and how well you hear ... and I wonder whether you truly want to know what it is we are talking about or whether that becomes a kind of disturbing knowledge.

If you think about ideas in the four corners of the quarters of your brain, the things that come forth from these let you go forward pretty well. Three fourths of what we think is not truly intellectual in the hemispheric sense, because if you think about the right hemisphere as having a front of the brain as well as a back, you have one in the front and one in the back ... and then you have the left side, which is the one that is left, and you take the one and the one there, and you add that one and one and you get two. Then you take the two on that side that is left and add it to the two on the side that is right, and you get four. You can look forward to an additional gain from this kind of addition because when you add things up in that way, one is when you win, and when you win it means you gain. But sometimes the only way you can gain is by losing. When you lose, are you really gaining? ... Because you win only what you gain by losing, if you understand that some losses can be very positive gains ... especially if you do not need to have it all add up ... because if it does, and you think you know what you are really listening to, then I suspect that what you do know is not what you are willing to know that you know. If you compare that to what you do not know that you know, you find out that the three fourths I mentioned earlier in adding up the gains and losses is reflected in the kinds of things that you think you see when you look in a mirror or when you look through a window pane. I wonder, when you look into that pane, whether it is very painful to see what you see in that sea of scenes that you see: do you seize the scene that you particularly want to see ... do you see where you were, and when you were where, and where you end up in that particular scene. I wonder whether when you look at it through a very clear glass, seeing the reflection lets you understand where you can go. When you take any kind of pane you can see through ... and you wash it with any kind of fluid that you have available ... I wonder whether it lets you merge the mirage of wavy lines in our lives that come through there into a marriage of past events which have shaped us, present events which surround us, into a future which adds up.

Just by knowing that we do know that one ... on one side ... and one ... on the other side ... is a gain, so it is okay to finally win by understanding that you can learn to gain by losing ... and still know that you know everything that you need to know. Because by doing ... you can be what you are and what you want to be ... which is the sum total of those four quarters of the brain. But if you choose that, it involves a risk ... and it demands expansion of those very comfortable kinds of walls behind which many of us hide and through which we refuse to see ... or be seen. If you can confront that fear ... if you recognize that it is okay to be afraid, and to go ahead anyway ... then the good feelings that make it all worthwhile are the kinds of additional positive responses you get from a recharging of enthusiasm and a renewed look at the language. And so you go on from there.

Some of us are going to go on doing things that other people do not really understand and probably do not approve of, since we have tried to work within the system and found that it did not give us everything we wanted. We keep trying to explain to the people who will listen and will carry on, but we accept the fact that at any given time many people do not understand the language of hypnosis. We rely upon our students to surpass us and to excel in ways that we do not really understand. Every teacher should be surpassed by his students; otherwise, he is not a very good teacher. The potential is always present; it only needs to be activated. Louis Thomas (1974), president of New York Memorial Sloan-Kettering Cancer Center, said:

> The real amazement is this: you start out as a single cell, this divides into two, then four, then eight, and so on, and there emerges as the cells differentiate one cluster of cells which will have as its progeny the human brain. The mere existence of those special cells should be one of the great astonishments of the earth. One group of cells is switched on to become the whole trillion-cell massive apparatus for thinking and imagining. All the information needed for learning to read and write, playing the piano, or the marvelous act of putting out one hand and leaning against a tree, is contained in that first cell. All of grammar, all arithmetic, all music.

One does not need to stop there; one can go on to all of the uncon-scious learning and responding and thinking and feeling that the individual is capable of doing unless he chooses to switch it off. Every time I start with a new patient or with something different, I have some real concerns because I am never exactly sure what is going to happen. I do know that the more I travel, the more people I find who want to listen, hear and understand the kinds of things Erickson teaches and taught. In Scandinavia and the Netherlands and in Singapore and Australia, people want to know about this very special way of working with patients.

I recently returned from a trip to the Netherlands, and the people there learned the most when I was able to tell them that I was afraid when a 13-year-old girl was brought in with a dental phobia, and she did not speak English. I was supposed to work with her. I would have been out of my mind if I was not scared, but it did not stop me. I was willing to confront that fear and go on, relying on the patient's ability to understand. In that sense and for the future, I am not really worried. I may be scared, but that is different from being worried.

When Erickson picked me out and began working with me, the thing I learned to believe in was the patient. I learned that the task of the hypnosis facilitator is to activate the wealth of potential in the unconscious of that other person. That is, to all those who will never be able to understand it, what is so mystical about the Mythical Trance.

References

Watzlawick, P., Weakland, J. H. and Fisch, R. (1974). *Change: Principles of Problem Formation and Problem Resolution*, New York: Worth.

Thomas, L. (1974). *The Medusa and the Snail*, New York: Viking Press.

Chapter Twelve
Dual Induction

Introduction to Dual Induction

James Auld

It is with great pleasure (and some trepidation) that I write this chapter introduction—pleasure, because of the opportunity to give something in return for all the gifts bestowed by Kay, and trepidation in that I might not do justice to her memory and skills.

I first met Kay Thompson in Melbourne, Australia at the 1979 International Society of Hypnosis (ISH) meeting. My reaction was, "Wow, this lady speaks my language!" I was "mesmerized" by her use of language and her ability to deal so elegantly with so many problems which are frequently the bane of dentists' professional lives. I recall she visited Adelaide, Australia two years later, when two parallel workshops were offered. There were about 30 delegates in each, but, after lunch on the first day, the other poor fellow was left with only three! The rest of us crowded into one small room, such was the charm and skill of this wonderful lady.

My first experience with the dual induction was in Glasgow at the ISH meeting in 1982. Kay asked casually, "You wanna do a dual induction with me tomorrow?" and explained that all would be well if I just kept talking. It worked! We met again on five or six visits I made to Ericksonian meetings on the West Coast over the following years, and on several of these I was fortunate enough to share the stage with Kay.

She mentions on this tape that she wishes I lived several thousand miles closer, a sentiment wholeheartedly reflected by me. The infrequency of our association probably serves to highlight the fact that the dual induction is not a sophisticated technique that requires a great deal of practice. Rather it emphasizes that two (or more) clinicians with a reasonable grasp of hypnotic language can use the technique very effectively. In fact, I have done so, with one of my postgraduate students being the other clinician, and reading from a script while I provided the counterpoint.

On this tape, Kay provides comments on the origin and development of the dual induction technique. It does serve as a potent technique for assisting listeners to overcome blocks they may have about achieving their trance potential. It also serves as an excellent training tool to assist clinicians in becoming fluent and flexible in their use of language. It is difficult, if not impossible, to maintain a flow of words in this situation without being in your own trance. If you focus on the other person's language, the confusion and distraction produced often results in a "yes set" type of response, with trance and silence following. Once you are able to maintain the flow of your own "story", monitor (but not listen to!) the other person, and observe members of the group, you know you have achieved a significant level of mastery in the use of hypnosis, not only at a clinical level, but also on a personal level.

Kay was an excellent teacher: she used example, anecdote, participation, and experience, and repetition. Sometimes the experience was a little uncomfortable, as the "yes set" induced in me and described on the tape, but this was never done with malicious intent. There was always a gentleness and profound understanding of people's needs whenever Kay acted. She knew what it meant to grow, personally and professionally. One of her stories about herself was: "You think I was always like this? Well, at university they said you could always find Kay by feeling along the wall at the back of the lecture room; when you come to the bump, that's her!" Dr. Erickson saw the potential, and perhaps the need, and helped give us the person we knew and loved. I believe Kay also worked toward unlocking this potential in every person she worked with.

For this 1992 workshop, Kay asked me sometime during the previous evening to work with her the following morning "around ten". I had a message waiting in my room saying the workshop started at 8:30. I called Kay at 8:00 the next morning and woke her! We both made it by 8:30, and the result is what you hear here; it really was unprepared.

The comment at the end of the tape deserves some explanation. About 1988, Kay had related a story to me about a colleague. When asked how he knew he was in trance, he replied, "I think differently when I'm in trance." Kay said to him: "Bob [Bob Pearson, one of Erickson's earliest students and a renowned teacher of hypnosis], think like you're not in trance." At this point, Bob went "out to lunch". That afternoon someone asked Bob, "What did Kay say to you this morning?" As Bob reviewed the morning's question, he went into trance again! At dinner with a group of conference people in 1989, someone asked Kay, "How does someone put you into trance?" Kay's response was to sit very erect, and say, "No one puts me into trance!" At the end of the tape, I rather innocently asked, "How does no one put you into trance?" Kay's response was similar to Bob's—but only briefly! When you listen to the tape, there is a long pause after this question by me, as Kay again does the search for meaning and association. It is this search for meaning, and the many linked associations that are explored, which make indirect hypnosis such a powerful tool.

It has been my privilege to know and work with Kay. I profoundly respected her knowledge and skills, but even more her humanity. I trust this present book will preserve, in some measure, the lifetime of accumulated knowledge and clinical skill with which she has endowed us.

Kay Thompson

The dual induction is something I have a lot of fun with, but don't get to use a lot except in workshops and since Jim is a dentist in Australia, he's a little far away to call. It's a little bit different than the kinds of things you are generally exposed to here.

I take one third of the credit for developing the dual induction. Bob Pearson, Ray Le Scola and I, back in the early 1970s, were at a workshop in Banff. Ray couldn't go into trance and hallucinate. This man could do anything else. He could teach me to bleed in alternate inches on a scratch down the arm. I believed that anyone who could bleed in alternate inches, could hallucinate.

We were sitting in a room, just kind of talking after one of the sessions. We were triangulated and Bob and I started talking and we watched Ray as he started to go into trance. We were talking in turn about the same thing and then we started talking simultaneously about the same thing, because something seemed to be happening. We didn't know what it was but we were going to find out. Then we started talking about different things simultaneously and Ray had this absolutely gorgeous hallucination of Christmas in Mexico. And we thought, Oh! This is kind of neat!

So for quite a while we thought that it was only going to be useful for people who had trouble achieving some particular phenomenon, and then that became very obviously selfish. And we started expanding the utilization and now it has become apparently very popular. At the time, Jay Haley watched a tape we did with a man down in Savannah and said it was the first new thing he had seen in hypnosis for 15 years. And looking back I can't understand why it took so long! Why didn't we do this 100 years ago? Because it's so natural.

Jim and I didn't know that we were going to do this until a couple of days ago. We don't preplan this, we had not talked about it, we came in this morning and said, "Whatever happens." That's a real important part of my belief about the dual induction. I don't think it can or should be scripted or preplanned; you've got to go into it with what you are given, and that's with the two of us working together.

J: Our focus is on giving you something worthwhile, possibly a retrieval of resources, ego strengthening, giving a nice time to get in touch with yourselves …

K: This is not intended as a therapy session, this is a demonstration. You can learn a lot from this, if you choose to. The only requirement I have is that people keep talking. Sometimes, I find myself up here by myself.

J: It's quite difficult to stay out of Kay's trance. When you finish a phrase, you are suddenly listening to the other person's words.

K: We have to be in our own trance in order to pay attention to you, listen to what we are saying and sometime monitor the other person. The pacing is fun. I enjoy it tremendously.

First Dual Induction

K: You can decide which one of us is easiest to listen to *now*.

J: That may change as time goes by.

K: And time does go by.

J: Surprisingly quickly when we are doing this sort of thing.

K: This sort of thing means dual induction, because it is a little different from the kinds of things you are generally exposed to here.

J: In this sort of dual induction, no one is going to put you into trance. You have a choice of going into Kay's trance

K: or going into Jim's trance

J: or going into your own trance to stay out of the ones we are working on.

K: Since the objective is a demonstration of trance, it doesn't really matter whose it is or how you get there.

J: That's a nice example of a triple bind.

K: Triple binds can be nice examples; they don't always have to be home runs or flies out, assuming that you know enough about American baseball to know what I'm talking about.

It's interesting the clichés we use and other people really don't understand what we mean, because language is such an important part of hypnosis …

J: It's interesting to note the different idioms when I come to the United States. You pull down the shades, not the blinds, as we refer to them.

K: Pulling down the blinds has a number of meanings.

179

J: It gives you an opportunity to have a period of quiet peace.

K: It gives you an opportunity to close out the rain which sometimes happens in Phoenix when I arrive here.

J: The rain in the desert is kind of beautiful.

K: Rain comes and has its purpose. I used to really hate the rain.

J: It's a regeneration, a necessary re-giving of life,

K: an opportunity to make something new

J: and for things to start growing

K: and let them understand that they are only temporary.

J: The blessing of falling rain may be a disadvantage to some people

K: You look at the clouds that bring in the rain …

J: but to those dormant plant seeds—

Talking Simultaneously

K: And you think back to when the clouds were pretty, fluffy, white cumulus clouds, along with those … cumulus clouds you begin to see the stratus clouds, and you see the little horsetail wisps … of ideas … which come in … and when they get together you know what it is they are going to do

J: Lying in the ground it's a blessing of new life regeneration and invitation to push out and go foward it's a kind of like the initial decision to make on your career paths to … choose a particular direction which

to you ... and it gives you time to get ready ...

time to think ...

time to decide ...

and as you do this, let yourself, know that you are ready ... for whatever it is that these clouds will bring in ... this time, knowing that the regrowth and the regeneration of ideas ... that have been planted sometime ago, will grow and survive and expand with the rain, knowing as you look on that surface, that you can enjoy the understanding of that growth and the expansion of the ideas, as you understand that this is the greatest gift that you can give, even thought you may not understand ... letting yourself look into the things that have been planted, that have the ability, that understanding of how to grow, how to expand, how to become what it is that you know they have potential to become ...

watching that growth, reveling in that growth, into a wondrous time of magic, because just the right amount of sun and rain, and wind in that fertile ground lets that plant blossom and spread its

enables you to reach a destination that you hope to achieve
sometimes there will be particular facts ... particular people ... that give you that impetus to make that decision to push you in that particular direction and as you move along that path ... toward your destination it's like that plant throwing out its first shoots absorbing the blessing of the moisture in the soil seeking out nutrients anchoring itself firmly in the underlying substance to give its strength to resist those heavy spring rains and winds that it's going to encounter as it shoots eventually through the surface and that those stones that have been such obstacle to its growth can be used to great benefit, a protector from those little plant eating animals and the young plant can hide behind those protecting itself from those with greater strength, and as time goes by

leaves and its seeds far beyond anything that ever, ever wondered … and as you let yourself relax deeper, and deeper, and deeper, knowing that those seeds that have been planted that deeply sometimes take a little longer to grow and reach the surface … but you know that fertile idea will come out, will grow, will expand …

in ways that may be very unexpected for you,

being curious about why you might have chosen that particular direction,

knowing that all the reasons that you need not understand, at some point will make perfectly good sense …

and growth continues so that … increasing strength, increasing security … a developing stem that can raise nutrients from the roots to the growting tip, … and the growing tip that sends the energy of sunlight back down to the roots allows the plant to grow ever more strongly, tall and taller … and this may be kind of like where you are now seeking downwards for strength and security and anchoring yourself just where you want to be while you stretch out with another part of your being seeking that knowledge and inspiration and strength that to obtain from mixing with your colleagues … from going to seminars and exploring your boundaries pushing ever …

K: It's funny how long it takes some things to grow while others grow at a different rate …

J: Perhaps it depends on the amount of fertilizer they have.

K: Yes, but they grow in their own time,

J: and some needed more tending than others.

K: Yes, much more attention

but they can pay attention to that tension when they need to

J: and as they attend to the things that they need to pay attention to

K: they can tend to tune out the things that tone down that tendency to pay attention

J: even if that tension relies on a tendency for attention

K: and we all can take those gentle peaceful calm tenets and really tend to our tension …

J: and sometimes it's nice to have … a pleasant awareness of the lack of … tension, even while you … come back and pay … attention.

K: It's kind of like letting your mind and body be at two different places at once and slowly … watching them merge and get back together again …

J: Just waking up from the neck up, and that could be a new experience

Imagine … that you have come out of trance

K: and imagine how good the ground feels after the rain, when it's all clean and refreshed, bright and wonderful … I've got to believe more went into their own trance than went into ours … I'm jealous, I want to go down there and sit … or in some cases, stretch out … Aha! The noise level is coming up … Because it is your trance, you can take as long as you like to rejoin us … you don't even have to.

J: Or you can just simulate rejoining us …

Comment: Your voice qualities are so similar, and you paced each other so well, that you were able to work so beautifully as a team, and that seems to be the strength of the dual induction.

K: I've done this with a man who speaks faster than I can think, but it still works. The only requirement I have is that the other person keeps speaking!

J: It is difficult doing this at first because you have to stay out of the other person's trance while still listening to them.

K: We have to be in our own trance to pay attention to you, to listen to what we're saying, and to monitor the other person.

J: We did this some years ago in Phoenix, in the Convention Center, around midday, and the clock started ringing. This was just as we were running down at the end of the first half of the session. We looked at each other and we decided, we have to utilize. So it can be amazing how things can strike a chime in you memory, you would hear an unexpected sound which would ring a bell about this meeting …

K: It became really time for you to understand … Someone said "How did you manage to do that, how did you get that clock to chime right then?"

J: So utilization is important, and recognizing that, like you've experienced in sleep, when a sudden sound comes into the dream, but the dream seems to precede the sound, and then include the sound or body movement in the dream. In trance the same thing happens—you get this confusion about temporal positioning. Perhaps people were not hearing the chimes until we drew their attention to them, and then it seemed so wonderful that it was all there.

Question: Why does the dual induction work? and discussion about personal difficulty of going into trance during this dual induction. I couldn't manage both of these channels. Have you had this reaction before?

K: Yes, I think the reason that it works is because it is really pretty easy to defend against one voice coming at you from outside; it's much harder to defend against two channels, because when you are defending against one, the other one is getting through, and when you are defending against that one, this one is getting through. And I think one of the issues there is with traditional hypnosis you have more of a recognition of your control, and with this, there's the feeling, "Oh! I don't really have as much control over this and I'm not sure I can monitor both." What frequently happens is that after the first time that we've done it and you've gone through it and you've satisfied your curiosity and you understand what was happening.

Then it's easier for you to let it happen the second time because what you learn is that you can listen to both of us at once and you can hear both of us and you can respond to suggestions we both give. The people for whom it is most useful are those people who have had difficulty learning trance, for that reason.

Comment: I found it especially useful, because I went right back to when I was 4, 5 and 6 years old, to a happy part of my life when my parents used to have friends over, and I can remember I was back in my bed listening to all the happy voices in the living room. It was very pleasant, a strengthening experience.

K: Whose trance is it? No question, it has to be your trance. Both Jim and I firmly believe that.

Question: If two is natural and good, would three (voices) be better?

K: We did a quad once. I find it very distracting because I think I only have two ears. There are people who have taken this and worked with three. I don't know where you draw the line between ridiculousness and seriousness with the utilization. It does say that the person in the trance is certainly able to be in rapport with as many people as are talking. You don't have to do a triple or quad induction. You can choose to hear them or tune them out.

J: At a party, when you attend to one speaker, if you let your attention wander, you can hear the buzz in the background which is all the other people and quite a high volume and yet you are totally tuned in to the one person you want to attend to.

Question: You both are coming out of the same speakers. What if we heard each of you from different speakers, from one side and the other side?

K: We've hassled back and forth, right brain, left brain, right ear, left ear, stereo. When I had my auto accident I had a couple of my friends do a double induction with a speaker that happened to be stereo. One of them talked about the psychological impact and one talked about the physiological healing. It really didn't make any difference to me because I was so interested in both aspects of it. There are people who are playing with this and will give you all sorts of theories. I'm not sure that you don't choose to hear us in whichever half of your brain is most tuned into whatever it is we're saying ...

J: Don't think it would work in this (lecture) situation. You'd have greater volume from one speaker.

Comment: I had been given a tape of a previous dual induction by Kay and Jim and found it stressful, but while in this session found experiencing you in person as a totally different (positive) kind of experience.

K: I think if you've been here and you get the tape and it might be useful because it puts you back here. You were going into surgery and you had a specific need. And we were not addressing that need at all! I think you were absolutely right to get very upset with us because we were not meeting your need.

Question: Is it better to have a man and a woman doing the induction, or is it not important? I've never heard two men doing the dual induction.

K: Works any way. I have heard two men do it.

Question: I did choose to listen to Kay, but now and then Jim's words would come in like a chorus on a poem, but mostly I listened to Kay.

K: There's no wrong way to do it or to hear it.

J: We tend to draw words from each other any way. Part of the unconscious hears words and feeds it into our own pattern.

Comment: I'm just feeling awake from the head up, and it's very nice. I couldn't even raise my hand (to ask a question), I had to motion with my head—it's very nice!

Comment: (By a therapist who had previously heard Kay giving a workshop on the dual induction.) I used the dual induction successfully with someone who was dying and having trouble handling the pain. I asked my client's spiritual director to recite religious verses which the patient was familiar with for the background while I worked with pain issues. It worked very, very well. The patient could latch onto things that were familiar in either case and it helped him get though her pain. I wanted to let you know that you are still working ...

K: Thank you. I think that is one of the most useful things. I appreciate that. I also appreciate the comment from the gentleman whose body has decided to take its own time to (awaken). I put a specific suggestion in the end because of a semirequest about body-mind and that was put in for that. And you chose to do something for yourself with it.

Comment: (By someone who heard Kay and Jim at the previous Phoenix meeting and had a very profound effect from it, and took the tape home. She comments about the changes in her perception over the last 4 to 5 years.) First, I heard only Kay with Jim in the background. Then I was aware of my need to be more logical in my thinking, so I paid more attention to Jim. Now it feels real slowed down and I can hear both messages very clearly together. I've also used it with students, teaching right-brain, left-brain stuff, and they love it.

K: I think that's the tape where Jim was building a house, a framework, and that would fit your structure very well.

Second Dual Induction

K: It's time to do a second induction, and I know it's time to do that because my time sense says time is moving on.

J: Time sense is a kind of non-sense.

K: Nonsense makes sense when it's time for it.

J: Perhaps it's not yet time.

K: For the sense or the nonsense?

J: The sense of déjà vu that comes from reviewing the things you have done

K: or the essence of your learning ... what makes sense out of the nonsense that we offer you ...

J: Sometimes you have to ... go way back ... and look for some thing to latch onto that sense.

K: That sensation ... can be a very sensitive one

J: 'Cause many of you have come here with particular ... needs,

K: particular goals and ideas and mind and nobody else needs to know about

J: and ... perhaps with certain problems, that you want some help with

K: curiosities about the things that you can learn ... for yourself

J: and to let you go forward to reach your goals ... to assist those who depend on you

K: and it's nice to be depend-able ...

J: and it can be a problem ... remembering ... all those things that you really need to know

K: that's better … because it doesn't matter whether you know everything that you know that you know …

J: and there are many things you forget, that you're not aware you've forgotten …

K: as long as you know that you do not know everything that you know …

J: and I wonder whether you become aware of forgetting that you've remembered or knowing that you remember that you haven't forgotten things that you haven't thought about for so long … that they are just back there

| K: Knowing you do not need to know everything that you know means that no matter what the test or the challenge … you can rely … on what you know that you do not know that you know … let yourself listen to the part of you that reflects that particular illusion

and that you can allude to that illusion because the illusion … of that reflection … in that dream … lets you move on, knowing …

that this is kind of like Alice in Wonderland. You can go through that looking glass and take your own trip down whatever hallway and path-way is useful … as as you let yourself relax … your mind, knowing that whatever surfaces on that surface may | J: In the back of your mind … there for your own use

you can … reflect … on all those things in the past rather like looking in the mirror to see behind you

and when you look at that reflection in the mirror there is a large area behind you which you can never see

and sometimes that blocked reflection can be very frustrating, because you have the feeling that perhaps there's something back there are which you'd really like to find even with its distortions

and as you see through the glass and take that scene and seize onto the particular scene now that you see … in the glass |

be like a pond that reflects so perfectly the sea and sky and then you drop a pebble into that pond and that ripple that starts small and moves out influences a much broader expanse of that surface but it's even more important to know that that pebble that settles down to the bottom and stirs up the sand that's down there for just a moment

and you can strain it through a sieve and get rid of the things that are not useful,

the impurities

and be left … with a clean … pure … clear idea
that becomes so bright,
so shiny
and you look at that shiny clear crystal and it's like a prism and when the light bounces off that prism you know that it breaks up into the most magnificent colors and those colors represent the different strengths that you have and the red is the fire and the passion of your strength, the orange is that brilliance and the yellow is the sunshine that is always there above the clouds, green is for growth that comes from the rain and blue is the intensity of the perfection of the ever changing

you can examine in minute detail those things that are particularly relevant to you and it can be confusing sometimes to see the spreading ripples reflected from the obstacles and watch the fascinating patterns of the interactions of all the things you have known and experienced you can choose to examine in particular detail those areas which are of immeciate relevance, the things that are of immediate importance to you

and when we take those particulr points which are of immediate relevance
and examine those thoughts
and then take those thoughts inside yourself
and examine them for their deep inherent meaning
their deep inherent value

and you can gain a profound insight, as though you're able to see through the problems in the past that seem so difficult, so insurmountable, because in this state that problem can fragment into its particular parts letting you see the individual components so clearly that you can do with each one at its own level in its own way sky and sea and indigo the passion, the depth, the intensity of your commitment to yourself and your integrity.

The violet is the color that lets you understand the healing, the vibrations, the way that you need to know that those healing colors can be at your beck and call and that you find yourself like a bicycle wheel or a color wheel, you are the center, you are the core and each of those spokes goes out to a different part of you and you can give to each of those parts on that rim or that wheel but you maintain your strength, your integrity and your personal power. And a center of that wheel. It feels so good ... to know and under-stand

that you don't have to make it happen.

All the time you need in the time you have. But we know that knowledge is there.

and that can be ... a really neat experience in being able to examine those problems in that way, with the separate-ness, without being concerned at all about the hole that is left when the problem breaks up

and perhaps you can use this in ways in which you are not yet aware to help you in your future path, your future growth, and your future understandings

and the can be ways in depth of that pond of thought that will let you understand ways of going forth to your patients and allowing them to communicate to you so much-more clearly, so much more comfortably, really feeling deep within you things that you need to know, the feeling of great comfort and sureness deep inside being able to expand that feeling of comfort and peace in ways that will benefit you always that you just need to be ... there

just let it come to you because you know all the things that you need to know

and you just need to know that you no longer have to "no" them

J: and it's okay to take that time that you have to do the particular things that you want

K: and to make sense for what is important to make sense of

J: and if you are beginning to sense a solution, you can continue on the path that leads towards the answer that you want.

K: The process of growth and alertness need not be separate and as you rejoin all those parts that have done their thing and you integrate things you didn't even know you knew. It's kind of a smug feeling way down deep inside you.

J: As you begin to realize that profound power that relies deep within each of us but sometimes needs to be unlocked because we don't acknowledge it

K: but we know that knowledge is there.

(*Pause.*)

J: Some of you can continue on and enjoy your state of trance in whatever part of your body you wish to retain it.

K: You get what you want from what we do.

J: And you do it.

K: We do make an effort to keep it light and learning. It's what you are here for.

J: Decisions about rejuvenation after the heavy work from the other sessions we go to.

K: I remember having dinner with Jim in Toronto and I was literally falling asleep, with my face falling into my plate, literally. Seriously. Okay, are you all back here? Your bodies back here too?

Question: Did you ever make a double induction tape with yourself?

K: I have. And you can also make a double induction for yourself. I've always said, you know better than anybody else
what you need to hear, so why not make a tape, go into trance,
and listen to it. You can also make a music tape and play the
music. What you are doing is you are overloading the circuits
so that the important things can be heard. You give the ability
for your unconscious to do its own thinking and feeling
and organizing by giving these distractions to it in whatever
way.

Question: Speaking of colors. I noticed that somebody else noticed
that they were focusing more on you than Jim. I noticed in the
second induction that you were much more visually descriptive,
talking about colors and things like that. Is there a technique
when one person might emphasize an auditory, or visual or
tactile element?

J: If it were more preplanned we might incorporate something like
that in a session.

We've worked together like this four or five times. I tend to hear
Kay start a particular pattern; I had the ripples and interferences—
we sort of steal things from each other.

K: Whatever we're doing, we're not doing consciously. We get
along so well. I really enjoy working with Jim. I kind of trust my
unconscious. There's plenty in my unconscious for it to be spontaneous. You might, for someone who was differently oriented,
you might use different senses. There are no "no's", as far as I'm
concerned. It's whatever is best for the individual.

Comment: It was like listening to jazz improv.—really getting into
the experience of the whole, and being there. It was wonderful.

K: Thank you. In general we just wanted you to have the
opportunity to have an interesting and hopefully a fun experience that you can take back and consider using in the different
ways it would work in your office. That's the idea of the whole
thing.

J: If anyone is not out of trance, raise your hand *slowly*.

K: If anyone is not out of trance yet. That's one of those limiting words. Make it what you like of it, but like what you make of it. None of what we are saying up here is rehearsed. Playing with words is my thing. I know Jim does a lot of it back home. We both work solo back home.

J: One of the most difficult things in trying to practice, or put into practice, dual induction back home. And that applies to any of you, is finding someone who can do it with you, because the difficulty is in maintaining your own integrity in keeping the flow of words going, while you're listening to the other person, or for the other person to maintain the flow of words. Kay did that beautifully to me some years ago. We were playing with "left" and "right", and Kay ended up with a phrase like: "And if that's all right, what's left?" I was left standing with my mouth open. She knew where I was going, and led me right up the path!

K: One of the things you need to know is make sure the person you are working with can and will keep talking. The first time I do this with somebody, I will say, "What is a really comfortable induction technique for you? Okay, you do that, and don't stop talking!" Here I am supposed to do a dual induction and all of a sudden I'm solo. And nothing is happening with the person you are using the dual induction to help.

J: My experience was total elimination of the audience, the first time I did it. I had to focus so much inside that the audience disappeared. Now I find I can use my own trance. So I listen to Kay and what I am saying and watch all of you at the same time.

K: It takes all three parts of your brain.

J: All three parts. Kay, how does no one hypnotize you? … and you watch

K: (*Pause.*) How does no one hypnotize me? Where do all those little thoughts go when you don't think them?

J: That one goes back a long way.

K: It sure does! People occasionally, when asked questions like that kind of fall off a cliff into trance. That's the reaction to the circumstance when that particular question was asked. As far as we are concerned, that's it.

J: It's time.

Part IV
Suggestion and Utilization

In her commentary, "Healing Through Language", Roxanna Erickson Klein tells the revealing story of Kay Thompson's first meeting with Erickson. Through numerous examples, she then vividly illustrates Thompson's methodical crafting of multilevel communications.

In Chapter Thirteen, Thompson presents an original and provocative orientation to the subject of posthypnotic suggestion. Her playfulness and multilevel communications are especially evident as she challenges therapists to become cognizant that anything they say to a client during trance could be interpreted as a posthypnotic suggestion. She also explores the interesting similarity between posthypnotic suggestions and numerous experiences, such as prior learning and symptoms. This is a superb example of Thompson's smorgasbord teaching; she is thought provoking, challenging, motivating, and constantly intriguing the reader with hypnotic possibilities for communication.

In Chapter Fourteen, "Utilization", Thompson illustrates her distinctive "suggest, motivate, suggest, motivate" approach with clients in the section, "Utilization Techniques". Opening up possibilities through providing logical reasons for clients to change their perspectives, and thus behavior, is a fundamental aspect of utilization of trance, according to Thompson.

The second section, "Clinical Utilization", offers a broad spectrum of Thompson's key teaching about utilization, including central issues about the personal interrelationship in hypnotherapy; meeting clients' needs in metaphor; imagery and imagination, and memory and amnesia. Thompson also generously explains the construction of several of her favorite metaphors for clinical utilization and suggests various client populations for which they are applicable. The last section, "Balance and Control", contains an interesting clinical vignette with a difficult client and one of Thompson's favorite multilevel metaphors.

Healing Through Language

Roxanna Erickson Klein

Kay Thompson loved telling the tale of her first meeting with my father, Milton Erickson. She was a young dentist, attending a lecture with the hope of learning trance skills to help her dental patients relax. Listening intently and fascinated by the material, she embarked on what would become a lifelong path. Erickson addressed the group of professionals with a deep intensity, engaging various audience members with his well-known, captivating hypnotic gaze.

Kay let her shy habits prevail and concealed herself near the back of the room behind a large fat man. Intrigued by her evasive maneuvers, Erickson actively sought to bring her out of hiding. In telling her tale, Kay would mimic Erickson gradually easing his way about the lecture room to reposition himself in a place where her cover was lost. Each time, she would scoot her chair away, avoiding his penetrating glance.

At last, late in the day, Erickson walked directly to her. He greeted her like a long lost friend whom he was both surprised and delighted to see. Thus began a long relationship that involved a harmony of professional respect and loving friendship that endured for both their lifetimes.

The anecdote of the initial meeting contains glimpses of the unfolding of the many ways Erickson influenced Kay Thompson's professional development. Part of that story is of a painfully shy young professional with the guts and determination to combat gender bias in going to dental school. It is also the story of a lady who lost her own father and mentor, just at the time in her professional development when she depended on his unceasing encouragement to tutor and guide her into the tightly knit dental professional circles.

I learned about her father's powerful presence and understood a little about the friendship she shared with my own father. My dad had similar attributes of strong presence, enthusiasm for a challenge, and omnipresent encouragement. The relationship provided a continuum of many of the factors that had shaped and enriched her life, both as a person and as a professional. Her friendship with Erickson integrated respect, admiration and love with professional prodding, encouragement, demands, interests and mutual regard.

Lony Thompson had encouraged his daughter to break gender barriers and strive for accomplishment in the male-dominated field of dentistry. Erickson supported her in her reach beyond dentistry. One of Kay's favorite comments about dentistry, "There you are with your hands in a person's mouth—and in their head," reflected her view that in order to do good dentistry, one must work with the psychological orientation of the whole patient. Working with Erickson, Kay learned to develop techniques that moved her into realms that encompass facets of deep healing.

Therapeutic Language

Kay's methodology for eliciting healing from within was clearly enhanced by her appreciation for the value of collecting words. Kay delighted in language play and continually worked to enhance the communication skills that she credited Erickson for teaching her. She collected pairs of words that sounded similar and could be substituted, if appropriate, in the message: wait/wade, look/luck, near/here, mere/mare, read/reed, think/thing, classes/glasses, going/showing and bud/mud. Discrete substitutions were one element of more complex techniques of multilevel hypnotic induction and suggestion that intrigued her.

Undertaking her explorations with the revelry of a favorite game, she polished her abilities to a fine art, achieving a level of mastery and brilliance in her use of language. She jotted down lists of words that had multiple meanings, then practiced integrating them into sentences that would supply metaphorical, therapeutic messages to the unconscious. She entertained herself by creating phrases, sentences and paragraphs that utilized the flexible words which she practiced for fun: fan, well, fall, present, right, left, tear, rent, carry, store, might, wait, welcome, charge, bear, lean, pat, coupling, green, rail, hare, nun, pane, blew, weather and change. All these were a wee share of her repertoire. Kay carefully selected words, then precisely adjusted their punctuation, enunciation and emphasis. These techniques, especially when combined with trance phenomena, delivered indirect messages to the unconscious. For example, a benign account of "... a friend who went out on a day of pleasant *weather*, made a small purchase, and *waited* to get *some change* which resulted in being a *tiny bit* late for an engagement", is a little story replete with therapeutic messages, if given in the right circumstances and with the right inflections and intonations of voice.

She might begin a hypnotic trance induction about a walk through the woods, mention noticing the beech trees; then by substituting the word *sand* for *and* facilitate the building of an underlying deep layer of trance with imagery of a seashore. This duality could be reinforced and enhanced by further suggestions of "feeling the waving of the leaves, the blue of the wind, and a splash of color". The mismatch of tenses or sensory processes is a technique she often used to elicit curiosity to engage the unconscious.

Kay practiced the technique of interjecting unexpected words into everyday conversations with friends, salesclerks, and waiters. Watching responses, she was able to refine her techniques until her "choice" words were hardly detectable in casual conversation. Once she asked me the strange question, "How did you rent your dress?" and looked at me with her fixed innocent stare. I processed the question, and replied, "No, too unusual. The dog *teared* it." (using the pronunciation of *tears* from crying instead of "tore the fabric"). We both laughed at the awkwardness of the interchange. I noticed, with great admiration, that she later used the word *rent* in a context that capitalized on its unfamiliarity and facilitated the trance induction she was invoking at that time.

Instead of asking the usual question during a follow-up dental exam—"Well, I thought I'd ask about the toothache you had yesterday?"—Kay might ask, "Well, I think I see how that old toothache you had yesterday has gone?" The questioning inflection and emphasis bring a subtle but significant variation to the anticipated question. The awkwardness of saying "I see" where "I'll see" rightfully belongs, calls unconscious awareness to the question as a whole.

The question itself carries several imbedded suggestions, "I'm a professional doing an objective observation—I anticipate improvement—The toothache is a thing of the past—and—It went away." In the spoken delivery, she would emphasize "Well," while lowering her voice at the end of the question, giving additional suggestions to the unconscious. The credit for improvement was given to the patient, supported by smiles and praise for a job well done, again reinforced because she was the dentist who loved to see progress like this.

Erickson had a favorite induction technique in which he brought about confusion by giving direct suggestions pertaining to the "right hand" and the "left hand". Then he built intense confusion using "the right hand" to indicate the correct hand, and "the left hand" to indicate the hand not moving. It was hard to listen to the induction even as an audience member without developing trance.

Kay mastered that induction, and gave it her own special touch of lovely lilting melodies of alliterative phrases. Sometimes, when we shared breakfast on the morning of a presentation, Kay would jot on a napkin, all the words beginning with "m" we could both think of. Then during the demonstration, well after the subject was deeply in trance, she would reach into her pocket for the napkin and review whether she had omitted any choice words from the induction. Those moments, invariably coupled with a knowing look in my direction, affirmed that the little game we had enjoyed over breakfast had come in handy after all.

Kay was a unique and intriguing woman who presented a balance of frailty and fortitude, strength and gentleness, tenderness and endurance, courage and vulnerability, patience and productivity. The friendships, professional relationships, and interests that she nurtured illustrated some of the wonderful parts of Kay, but it was the harmony of her endeavors that most distinctly defined her. She was a professional who found fun in her work and brought hypnotic "languaging" to a higher level of understanding and practice. She was a dentist who reached so far into the scope of therapeutic communication that the gap between therapy and dentistry was finally bridged.

She was unwavering in her dedication to furthering the advancement of professional hypnosis. She was loyal in her friendships, in her affiliations, in her dedication to community, and in her spirit.

I dearly miss her.

Chapter Thirteen
Posthypnotic Suggestion

I can't quite figure out how I can take three hours to talk about that. But I'm sure you will find a way. I went to bed last night assigning it to my unconscious, and my unconscious went on vacation because when I woke up this morning there was this kind of vacuum that wasn't picking much up.

Posthypnotic suggestion is any suggestion after trance to be carried out after trance. It sounds like I'm saying the same thing, but I'm not. What that trance-lates into is any suggestion that is carried out after the patient achieves trance to be carried out after the patient terminates trance—any suggestion after trance to be carried out after trance. The words left out are the words assumed to be in. A great deal of the time we assume that posthypnotic suggestion has to be a much more blatant, rather than an assumed pose.

When we teach hypnosis for therapy and it is successful, isn't that by itself a posthypnotic suggestion? If you look at hypnosis with the expectation that anything that you say during the trance state that is accepted is in fact going to be utilized as a posthypnotic suggestion, then it makes you a lot more careful about what you say, which you should be anyway. People talk in fancy terms about amnesia for posthypnotic suggestion, and about whether you go back into a trance during a carrying out of a posthypnotic suggestion, and how long a posthypnotic suggestion is effective.

The only thing I find interesting about that is that in all of those instances, we, the therapist or doctor, are intentionally structuring what we say to be interpreted as a posthypnotic suggestion. Maybe that's our problem. We don't look at it from the viewpoint of the patient-client who may choose to accept everything we say as a posthypnotic suggestion. Just because we do not specify that those things are "posthypnotic suggestions", does not mean that they are not, or conversely, just because we say they are, does not mean that only those things are. I'm really curious to see where that came from. At this point it makes a reasonable amount of sense.

I get the sense that since this is an advanced group, it is essential you get some sense that there is more to it and that the sensation you get from it can be different. The posthypnotic suggestion is based first on how do you give a posthypnotic suggestion? The tongue in cheek answer is "very carefully". When you give a posthypnotic suggestion, recognizing that it is to be carried out at a future time, you need to put it in a framework to permit the individual to accept it on a level that makes it practical. A posthypnotic suggestion for someone who goes into a fairly good trance for maybe their first or second time may be, "When you leave my office today, you will find yourself compelled to buy a pack of Camels and bring them to me sometime before your next appointment." If the patient doesn't smoke and knows I don't smoke, that kind of suggestion will have a great deal of difficulty having any reasonable basis in fact.

Therefore, the individual would find himself in conflict because there would be this tendency to want to comply, "because if I don't comply I wasn't really in a trance and maybe the expectation that I have for help is going to be shot down. But that really is a stupid thing for her to want me to do and I need to show that it's really my trance and that I am autonomous so I don't want to do it." There is this conflict you read about and the person fights the suggestion and gets uncomfortable. They go home and can't sleep and finally get up and buy the pack of Camels and get even with you by bringing it to you at 5:30 in the morning because you kept them from sleeping. But this is game playing that doesn't do anybody any good. If someone really needs to have the understanding that they were in trance, playing that kind of game just isn't fair. There are so many other ways to demonstrate to them that trance is useful. You can have fun without having to play that kind of game.

The Ericksons[11] did a study about whether people can go back into the original trance state to carry out posthypnotic suggestions. If the person who originally gave the suggestion intruded upon the carrying out of a posthypnotic suggestion, which took a reasonably long time to carry out, would the individual regress to the original trance wherein the suggestion was given?

---

[11] Milton Erickson and his wife, Elizabeth M. Erickson, collaborated on several articles.

Maybe they do for something like that. I have difficulty under-standing why my two broken legs didn't hurt for the seven weeks it took them to heal, because I didn't appear to be in a trance state during that time, and nobody had given me the original suggestion. In terms of carrying out the posthypnotic suggestion, which it had to be of no pain, was I in a trance for the seven weeks or was I not? Looking at it from the fairly pragmatic approach I tend to take, I would say, "No, I don't think I was, but I think my legs were." And that was all that was appropriate. Maybe the kind of posthypnotic suggestion that we may structure for the individual lets us limit the area of that posthypnotic suggestion and also the area of the original trance state.

We give exercises, assignments, and homework to our clients, such as, "When you go home I would like you to sit down three times a day and write down for me all the positive thoughts you have had since the last time you sat down." If you do not say this is a posthypnotic suggestion, does that mean that the patient will not be carrying it out as a posthypnotic suggestion? Do we think of it as a posthypnotic suggestion? That depends. It depends on the way it is structured. When it is a specific assignment or specific exercise, then yes, we attribute it as a posthypnotic suggestion.

I don't think that the therapist wants to take the responsibility for accepting the fact that everything that he or she says may be accepted as a posthypnotic suggestion. I am coming more and more to the recognition that that fact is in fact a fact. And that people do need to think about what they say in terms of the question, what if the patient chooses to hear this as a posthypnotic suggestion? Would it be a good thing, in between, or inhibit the individual's progress?

I think there is another way to look at posthypnotic suggestion. That other way includes the idea of using past learning, and accept-ing that prior learning as a posthypnotic suggestion to be used for the recognition of a present skill. What do I mean? When you learn to ride a bike, learning to ride becomes automatic. When you get on the bicycle, you put yourself in a mode, and it becomes kind of like a posthypnotic suggestion. All of your prior learning will be brought into play in order to ride the bike. When you teach some-one else how to ride a bike, you utilize your skill and all of your learning to tell them what it is they need to do. Or you can use that skill to generalize to balancing on a tight rope, or playing tennis, or rock climbing or other active things that you do that utilize the same senses that you learned in that prior learning set.

When people come in and we ask them to go back in their memory and to remember, we think we are asking for a regression. I wonder, sometimes if we are not also asking them to utilize the skills we are asking them to remember, as if they were posthypnotic suggestions from some previous time.

"I wonder whether" is an interesting way to start a posthypnotic suggestion. I wonder whether when we say, "I wonder whether" to a patient, we realize we are asking them to weigh or we are asking them to balance or we are asking them to do things that we are curious about, not whether they are going to do them, but about the way in which they are going to do them. Then posthypnotic suggestion is nothing more than one big therapy session where they carry out the homework assignments that we give.

Question: Request for a definition of posthypnotic suggestion as any suggestion after trance to be carried out after trance.

T: When I say it that way, what it really means is any suggestion given after trance is achieved to be carried out after trance is terminated. You could still say it the same way depending on the emphasis you put on the words. I was emphasizing only the assumptions we make. I was asking you to tie in the assumption we make in that sentence—that a posthypnotic suggestion is given only when we are giving it and acknowledging that we are giving it. We need to look at it as if the patient might accept anything we say as a posthypnotic suggestion.

Question: Could you comment about your statement that exercises are posthypnotic suggestions?

T: I think that, frequently, we give exercises for patients to do at home. We say, "I am going to make this tape for you and I'd like you to listen to it every night before you go to sleep," and they take it home and listen to it every night before they go to sleep. Do we really acknowledge that it was in fact a very structured hypnotic suggestion? When we say, "I think you will find that you can be pleasantly surprised at how much more comfortable you are going to be when you leave here today," we are saying that as a reinforcing kind of statement, as an encouraging and supporting kind of statement. But it is in fact a posthypnotic suggestion.

Everything we say to a patient is something they take home and work on and do. In that narrow sense of the word, it is a suggestion or recommendation given during trance so they are going to carry it out. What it usually means is that they go home and work on all that material they have been dealing with, with you in that hour. All the work they are doing is in fact a posthypnotic suggestion.

You cannot not give posthypnotic suggestions, simply by virtue of the interaction between you and that person, who comes to you for whatever reason. Everything you do and say to them is in fact a posthypnotic suggestion with the possible exception of the things you get them into right now as experiences.

Question: What kind of failure experiences have I had?

T: I have had some dandies. The failure was for a number of reasons. This woman was sent to me by her friendly psychologist because the problem was oral and I'm a dentist and he wanted to get rid of her. She had an interesting habit. At least twice in every sentence with more than four words, she would grimace and her tongue would come out touch her chin and nose and every muscle in her face would contract and her tongue would go back in her mouth. It was pretty nauseating and revolting and I have a fairly strong stomach.

She learned to go into trance for me. She wouldn't do it for the psychologist, maybe because I was a dentist and not a shrink. It was safe and all right to go into trance in my chair. When the spasm is tension, teaching relaxation is a logical thing to do and it's appropriate. I taught relaxation and she quit having spasms. And I gave her all these proper and appropriate suggestions, about the understanding that she had needed this habit at one time and it served a useful purpose and it was no longer serving a useful purpose, which wasn't true. And she could learn how to carry on this relaxation when she left my office. She came out of trance and was fine, got out of her chair, and the grimace was back. I talked with the psychologist between sessions. She came back next time and sat in the chair and went into trance and stopped the grimace and I talked with her about things that were appropriate for support. She left the chair and the grimace was back. When she came back again, she stayed in the chair for two and a half hours and not once did she grimace.

I tried to give her other kinds of options to deal with it. When she left my office, the grimace was back. I called the psychologist and said, "I think this has to be dealt with." She was not willing to accept other substitutes using her skills. As long as she had the grimace, she could not go to work. Who would want her to work as a sales clerk? She could collect unemployment and social security. She couldn't go shopping so her husband had to go shopping. They couldn't accept invitations to visit friends and they couldn't invite anyone to visit. She had absolute control over her life and her family. They had to do everything for her and take care of her and all of the outside needs. She was not willing to even begin with me to give up that kind of control. She recognized that when she was in my office, that she didn't do it, but that was because she was in trance. She couldn't give it up.

The effort I made to have her go into trance and give up her symptom, and come out of trance remaining symptom free, and acknowledge that she was out of trance, did not succeed. She was not willing to accept that responsibility—yes, I am out of trance and no, I don't have the symptom. It was the magic of being in trance in my office. I sent her back to the psychologist who worked with her for a while. She went home and as far as I know, she is still grimacing.

We tried to shift the symptom to her hand so that could give her some of the helplessness and she could still maintain some control. There was a tremendous amount of anger and hostility that she would begin to get into and then turn off. It wasn't appropriate for us to go into that. The only reason she came to me was because I am only a dentist. I have been able to use that. As soon as she went back to the psychologist and was threatened by the need to deal with the psychological aspects, she was not ready or willing for other people to get her ready.

Question: Did I ask her for feedback?

T: On an ideomotor level she said she really didn't want to do anything.

Question: What about patients in trance who can get rid of severe pain, can get up and walk around, but when they "come out of trance", the pain comes back?

T: I think there can be a number of reasons for that. One way I approach it is with posthypnotic suggestions. The patient really had a reason to have the pain. Pain is a danger and warning signal. I say, "But in your case, the pain is kind of like a hysterical child syndrome. And you know how sometimes the hysterical child gets started crying and even when the reason for the crying has been removed, they keep right on crying. And so, I would like you to look at your pain that way and realize that even though you had a valid reason for it, now that everything that can be done and should be done, has been done, there is no longer any reason to have it. Your hysterical child part of you has not had something to interrupt it, so that recognition can come true."

And I give the suggestion that the feeling of pain interferes with healing. "As long as you have this kind of pain, you are not able to discriminate whether there should be any other kinds of feeling there. You need to have feeling, but feeling is not pain. You need to be able to have feeling in order to discriminate that from the pain, that you thought you needed to have in order to assure yourself that you had feeling."

Question: When I give the suggestion that part of the patient's body will remain in trance, do I delineate it in that fashion?

T: Yes, I think I do. I see no reason not to clarify for the patient the fact that they know and they have the ability to do everything that they need to do. The basis on which I would give that suggestion in a posthypnotic sense, would be to talk with them in trance about the fact that their heart knows how to continue beating and that their blood pressure knows how to maintain its appropriate pressure. And they know how to breathe without having to pay attention to it because they have learned those things, and because they are appropriate and the autonomic nervous system takes care of them.

I say, "I think it's appropriate for this part of your body to permit itself to function on this same automatic principle. There's no real reason, once you have taught it that it knows what to do, to have you do this constantly on a conscious level. Simply, *let it happen.*"

Question: What kinds of suggestions did you try with grimacing client?

T: I think that this lady who would not grimace when she was in trance and would not *not* grimace when she was not in trance, would not accept any of my suggestions. I did a lot of suggestions, like, "In a minute I will terminate trance," and when she dropped her defenses, I made a powerful suggestion about next time, but it didn't seem to have any effect.

This is what you do with very resistant patients. At the end of trance, say, "I'm going to terminate this situation, this experience or trance," and at that point when they drop their defenses, you have a limited time to insert a powerful a suggestion, like "and when you come in next time, you will find you will accept these suggestions for your own good". Working with that with her got me nowhere. I would have liked to have had 20 sessions with unlimited amount of time, but she would not make that kind of contract.

Question: If I had seen this lady with the grimacing spasm as a long-term psychotherapy client, would I have been able to use a paradoxical overload so that it would have no longer been an adaptable symptom?

T: I don't know, but I'm going to say something anyway. I think I would have liked to have gotten a contract with her to involve her doing things with the symptom. I would have gotten a contract that would have made her go out and would have put her in embarrassing positions. The overload would have been in her not liking herself in the situation, more than she disliked being in the situation. That would have been the paradox I would have liked to set up. I think it could have been fun to do that. It would have taken a long-term commitment and required cooperation of the family and some of the other people with whom she dealt. That is my instinctive reaction.

Question: Did I know the precipitating event with the woman with grimacing spasms?

T: We knew the precipitating event. She had it for about seven years, long enough that it was useful and part of her life. We did deal with the question, what will you do with your life without the symptom, since you have built your life around the symptom? The psychologist and I covered what we thought were all the bases at that time.

One of the things we don't hear enough about was that Milton Erickson did not accept every patient who came to him. Milton Erickson did not succeed with every patient who came to him, because there were patients who came in and did not come back. What we hear and what we see are the cases who came back, the cases he accepted and the ones that were very powerful, very dramatic, very long term in many instances and some that were very tough.

We need to remember that hypnosis is not a panacea or a cure-all. Sometimes people just are not ready! They don't want to get better. I had a young woman who was a dental patient of mine who had a needle phobia and it was a long-standing serious needle phobia. I worked with her about four times to cope with the phobia and it did not work. I was able to use trance for her dental work and it was effective. I gave posthypnotic suggestions for giving reorientation, perspective, such as "you are now grown up and can look back", but none of those kinds of suggestions did anything for her at all.

Finally, she went into a hospital to have her four molars out and needed the preliminary injection. She panicked and got hysterical and regressed to the 4-year-old age. She called me on the phone and said, "I'm ready now," and I said, "Fine." We talked for about 45 minutes and there was no more needle phobia.

Maybe it's like the alcoholic who has to hit bottom before he is able to come up. As long as she could survive in her world without dealing with it, she didn't want to deal with it. And then it hit a point where she was ready, and that's when the hypnosis can be effective. Until that time, we are beating our heads against a stone wall.

Question: On the needle phobia, did I try to inject her when she was in trance?

T: I maintain that try means fail. Yes, I did. Every time we went in the phase when we were going to try and give injection, she would break trance. She would terminate trance and cry and say, "I can't do it" and go right back in trance. I learned more from my failures than I did from my successes.

Future Orientation

Question: How does one plan a strategy for dealing with future problems you anticipate for the patient-client you are seeing on a long-term basis?

T: The example is a young boy, and the therapist sees the person coming back at every major step of his life until he establishes an intimate relationship. I don't see why it should end then. My expectation is that in the instance where these people have no other appropriate support system, you are serving as their role model, their mentor, their family, their alter ego, and you are providing them with the reassurance that the life that they are living is worthwhile. It is perfectly appropriate to talk about how much that person has changed and reflect back to where they were.

And to be able to say, "Isn't it interesting that back *then* when you thought you wouldn't be able to do this, and now that you have done this and you look at it back then, you wonder how back then you ever thought you wouldn't be able to do it now. And I wonder how many times in the future there will be things that you will think looking ahead now that you couldn't be able to do then, and when you look at those with the eyes of looking back from here to the things you couldn't do, that you have done, then you know that you will be able to do the things then that now you don't think you could do."

And I would give "for instances" and "as if's" and those sorts of relationship equivalences. And I would say, "I wonder whether you are really going to need to call me or whether you are going to talk with me in person and I wonder what you are going to report back to me after," and put time frameworks with different options. It's not that they are coming to you because they need to come in. They are coming to you, because you have suggested you will be curious about how they will have dealt with those kinds of things.

Erickson realized that he was not going to live forever, and that some of the patients he had accepted as extended members of his family, would need a lot of support after his death. He dealt with one of them by sending him postcards that were future oriented, that dealt with feelings, that he knew that the person was going to have when Milton was no longer there to help him deal with them. He knew that this person would make a notebook of those postcards and keep them.

He gave him the ability in trance to fulfill the posthypnotic suggestion of going through the notebook. To idly leaf through the notebook and coming to a page, and wonder what was on this page and read the postcard and on some level somehow understand that that was the letter and message that he needed at that time. And he could read it and let that help him. He spent years creating that situation and what you are talking about is years with the patient.

Every once in a while I have this, "Oh! That's where you got it," kind of phenomenon. I have an absolutely voluminous collection of cards with nice little messages and I do a lot of that with people who have been patients of mine. I have one with an ethereal scene and on the front it says, "Believe in yourself," and you open it up and it says, "We all do." That kind of thing can be very interesting when you know there is a traumatic situation coming up. When you have established that kind of relationship, the message doesn't have to be in the personal contact. All the message has to say is, "I'm here." I have one I'm going to send to someone who couldn't be here that says, "I'm here. That's not as good as being there, but it's the best I can do and so it's all we need for the moment"—that's sort of an interim support, without necessarily waiting for a crisis.

The posthypnotic suggestion effect of that says, "I am always available and I trust you to do the right thing, to know when you need to come back, to know when you need to be in contact, and to know you don't always need that." It's like mountain climbing. I'm a rock climber and I hope to heaven I'm not going to need that rope around my waist, but I'm awfully glad it's there.

Personal Biases Affecting Our Suggestions

Question: To what extent do we let our own subjective biases influence the suggestions we give our patients? If we are aware we do that, how do we protect the patient and ourselves from that kind of influence?

T: When I talk to patients, I do *not* have the ability not to permit my own biases with my experiences of hypnosis to interfere with my suggestions. I use them for the smorgasbord approach that I utilize for the people I work with. I am prone to say, "When I had this," or "I had a patient who" and Erickson used that a lot. And I say, "It's amazing because each individual can find his own way and it isn't necessarily the same way. You can go the straight way or drive over somewhere before you go to your goal, but the ultimate goal is to get there. It doesn't matter what route you use as long as you recognize that that's where you are going to get. Some people may choose to stop here and there along the way." I'm using the metaphor to explain to the patient that there are multiple ways to get places and they don't have to do it the way I do it.

I need to be clear about this. I am sometimes very directive. I worked with a young woman who had a fear of dentists because she had been inadvertently badly abused by them. In that instance, I wanted to get her to really feel the anger, hostility and hurt and pain. There was none of this, "You can do this if you wish." There was, "I want you to!" I don't care if my biases have come through. "I want you to deal with this my way, right now!" It was not indirect. It was a deliberate, very strong suggestion. My biases were way up front that this was exactly the way I wanted her to deal with it. After that, then we could negotiate about what she is going to do with it if she wants to. It was a strong posthypnotic suggestion including my own personal biases.

Amnesia

Question: About creating amnesia as a posthypnotic suggestion.

T: Creating amnesia for a particular symptom is one of the things Erickson did. The case written up most frequently was about a man who was unable to go to a restaurant for dinner. When Erickson went out to dinner with him, it became, "Should you get sick as we are in the car going to the restaurant," or "Should you wait until we get to the door of the restaurant before you got sick enough to throw up?" or "I think it would be more effective and I would be more convinced you really were sick, if you waited until we are inside the lobby where we are actually going to be taken in. Maybe you could really get very sick until we get to the table and look at the menu." There was a postponement in that particular symptom. "Maybe it could be stronger, maybe it would be more effective. Maybe this isn't the best time to do it. I don't want you to give the symptom up. I want you to pick the absolutely perfect most debilitating, most incapacitating time to do it."

So that thinking about how and when to do it was what kept him from doing it. Carrying posthypnotic suggestions out in the semiconscious or unconscious state was done more in the demonstration situations than was done in actual practice. We need to realize that much of what he demonstrated was in the teaching mode and not in the therapist mode.

Question: About amnesia.

T: One of the things that Erickson did so very effectively was talking to somebody about something inconsequential, and immediately changing the subject to the particularly significant item. When he was through giving the strict standard direction about it, he would stop talking about that and pick up with what he had been talking about immediately before the suggestion was given, thereby suggesting to the patient that the intervening period of time had never happened. Anything that didn't happen you have to have amnesia for on the conscious level, so when the posthypnotic suggestion is carried out, you simply have no memory of it. He used it in the case of the erection, to help people avoid the frequency of urination, and to experience pain without having the anticipation of the next pain or the memory of the last pain. In those cases, amnesia as a posthypnotic suggestion or incorporated in the posthypnotic suggestion can be particularly useful.

T: "Did you watch that ball game on Sunday? I really thought we were going to win that game and *go deeper and you will find that you will be able to do whatever you want to do.*" Give the suggestions in any degree of detail that you choose and when you are through giving the suggestions, go right back to the same tone of voice, "... and in that last 30 seconds I almost died when they kicked that field goal." So what happened between, "Did you see that game on Sunday, I really thought ..." and "... in the last 30 seconds?" There wasn't anything in between there, certainly not!

Question: Suggestions about how to tie posthypnotic suggestions into ordinary activities.

T: "And when you sit down in that chair, it will be absolutely fascinating to you to discover the feeling against your back. As you lean back, you can remember ..." and the reference there is "back". And, "As you lean back, you can remember back to the time back when," whatever it is that what you wanted to institute has been instituted. It isn't only the activity of sitting down in the chair. It's the leaning back that lets you go back to the time when the suggestion was made.

"And when you reach your hand out to touch the door knob, any number of interesting things can happen, because it's almost as the spark that connects when your hand touches the door knob." Giving a semilogical or a quasilogical reason to trigger a posthypnotic suggestion can make it very useful. Giving a pure posthypnotic suggestion for the sake of giving a posthypnotic suggestion that doesn't have any logic or rationality, has to be done in a very direct, very authoritarian manner. In order for it to be successful, the person has to be clear that it serves a useful purpose for him. That useful purpose may be to convince him that he cannot ignore or deny any of the suggestions that are given.

If a person wants to get well and he has tried absolutely everything he knows how to do to get well, he wants to be overpowered. The way to do that is to give a posthypnotic suggestion that is so strong and yet so irrational that when he does it, he is aware that if he can be made to do that, he can maybe have the hope that some of these other things that he hasn't been able to do can also be done. That's why the ridiculous contracts that Milton made with people were carried out. They needed to break through their set by having some really ridiculous thing happen. When that happened, then maybe something equally astounding could happen, like getting rid of or overcoming their symptom.

Question: What do you do if you run into the patient?

T: I say, "Excuse me!" (*Laughter*). That shows I'm being literal, therefore I am working in trance. What do you do with a patient who has had detrimental suggestions given? I don't think it really matters whether those suggestions were given in a formal recognized trance state. We can't dictate when people shall not go into trance. We can make the effort to direct when we would like them to go into trance. We cannot direct when we keep them out of trance. During any stress situation or any trauma situation, it's very natural and automatic for the person to go into trance, such as after a statement like, "You are just going to have to learn to live with that pain."

All of us, physicians, dentists and psychologists have made inappropriate and inadvertent statements. The one I remember most clearly, David Cheek, an Ob-Gyn physician from San Francisco wrote about when he first talked about patients hearing under general anesthesia. He had done a gynecological operation for a friend of his and after the surgery, during some of the follow-up work, she finally said, "You know, David, I really don't like you. I have this tremendous feeling, I don't know why, but I don't like you." He said, "Oh, let's use hypnosis and you go into trance and we'll find out if anything happened."

Using ideomotor signaling, he asked her to remember through the general anesthesia surgical procedure and if anything came up, she should wiggle her finger. And she wiggled her finger. What she heard him say toward the end of her surgery was, "If she weren't so damn fat, we would have been through here 45 minutes ago." That had enough impact that it worked as a posthypnotic suggestion. She didn't recognize it at a conscious level. All she knew was that she no longer liked him. Recognize there are a number of operating rooms that now have a statement on the door: BE CAREFUL, THE PATIENT IS LISTENING. I think this is extremely appropriate.

Question: Using hypnosis with children who are incest victims and are told, "Don't tell," or "Don't tell or I'll kill you."

T: Recognize that that was a posthypnotic suggestion. I think that hypnosis can be used for that circumstance and they can learn to neutralize that prior learning. I think that not only the posthypnotic suggestions that we are giving are important, but what has happened to the individual that brought them to us that may have acted like a posthypnotic suggestion. A dentist who uses a general anesthetic and mask and the child thinks, "He is going to kill me," serves as a posthypnotic suggestion, any future time that person has a mask put on. That may surface when the person tries to learn scuba diving to be able to go under the surface. You have to utilize the recognition that you may be dealing with prior posthypnotic suggestions.

We need to recognize simply that we are constantly dealing with the person's adaptability and their recognition or remembrance of prior experiences as fact. Our ability to utilize hypnosis is to reframe and look at their prior experiences in a new way, by superimposing a new set of suggestions, stronger than the old ones.

Question: About posttrance return of terminal cancer pain.

T: Posttrance return of terminal pain does not necessarily have to do with the inability of the patient to accept, or the lack of strength of the posthypnotic suggestion. It frequently has to do with the ability of the individual to understand that he doesn't need to have pain to convince himself that he is still alive. He doesn't need to have pain in order to convince himself that he is remembering whatever he needs to do to deal with the terminal situation. He doesn't need to have pain to hide the fact that he has not dealt with the psychologically painful feelings surrounding that kind of thing.

I say, "Feeling in itself need not be painful. You can use real pain to hide painful feelings. When you learn you can utilize feelings other than having to have painful ones, than you no longer need to have so much real pain." When you talk about it as a posthypnotic suggestion, you want it accepted in that way. You don't have to say, "And when you come out of trance, you will find …" because then the walls go up. You say, "I wonder how, I wonder when and I wonder how much, do you suppose it will be possible for," questioning kinds of things and leaving the options open.

Question: About dealing with emotional aspects of a problem.

In my office I would say, "Right now, I don't want to know. Right now, it's still not any of my business." Did you hear me say "still"? That says in the future it will be. That was a posthypnotic suggestion. When I ask you to go into trance today it will be to give you tools to handle it. When I ask you to go into trance, today. When I ask you to go into trance some other time, it may be for a different contract. That was a posthypnotic suggestion.

You don't really think about them in that way until you start taking these sentences apart. So I structure it with, "Today, you are going to learn hypnosis and you are going to be given some tools that will help you be more comfortable." Maybe some other time we are going to ask you if it's all right to talk about these other things. Today you are safe. You can do anything you want to freely.

Erickson would teach people hypnosis very deliberately before he would teach them utilization. I will frequently say to my patients who I think are showing resistance or hostility, "Today you are going to learn hypnosis. Next time we will talk about whether you want to use it with your problem." What does that do? It wipes out the need for the patient to resist the hypnosis because there is no commitment, that if I learn hypnosis I will have to learn to stop whatever.

The posthypnotic suggestion is that you can decide after you learn hypnosis whether its going to be useful for stopping whatever. It's up to me to make the hypnotic experience so good and so clear that the individual is going to want to use it to help stop the symptom. They don't understand that part of the contract which tends to be unwritten, but it's still there.

Question: How do you frame that pain is a signal? When everything that can be done and should be done has been done, that the pain will be gone.

T: No, I didn't say the pain will be gone. I said there will no longer be any reason for the pain. I think that it's important the patient know that's how I regard pain. That's how I regard most things.

I think it's important for me to make it clear to patients how I feel about things and why I expect that when they learn these things, they are going to be able to do them. And then the patient has the ability to have a foundation for believing in the potential for change. I can't just say, "I want you to change. Go into trance and you will!" I want to give them the foundation that says there is the possibility for change. Once they have that foundation, then the posthypnotic suggestions for change are more likely to be effective.

I believe that everything that I say, once the patient walks in that door into my office, is leading toward the ultimate goal. And everything that they say that can multiple meanings does and everything that I say that can have multiple meanings does. That's when I start playing with words.

Question: Can I use the same format or the same sense for other symptoms such as psychosis and depression?

T Yes, I believe that I not only can, that I do. This is a basic philosophy of life under which I operate. I'm sure I generate that same kind of positive potential to eliminate the kinds of negatives that they have been utilizing. Blow their fuse in terms of negativism if you will.

Question: When I use a word that has multiple meanings and I am playing with it over and over again, am I teaching the individual that the word could have many meanings, many feelings?

T: Yes, but it not only has that. It has more than that. Let me take a real blatant one. That involves the use of the word back with someone who has back pain. I'm just talking to them. "If you think back (my signal to the person to regress) to the time when that back was no longer bothering you and you found out you could be comfortable back then. You didn't have anything you had to back down from or back away from. You could back out of things without feeling bashful about it. You weren't backward saying you wanted to back into some other kind of situation."

Every time you say it, you are not only referring to the organ, back, but you are giving different connotations to the word, that would give them reasons for having focused on the word *back*. To back down, to back out of, to back away from, to back into, to look backward all have slightly different manifestations, that could very well result in back pain, as a means of letting them back away from all of these things. I'm not going to do it quite that concentrated, but I'm going to work it into the discussion we are having.

Then I would go into simply carrying that conversation forward with the word *forward*. "I wonder as you look back on those things and you realize how much they influenced you back then,

221

and you recognize those were appropriate behaviors." I might use the hysterical child syndrome or I might talk about the house you grew up in and how much it has changed. "But the house really hasn't changed, it's the way you look at it that has changed. And it's time for you now to move forward."

And I would start future orientation, so we could get rid of the background, and start looking forward to the foreground, moving forth, putting forth effort, that kind of thing, if I wanted to continue to just play on the words. Mostly, I want them to get it in perspective and recognize that the things that happened back then do not have the *right* to continue to interfere with their future.

Question: Was your use of the phrase, "when your back was no longer bothering you", intentional?

T: Yes, the use of tense, other than in the word, tension is a very significant kind of thing. "Where are you now?" can produce the nicest regression, rather than saying, "and I want you to go back to being a little girl", or "and it will be interesting to think about that pain (in the future) as being something different, from what it was only because you hadn't thought about it as being what it had been, when it wasn't that way". You are taking a bunch of tenses and jumbling them all up and letting the person recognize that it is mobile. That you can change, you can alter your perception, because it didn't use to hurt and "maybe now it only hurts as bad as it was hurting, when you thought it couldn't hurt any worse. And it isn't as bad as it would have been if you hadn't been able to make it worse."

Question: If I had the time to work with someone and it was not a real pain problem, how would I work with it?

T: I would work with fear in very much the same sort of way. I would start with the word *fear* and then I would take the word *fear*, and I would start to use "interfere" and I would take the "inter" and say, "and that interference has interrupted the ability to deal with that fear and as we enter into ..." And so all I am doing is using a diagram for the patient that this word then is carried over into this phrase. And in this phrase, it's used in a different way, and we will take the other part of the word and carry over into the next one.

It is almost like what Erickson did with so many of his stories. It's to disarm the patient. To get them involved in thinking about something else, so the meaningful suggestions you give them can be accepted without the conscious walls that they need to have. The word games that we play do not have to be the unconscious message. They can be very blatant word games so the patient can be involved on the conscious level to follow the word games and on the unconscious level can accept the meaning of the help that has been offered.

Question: Could you talk about the effects of various medications to induce trance, in particular minor tranquilizers and major tranquilizers? Could you give some case examples using psychotic patients?

T: They don't and no (*Laughter.*). I happen to believe that I want the patients' highest potential readily available when I am going to work with them with hypnosis. I would prefer they not have any medications that would interfere with their ability to use their mental functioning. Antibiotics or chemotherapy is okay. I would prefer if they are not on any other kind of medication. If they are, I would like to work with them right before their next dose. I will say to the patient, "It is going to interfere with our ability to communicate if you are zonked on your medications. I would prefer that you be willing to work with me on as an alert level as possible."

That extends to lithium. I would prefer that I see them as far away from the administration as possible. I don't have a problem with dilantin or insulin. I do work with psychotic patients. They get toothaches. Somebody has to deal with them. The neat thing about being a dentist is that I can retreat into the dentistry when I am teaching a psychotic patient about hypnosis. We are going to use the hypnosis with dentistry. They learn hypnosis very well and they use it for the dentistry and it gets them through the dentistry. It's always been clearly specified that they are not to play around with it with anything else.

If that patient is truly psychotic, it's my obligation to get them to someone who's able to do the long-term therapy necessary. A psychologist and I have worked with many patients who have exhibited various types of psychoses over the years. They have been able to utilize trance very effectively. A significant number of them, particularly the schizophrenic types, are on some sort of drugs. I evaluate if they can communicate and learn. I'm more uncomfortable with fairly heavy doses of tranquilizers.

Question: About deciding what kind of approach to use.

T: That's not hypnosis, but using your sense of observation to determine those kinds of things. That is the responsibility you have. Erickson said, "When you teach someone this kind of skill, you have the obligation to teach them how to handle it."

Question: About the belief that he would give suggestions and right away people would take them.

T: The belief is nonsense. It took him 200 sessions to get that one gal to go into trance. He had a woman who put him in the most beautiful double bind in the world. She said she couldn't be hypnotized and she wanted to write her doctoral dissertation on the subjective experience of hypnotic trance. He agreed to be on her committee and teach her to go into trance. She resisted this for 200 hours. How many of us have patients who could pay for 200 hours to learn this?

He used to spend a lot of time before he saw the patient. He used to sit down and write down his induction approach to patients and would practice the gestures in front of the mirror and do the voice. The man was so dynamic and so impressive and he had these John L. Lewis bushy eyebrows and, as Jay Haley said, "this ocular fix stare". If he were doing a demonstration, he would just look at you and you would get uncomfortable. And you knew you were up for a demonstration, he hadn't said anything and how were you going to get out of this uncomfortable situation and you would go into trance. He didn't do anything except have the expectation.

That is so different from a person who has a problem and has tried everything and is so desperate. Erickson would spend three, four, or five hours teaching a patient trance because the patient needs a wealth of experience in this neuropsychophysiological reorientation before they are able to understand how good they have the potential to be. If you could get them to recognize their prior learning and experience, which would be incorporated, they could do that quickly, in an instant. If he had to teach them all over again these things they didn't know they knew, it took time. If all he had to do was trigger prior learning sets that were already there, those were the people that would get those kind of quick results.

Remember, in teaching demonstrations all of you are set up to learn. The best way to learn is to do it. You have something to gain from that which is different from the commitment the patient makes. The posthypnotic suggestions are different from the way you would do it your office. Yeah, after 30 years, I can access my unconscious. The main thing I learned from him is to trust and rely on my own unconscious but there has got to be an unconscious to trust and rely on.

Question: How did he finally manage to teach that woman to go into trance after 200 hours?

T: He used many techniques and approaches and eventually was able to convince her that she was not giving up control. That was the issue, it was a control issue. He taught her by demonstrating to her that she could basically spit in his eye and still demonstrate trance phenomena.

I'm not sure that this was not the same woman who he taught amnesia for a day's trance experience. She wanted to have the experience of getting up some morning and going into trance, not knowing when she would do it and spending the whole day in trance, and not realizing that she was in trance until she got home and came out of trance. If she realized she lost a day, amnesia for that trance experience would be very reinforcing that the trance actually happened.

It was set up in the way that it was extremely permissive for the unconscious. "I don't know when you are going to do this. You don't know when you are going to do this. Your unconscious will select the day and the time and situation. When you are doing it, you won't know you are doing it on an unconscious level. It will not be until you have terminated the trance, that you will realize that you don't remember anything that you have done that day. And that will be the impact that you recognize that you have in fact had amnesia for having been in trance for this whole period of time."

Question: Whether I programmed my unconscious with the kinds of things that are now in there that I anticipate I can access?

T: I am scanning. I think I did. I'm very aware of having written down many of the approaches that I would use for different patients and I would have two or three options. I would take parts of one and put it into the other one. If the individual threw me a curve and changed their behavioral response, I would be able to modify my response. When I come to lectures, I bring volumes in with me. We're back to the image of the rope around my waist (when climbing). I very rarely use those written notes I have. I suspect my unconscious is in that situation. Yes, I worked on it. I did write it down. I didn't practice it in front of a mirror.

I would suggest that anybody who has not done it, up until this time, go home and tape record sessions, so you can later on, go into trance and listen to what you said with the ears of that patient. You will discover that there are many things that you didn't mean the way you said them. The message becomes very different. You can start playing the tape ahead of time in your mind, listening to the things you are going to say before you say them and hearing how they really will sound, and if they don't sound correct, you can rewind the tape and let them come out another way. Using time distortion lets you do that in a fraction of a second. And posthypnotic suggestion works for that.

Chapter Fourteen
Utilization

Techniques for Utilization

People seem to have trouble with what you do with transitions during structured inductions. I use the expression a lot, "When this happens, then that will be the signal for this," so it is real clear to the patient, and they are not left hanging with their arm up in the air, not knowing what to do with it. The same thing applies to the sand bucket (formal induction technique). When you see the arm starting down, the patient needs to be programmed, so that they understand that when the arm touches, that's the signal for the bucket to dissolve, disappear, roll off etc. And for the other arm to relax into their lap and for them to go, wherever you have expected them to go when this happens.

Patients who are just learning about hypnosis don't know what they are supposed to do. If you have somebody who has been sitting there for 20 minutes waiting for that arm to go down, and it goes down, and you say, "And now I would like you to take a deep breath and just let yourself relax," the patient thinks, "Icchh! I have been working 20 minutes to get this down and she hasn't even acknowledged it!" When they have been working hard to do something and they achieve it, put that gold star on their forehead so they feel it. Good! Now! We'll go on to the next step. This seems like such an obvious thing. I hear people who do not do that. You don't just say, "That's right, that's good, you are doing nicely." When something significant is achieved, you say, "Fine! Great!" Now that you have achieved this, we can put another carrot on the end of that stick. Because that's what you are really doing. You are continually *motivating* them.

I talk about people getting stuck for words when doing induction techniques. This is one of the two things I think I will have contributed to hypnosis when I leave this "mortal" world. When you are talking with the patient and you ask them to do something, ask yourself, "Why did I say that?" and then answer your own question out loud: "So that …" If you do that, I promise you that you will never be at a loss for motivation of the patient. "Your hand is getting lighter and lighter." Why? "So that your fingertips will rise off your leg." Why? "So that your hand can lift up in the air." Why? "So that it can find that pillow of air." Why? "So that it can rest on that pillow of air." Why? "So that your unconscious can know everything that it needs to know." Why? "So that you can develop a hole in the pillow of air." You see how easily that flows. You never run out of words with the "Why? So that" philosophy.

There's something more to it than that. When you are working with hypnosis, you should be constantly motivating the person you are working with. You should be constantly giving them a reason for what you are asking them to do, so it will help them achieve their intermediate goal in order that they can achieve their long-range goal. Hypnosis is not something you apply and then you stop and go to the business of why they are there. When you are doing the hypnosis, you are teaching them so much that they are going to be able to utilize in the second phase of working with their problem. That's what we need to understand in this utilization as part of the trance.

I've already talked about the lady with a weight and the sand bucket induction (see Chapter Six), where all we did was a hypnosis induction technique. But the utilization was so integrated in that particular induction that we ended up with a 14-page transcript of that weight loss, sand bucket induction. It was a constant Why? So that: "Your arm is getting heaver and heavier." *Why?* "*So* that it is going to go down in your lap." When you are doing this, the suggestions you are giving for utilization are disguised enough, so that person who has put up all kinds of barriers to direct suggestion and diet, can utilize the indirect approach for learning hypnosis to be successful for weight loss.

A logic the client can accept

I talked about reasonableness for giving suggestions. I worked with a young man with sleep apnea. He had had a sleep study done and he was borderline; they weren't convinced he needed a machine but he was not able to function appropriately. He was falling asleep at work. He came to me. "I don't want this nonsense. Do you think hypnosis could help?" I said, "I don't think it could hurt." We worked with him. The thing that was so surprising to me was in as many years as he has known me, he should have expected what he got. Apparently, he didn't. What he got were very logical kinds of comparisons about why this should work. All of the physicians had told him that sleep apnea was beyond his control and that this was something that happened with his autonomic nervous system and these muscles. And that there was nothing he could do about it, except consider using this machine.

We began to talk. He had never achieved trance without closing his eyes. He was busy trying to figure out whether he was in trance because he hadn't closed his eyes. The suggestions I gave to him were reasonable, normal, and expected. Unexpected, in a way for him. All I believed was that this idea of sleep apnea as beyond your control was nonsense.

"You have control over these muscles, of this warning system. There are a lot of other things you have control over when you are asleep that are also part of your autonomic nervous system. For example, if you didn't have the ability to control these muscles, you would probably wet the bed a lot. If you didn't, you would have to worry about your heart not beating. I think this is really ridiculous.

"You have all these years of having known how to sleep without any problems. Now you have this couple of years with this problem. I don't care why you have this, I could care less. I know you can get over this. Because it's very logical that you have the ability to be aware of this unconscious need you have. If you didn't do that, your bladder would give you a difficult time every night." Every time I came back to that, he would get a big grin on his face.

When we finished the trance induction, he said, "You know, that makes such good sense. I don't wet the bed. I do have control over my bladder. It's a very similar phenomenon. I really like that!" He went away.

At the next session, he said, "Oh, boy! The first night after you talked to me, I spent the worst night I have ever spent in my life."

I'm thinking, "Oh, Lord!" He said, "I was awake every 15 minutes. I was so restless. I tossed and turned. There was no way. I spent a miserable, miserable night. But I have slept every night since then."

He said, "You gave me this logical reason why I didn't need to have it." That's a key ingredient in most of the things I talk with my patients about. Sometimes, it's not real logical, it may be just pseudological. But if it's a logic that patient can accept and under-stand, then that is enough. That's what we are talking about in terms of utilization of trance. He has maintained his correction of the sleep apnea for five months now. We are trying to get another sleep study to see whether there is any physiological change. It is so fascinating and so interesting, if we can demonstrate that somebody who has been diagnosed and has physiological data, can learn to control this with hypnosis. Just by someone giving them a reason to. Come on! But, if it works, it works and I'm not going to fight it.

Question: It wasn't the discussion before the trance?

T: One of the things that he said in the follow-up was that it took a long time to decide he was in trance, just because his eyes were open. It was the reason that I gave him regarding the bladder that *really* was the decisive thing for him. He thought, Oh, of course! If I can control that, I can control this too. That makes perfectly good sense. If I can get the patient to say, "That makes perfectly good sense," even when it doesn't, then we're home free.

Question: Do you have any sense about why he struggled that one night?

T: I'm not sure. I think it was just the reorientation that he was going through. Possibly, the competition between me, he had a lot of respect for all the work we'd done, and he had all this data that he had a sleeping problem and a breathing problem. There was very probably a disorientation going on for him. He doesn't know.

It very clearly points up this desire I have to connect to a logical reason for the individual. Remember when I said, "You don't need to have those headaches anymore"? The patient may have had a reason for migraine headaches at that time. When I talk about habit problems, I talk about it as a habit problem. And acknowledge that when the habit developed, there was a reason for it and a need for it; at that time it was appropriate. Let's look at it from today's light to decide if it is still appropriate or whether it has become more trouble than it is worth. We may get into secondary gain but we know how to deal with that. We don't have to worry about that in hypnosis.

One of the comparisons I use when talking about habits is based on my knowledge of the kind of background they have and childhood they had. Let me give a verbalization for a reasonably normal happy childhood. You can fill in how you would change it if they didn't have a normal happy childhood.

"If you think back to the house you grew up in and remember when you came from school. Remember how big and bright and shiny the rooms were and how good it smelled in the kitchen where dinner was being made. Remember that field out back where you used to go and play. The field was so long and it took you forever to run across the field. You also know if you went back to that house today, those rooms wouldn't be nearly as big and bright and shiny. And that field out back really wasn't very big at all. It's the way you looked at it. If the way you looked at those rooms and field has changed, maybe it's time for you to change the way you look at some other things too."

A woman who was in my workshop came in the next day and said, "You know, I went back last night and looked at the house where I grew up and I couldn't believe how little it was." Most people recognize and identify that that's what is going to happen and also remember how it looked when they were little. How it looked when they were little might not be big and bright and shiny; it may have been big and scary. You can talk about that and how that has changed as well. When you do that, you give them the option to recognize that many of the facets of their life have changed and improved.

If they could have changed those things, there's always the possibility with learning and practice, they can change these other things. Given a quasilogical or logical valid reason to change a habit, it is possible for that change to occur. There is no real way that people cannot understand that they do not stay in the same place forever. You are there to help them move on.

Question: How complicated is it and how much should you get involved?

T: I don't do any more than that with people who have habits. I permit the patient to do the reorientation. I certainly see that psychotherapists may get more involved. I see myself as a stimulus to give you a lot of ideas and then you are going to take the ideas and work on them and elaborate on them yourselves. I serve as an overview of things that are possible and potential and I hope I am going to stimulate your ideas and your own mind.

Although handouts of my metaphors are available, I would be very unhappy if anyone took them home and used them as a script. You are not me and cannot say my words with my inflection and tone of voice, the way I do. You can use them as a base from which to start. You devise your own way of communicating those same kinds of ideas. We all do that.

People talk about me being Ericksonian. I have never given an Ericksonian workshop. I can't. Erickson was the only one who could. All I can do is teach you what I think I learned and am learning from him. You are not going to go out and do Thompsonian hypnosis. You are going to do your own individual trance work. Maybe, if I'm lucky you will use some of the ideas from what I am talking about here.

I make a real effort to be creative in this bright-eyed bushy-tailed way, because I know that most of the people who teach, teach traditional hypnosis. I want to say, there is another way, there is another idea. These are some of the things I would like for you to consider and maybe utilize for yourself. This is a scan of 40 years of my own learning and ideas that have come to me, that seem most consistently to be useful in my practice and in my teaching. That's the only thing I can do here.

I mentioned that I am in trance most of the time I am up here teaching. I have worked with hypnosis for so long and been able to practice it and been helped by some really marvelous people, so I can trust that my unconscious, when I need to go into trance, will permit me to do that. When you see that I can be in full conscious contact with my surroundings, that this is a possible utilization of trance, you go home and think, maybe I can learn something from that. People who really know me well can tell when I am in trance.

When you become comfortable with word play is the time you start managing to maneuver to manipulate the motivation of the men and women you are working with. Now, it's okay to struggle and try to be clever. After you start listening to the words and really hearing them, what happens is you will have a word charge out at you from what a client said. You will hear four or five permutations or meanings of that word and you will feed them back to the patient and then drop it and keep going. It doesn't have to be the entire trance. We have to remember that we can't get so involved in the word play, that we forget the person is the really important individual we are dealing with.

When you start working with metaphor and analogy, I think the word play falls into place. It's very difficult to do word play without doing a story and learning to utilize the words and integrate them into the story.

I am a dentist and most of the work I do is sitting off to the side of my patient. I really like that because I can observe them and they can't watch me. In the teaching situation, we end up one to one. That makes it difficult for us if that individual chooses not to close their eyes. We are sitting, looking at them "afraid to breathe, afraid to move, afraid to blink, for fear it will interfere with the space that patient is in". I ask you to consider if it might be easier if you are off to the side.

If you are off to the side, it doesn't mean you can't have an intense involvement with the patient. I use my body as this instrument I tell you it is supposed to be. When I lean forward and I look at you, I really look at you, it is very difficult for you not to look back; it's hard for you to look somewhere else. This kind of intensity with the individual, when you are going to make a significant statement, is very important and that you use all of yourself. And, "Do you really need to have those headaches *anymore?*" You get the tone of voice and the non-verbal communication that gives the entire message to that person.

This is hard work. I don't understand how some people can do hypnosis for six or seven hours a day. I would be so rung out by the end of the day. If you are going to do this, you owe it to that person to give it your best, and to give it the intensity that you recognize that it deserves, not just with your voice. And to watch the individual. I don't see how you can talk without looking at the patient. When they wiggle or when an eyebrow goes up or when they swallow, if you don't see it, you can't use it as part of the enhancement of the approach you are using with the patient. There are times when people need, want, and deserve basic standard induction techniques. (Thompson tells a clinical vignette about using the sand bucket induction with a patient with a gagging problem; see Chapter Six.)

If you are the last hope that the patient has, we owe it to the patient, as long as they are willing to come and work. Just like Bob Pearson, I will delight in working with a resistant patient, but not a defiant patient, who wants to put another notch on his belt. Distinguishing between those two is sometimes difficult. The resistant patient is the one who is scared and wants, but doesn't know how. And it is my job to teach them how.

Clinical Utilization

Highly Personal Interrelationship

I am demonstrating where my belief in the potential of the individual comes in. Bob Pearson and I were involved in a Miami workshop and it was the first time we ever had small groups. We were approached by two psych residents who said, "We'd like to learn anesthesia and control of bleeding." And so we said, "Fine." We taught them hypnoanesthesia and control of bleeding. Anesthesia is really a pretty straightforward kind of thing to teach and I carry around this bunch of sterile 20 gauge needles. The way you test hypnoanesthesia and control of bleeding is by sticking a needle in the back of hand and it doesn't hurt and then they don't bleed when you take it out. I was being very fancy that day and I got a vein. I didn't really intend to but that's because I don't know what I am doing. The blood was dripping out of the top of the needle and I very calmly, on the outside, said, "And now, Andrew, it's time for you to learn something about control of bleeding." And the next drop didn't drop.

And Bob and I sat there, saying *wow*. Every time that a person does something like this, even though I have seen it so many times before, I am just astounded with wonder at the marvel that the human body is. It's like it doesn't matter if you have 11 kids, when your eleventh child takes his first steps, it's just as thrilling as it was when your first child took his first steps. That's how I feel when your patients learn these things. It's so stimulating and exciting to me when they have learned something. After these two people learned hypnoanesthesia and control of bleeding, they then told us that they had taken a hypnotizability test and both of them had been judged unhypnotizable. They said they really didn't think much of the test.

That says a lot in terms of where I come from in terms of hypnotizability, susceptibility and suggestibility tests are concerned. I look at them as good induction techniques; if you use them to help the patient go into trance, the various hypnotizability scales work well. I refuse to restrict myself and the patient to their ability to learn based on some artificial criteria determined by somebody, when the individuals who established those criteria really didn't have any motivation to go into trance.

What we are dealing with is a highly personal interrelationship. Each one of you has his own way to reach people best. You need to know what that way is, you need to enhance it, to capitalize on it, and to have an approach that you like and to be able to vary that approach depending on the individual's needs.

Transition

I talked about the separation of the induction from the utilization. In your own head, sometimes you need to know when you have made that transition decision. You move over to the other idea that now we are going to start doing the actual work. I think we need to do that because I am convinced that we listen differently when we are doing the work with the patient and when we are doing the induction because we observe different things. When we are working with the induction, what we are observing are the physical kinds of signs that the patient is giving us about their ability to go into trance, about their pacing and about their timing. At that point, you are starting to figure out how to interact with the patient and you are slowing yourself down to meet that patient's needs or you are slowing the patient down, if they come in wired.

Going to where the patient is

I talked about Erickson going to where the patient is. We need to broaden our own base of experience and be able to communicate about absolutely any concept. If you can't do that, you are going to be left foundering while the patient has given you the kind of cue that you need and you simply don't pick up on it. If you don't know anything about gardening, you have to be astute enough to ask the right questions or make the generic comments or to be able to make the transition.

Suppose you are an artist and this person only knows gardening. She is a 70-year-old woman who has spent her life growing chrysanthemums and you wouldn't know a chrysanthemum from a daily lily. You have to be generic enough about her ability to grow chrysanthemums and be impressed enough about the various skills she has in working with nature that she can think you know where she is and that you have joined her there. Or you have to give an impression that you understand by taking what she does, which is gardening, and then saying, "I've always thought gardening is like creating a painting."

You can draw some similarities between what you know about gardening. Everyone knows a little about dirt in the ground and putting seeds in the ground and getting water and sunlight. You can always assume there are bugs and insects that will make an effort to eat at the particular thing. You can take your particular expertise which may be painting and make a metaphor that utilizes her basis or her foundation with your understanding of painting. She thinks you are absolutely wonderful because you have tied in her skill at raising these flowers to the artist creating this magnificent painting.

You can talk about the effort that goes in it and the creativity and the different kinds of paint you can use, the medium you decide that you are going to work in; are you going to use canvas? Every once in a while, all you have to do is relate that a little bit back to the flower growing. She will then make the connection broad enough so you don't have to think you have to talk about things she knows more about than you do. When you do that, you are on safe ground. I think it is really important that we be on safe ground in terms of your need to be in control with that patient. If the patient does not assume or reasonably expect that you know enough that that patient can trust you, then you are in deep water.

Yes, but ...

When we are working with the patient, in talking about resistance, I think it is so important that you adopt the "Yes, but" philosophy. When the patient gives you some problem, you can agree with them, "*Yes*, it is a problem, *but*" and then you present a different perspective, one which they may not have thought of before. I think I am particularly good at that. When somebody gives me a really really significant obstacle for them, I'll say, "You know, that's really true, but I wonder whether," and I'll come up with something that will demand that they change their perspective.

It's the idea that, well maybe there is hope, maybe this "stinkin' thinking"—I have a friend who calls it that—can change in some respect and maybe this is the person who is going to be able to help me make it change.

Obesity

I think the "Yes, but" philosophy works very well with obesity. These young people have this fat image. When they look in a mirror I think they are looking at themselves, as they have learned to see themselves. One of the more interesting concepts that I would do with people with weight problems is using mirrors from a fun house. We could have people stand in front of them every time they come in and see themselves from a different perspective. They could get used to seeing their image in different ways. It is very safe to see your image in a different way in a crazy mirror and you can laugh about it. As you learn to get used to seeing your image in different ways, what are you doing? You are building up the experience of learning how to perceive yourself in a different image.

It may be done initially in fun, in the same way that metaphors are done initially in fun with no threat to the patient; they are able to listen to the story freely. The underlying message in this particular instance is, "Okay, it is possible for me to see my body image in a different way." At some point, you can then incorporate that different perception that they have of themselves when they look into these funny mirrors with the kind of perception they have of themselves when the look into their heads and see themselves in the way other people have made them perceive themselves. And then you have the structure for change in that particular instance.

Utilization with Metaphors

Double Meanings. People often say that some metaphors sound confusing. Inhibitions are tied up in nots, "n-o-t-s", aren't they? And we make so many things knotty, "k-n-o-t-t-y" or "n-a-u-g-h-t-y" depending on whichever way the person wants to hear it, rather because they are knotty, meaning difficult, "k-n-o-t-t-y", not just plain knots, "k-n-o-t-s". And we do not know about the things we no, until it's too late, to go back and pick up the pieces of the rope that got tied into the knots, that we didn't know how to unknot. But with patience and persistence, you can pick at the most painful knot, tie it into a bow that can bow, to the need to remember that is, was once, a not, "n-o-t".

When you say it, you hear what it says when you would expect what the normal spelling would be, but the unconscious hears all the possible meanings of the word *n-o* and *n-o-t*. In terms of derivative kinds of things, this is what we are working for when we use double meaning words, and this is the way double meaning words work for us, and the way we need to be aware of them.

This metaphor is a very good one because our world is made up of "nots". It would be very easy with children, particularly, to have a piece of string or rope and use the word *bow*, meaning the bow that you make out of rope, but what you are really talking to them about is the nots their world is made up of, meaning, "n-o-t" and "n-o".

It's really fun to listen for other kinds of messages in the words that we use. You can look forward, "four" or "for" and when you add two to two, too, you have to figure out how they are spelled. When two and two mean you go forward rather than back into the things you had looked forward to getting out of. You start being very much aware of the kinds of language that you are using all the time, that you have really not been listening to.

My patients tell me what metaphors to use. When I am talking with them, they will hear something I say or I will hear something they say that turns into the need we have to talk about the things we ought to talk about.

How many of you think about the word, sections being spelled "sextions". It really is when you talk about it. I could not not divide the word, "painting" into "pain" and "ting" when I heard it. If I can do it, when I'm not having the pain and if I can do it, when I'm not the victim of the incest, then how much more significant are those kind of words going to be with the person with whom you are talking? They are already the charged words. When you use them, and see your patient do something, go back and listen to what you just said and sometimes you will be astounded at what your unconscious can come up with.

Hemisphere Metaphor (see Chapter Eleven). When you look at pain and you are able to see through the pain to the other side. If you can get the person to spell their pain as a "pane", it is possible for them to wash the dirt on their pane clear enough with any kind of liquid they can produce, especially tears, so they can see through the pane to the other side. Seeing through the pain to the other side is kind of like talking with a patient going into surgery about when they are going home, rather than about the surgery itself. Talking about when they go home implies that you believe that they are going to survive the surgery, which is a very important point for many people. Really, it is a very nice way of saying to the patient, "You are going to be okay, you are going to make it, you are going to go home."

Rose (see Chapter Twenty-two). The Rose or the flower metaphor was developed for dental students. They need to take clinical state board examinations and that means for a couple of days they have to work with patients, do a gold casting, make dentures and prophylaxis for periodontal problems. This is extraordinarily stressful because there are so many things outside of your control that can happen. And you have to wait six months to take them again. Your debt and new offices you have contracted for have no bearing on having to wait six months. By the time of state boards, the students are up on the ceiling, permanently.

I would run sessions with this metaphor because it was the one they found most successful. Dental school is extraordinarily degrading. The faculty is the rock that obstructs you and you are so tender. The other instructors try to eat you up and they are the green sprout eating animals and all the tests are the rain that beats you down. And finally you develop thorns that protect yourself and you come out in the sunlight and you can develop into this absolutely spectacular flower. And you can also see how someone has had overprotective parents and may have been abused by those parents or someone in a job situation they don't like who had a boss who had a lot of power over them could use this. That could be used for ego strength or tolerance.

Orchestra. I heard someone who said the patient does not make the music but he is the conductor of the music. I really liked that and went off into a symphony orchestra metaphor. Each part of our body is like one of the parts of the orchestra. You can use this either physically or psychologically. What you are doing is listening for and looking for the discords. It's up to you to get that body back in harmony by finding the discords and correcting them before they pull off all the other parts of the orchestra.

That was developed for a patient who had a physical problem. It could also be used with someone who has cancer. The broad-based use of these is fairly straight forward.

Orchestra Metaphor.[12] And as you listen to that music with your mind it's like listening to stereo. All that time you thought you were listening to one instrument, other instruments were playing which you haven't been paying attention to, and now it's important to pay attention to the other instruments of the body of the orchestra. And you begin to know when there is a discord. It means you need to hear and adjust that tone because each part is necessary for every other part to be at its best and that instrument has the potential to help all the other parts of the orchestra to produce the right sound.

If it's a discord, the harmony is gone, the harmony is lost and you want to be able to tune in the discord. The way you do this, because the discord is a learning kind of situation, is all the other parts of the orchestra say, "Hey, shape up." Because if it's a violin which is out of tune and the violinist came in late and didn't have time to tune it and he runs his bow across one string, there's no sound at all because it's too loose. And he runs his bow across another string and it goes GHEE because it's too tight. You know that if the middle string is just right it doesn't matter because if the other two are out of tune you can't play the right kind of music.

And you are going to take all that discord and you are going to relax and tune it just right so the violinist can play the right kind of music. It's going to be fascinating because as he modifies his music the other parts of the orchestra can relax and play by automatic memory by paying attention to the music. When they heard that

---

[12] Transcribed from a student's tape of Dr. Thompson's clinical work.

discord they had to focus and tighten up and become much more tense in order not to be pulled off key and now that everything comes back in key, the rest of the parts of the orchestra can relax too. And it's lovely because you can shape and permit the other discordant sound to be modified by hearing the kinds of things it needs to hear and do and be. And you let yourself float along as you are surrounded by that glorious sound, recognizing the value of your contribution as the orchestra conductor.

And as you conduct the music of your mind and your soul and your body and you modify and shape those discords and you let yourself relax, let yourself know that you are no longer running and searching and making noise instead of music.

You have a measured sound and stability and you have the time and capacity to make the appropriate kind of music because there isn't too much or too little tension and trying to play is no longer a discordant shriek. And you know you can walk around with just the right amount of tension and tuning and you can learn to let yourself blend the kind of notes which produce the perfect mellifluous music which you want to hear and enjoy.

The senses are so marvelous in our body when we listen and are not distracted by other things. And you want to protect and support your body. You listen to the beginnings of any discordant notes. And you pay attention and you release the tension that comes from the tension from the beginning signal that triggers the impulse to the stimulus. Gradually, the notes and the instruments around that discordant note become stronger and stronger and that discordant note can rely on them and trust them to be relaxed and helpful and supportive. And it's so wonderful to have that sense of music that fills your body and lets your ears ... let it flow throughout your system, so wondrously.

Community of Cells. I talked about needing to talk about logic in terms of giving people a reason for things to work the way they do. I heard someone talking about the community of cells. That is particularly good for anybody with a serious illness. They need to understand that their body works for them in the same ways as a community works together.

Winemaking Metaphor. I think the winemaking metaphor is really kind of neat. All of us have a lot going on inside our heads. You talk about the way that things are developed and nurtured very carefully and you have to crush these grapes in order to get the must in the outside of the grape in connection with the inside of the grape so that the fermentation process can begin. We are expecting from you people that the fermentation process is going on during this workshop and we are going to separate out the good and bad and we are not going to get to the point of bottling all you are learning before you go home. I expect you will let the things you hear here ferment and when you are ready to use them you will discover that they are good.

The thing I think is important about this is that you know that every year's grapes are different. You can plant the same grapes in the same field year after year and you get a different wine every year. The nice part of it is the wine can all be drinkable; it is just different. It just makes it distinctively your own. Isn't that what we are after to make this our own and to have the kind of fermentation that will help us to appreciate what we have, after we go through the racking and the bottling and the waiting kind of procedure. That applies to a broad range of emotional problems that people can deal with in terms of their adjustment to living.

If you have somebody who drinks wine or from any place where the winemaking industry is really useful, it's easy for you to talk about winemaking. Tying into something the person knows about, likes or is willing to do is particularly useful.

Wine-Creativity Transformation[13]

And it's so wonderful to have that sense of music that fills your body and your ears, let it flow throughout your system so wondrously. It's kind of the other senses we don't pay that much notice

---

[13] Transcribed from a student's tape of Dr. Thompson's clinical work.

to, "the sense of smell, the sense of sight which we use all the time and it distracts us; the sense of taste".

If you think about drinking wine. Do we take wine as a matter of course until we are no longer able to take it, or do we think about what goes into making it? Because it is truly an amazing procedure before it gets its nose and its taste. Because the grape vines have to be planted in the proper place so they will have a *ground neither too acid or base*. And then they need the right amount of *moisture* and the right slope of *sunshine* and the *cold nights* which come in at the end of the growing season.

And all these things go on without you really having to notice and then nature does its work in growing the grapes and then man steps in and starts the process that results in the wine. And then an expert who knows when the grapes are in the perfect stage of readiness, sweetness and ripeness, perfect to be picked, teaches the people who are going to choose them how to select each grape. And as the pickers pick the grapes, you know how carefully they pick each bunch? You know how carefully they put them in their baskets, being careful not to mash any of them and what do they do?

They go ahead and mash them and get them all mixed up together because only in this way can they start the *fermentation process which happens when the natural yeast which is always present on the grapes* has the opportunity to come in contact with the *must that must be inside the outer skin of the grape and if the grape has this outer skin like you have and you look at the fermentation process which goes on.*

It's absolutely amazing, because you make a decision at this point whether the wine will be white or red, because for red wine the grapes are permitted to ferment with the stems and the skins but for white wine only the inside of the grapes are used. And when the primary fermentation process is complete, you have to press the grapes but you also, as the fermentation process continues, you have to keep the air, the contamination out of the grapes.

And so you don't really have to pay attention to what I am saying because the message is what you mean to hear and you know that you can hear that and do your own thinking and feeling and organizing.

Utilization of the air trap lets the carbon dioxide bubble out through the water without contamination by air and the bubbling lets us know when to rack the wine to get rid of the sediment, the undesirable byproduct, which settles to the bottom of the container. And we get into another container to get a new start, which is what you have, and this racking process and the aging of the wine lets it *purify and clarify, [name] and, as long as it's really working, you let it go on*. And then you stop it by running the must through a fine filter and you can be excited about what the must may become and how it will change and be creative. And there will be a fine final product in individual bottles, and the fascinating thing is that this product, as you know, is so very different from year to year and it's also very good.

And you know that you can smell and distinguish the aroma and nose. And you can roll the wine around your tongue and mouth, and you can feel the *explosion of the quality*, and when it's absorbed, you can permit that warmth to permeate your senses. And you know it's been worth all the growing pains, bruising, all of the pressure and fermenting, all of the trouble, because the final product is so enjoyable and the growth of the aftertaste lets it happen and you know and you understand. [End of metaphor.]

It doesn't make any difference what you use, as long as the concept you are working toward is down the road. The ability to start into it and be well into the metaphor before the person really has gotten sure what I'm doing is the advantage of telling stories. By the time the person realizes they have been had, they are so far into it that they don't care and it's all right. Giving them the opportunity by saying, "Now we are going to teach you hypnosis," to say, "No, I don't want to learn," is much easier to do than to resist my saying, "That reminds me of." I'm just talking. Are you going to be so rude that you are going to get up and walk away? Most people don't and so you have them.

I know enough about the things I talk about to have the ring of authenticity in it. If it is something I don't know about, I'm going to do a generic discussion and get them to fill in the blanks. You can turn almost any conversation into an induction and metaphor.

Imagery and Imagination

Imagery is based on previous kinds of pictorial kinds of experiences and learning. Imagination uses imagery to create nonreal kinds of functions and things. To do imagery you do not have to use your imagination in the same sense that using your imagination uses imagery. People get hung up with saying, "I can't use my imagination." What they think they are saying, is "I can't use imagery." My effort is to get them to separate the two and realize how easy it is to use imagery without having to use your imagination.

When I say, "chair", "school-room desk", or "bus", in order to understand these words, you get an image in your head. Looking at the fact that they had to learn the image before they could learn the word, automatically means they have to know the image, doesn't it? None of us could deal with words until we first had the images to go with them. Talking like that to people who say they can't image, or have any imagination, breaks down their resistance.

You may have to say to them, "Sure, now you are so good with it, you don't understand that you still do the imaging with these objects. You have to tap into the part of your brain that stores this kind of knowledge. Using your imagination is simply adapting your ability to use imagery of real objects and applying that to things that may not have happened. It still uses the same objects in a way you may not have experienced them." You can use logic with most of the people who say, "I can't use imagery."

There are people who do have trouble with using their imagination because they want the concept they see to look exactly like that chair right there, rather than having a concept of something that supports you. There are all kinds of ways of dealing with constructs that are permissible because the end result is what we are after. It doesn't matter how we get there because once we get there, the means we use are not important.

If necessary, you stand on your left ear. This is the way Erickson differed from the people of his time. One of his stories was about a young man who couldn't go out to dinner because he kept throwing up, so Erickson went out to dinner with him. He said, "Should you throw up in the car on the way to the restaurant? Or wait until we get to the foyer? Or should you wait until we get to the table?" With all these options, you got to do it at the best possible worse time. By the time the worse time had passed, because there was always going to be a better time, there really wasn't any time to do it.

How many people are willing to go to a restaurant with their patients? How many of you work with agoraphobics? How many spend time a lot of time outside with agoraphobics helping them do things they normally couldn't do? A therapist can get in a car and say, "Today is the day we are going to go through the tunnel."

Memory: Remembering and Forgetting

For experiences that people may not know they have forgotten, I like to do kinds of generic things because I don't think that I know what that person needs to recall. Doing it in a way that they can be protected is so important. Sometimes they have resistance to trance because they think it means they are going to have to remember things they may not want to remember.

And you can say, "It's really interesting that when you are in trance, you discover that you can remember anything you want to remember." The opposite is that you can forget anything you want to forget. You are giving the patient a lot of permission. "You can remember to forget and you can forget to remember," is a saying by Bob Pearson, and you can play with that in a great many ways.

I think it is important that we give people experience in forgetting before we ask them to remember. People who are going to be asked to go back and remember traumatic experiences or remember forgotten experiences need to have demonstrated to their satisfaction that they have the ability to forget other things, so they know it will be safe for them to remember these things, because they have already demonstrated that they will be able also to forget these things, since they can forget other things.

Milton said the patient needs a wealth of psychoneurophysiological experience in order to know he is as good as he can be. I think that this is one of those times that this is very important. Experience with the phenomena of hypnosis is very useful. Automatic writing helps the person know that there are different ways of remembering. They can remember in bits and pieces and they can remember in dreams that are so obscure initially that they won't be able to figure them out and they have to work on them slowly. They can remember in many different ways, in any way that is appropriate for them or that is necessary for them to handle, deal with and to heal from.

It isn't simply "go into trance, go back and remember". I don't like using the technique with an image of a movie camera and winding it backwards. I would rather talk about more recent experiences that I know are comfortable. "Where did you have dinner Tuesday night? What did you have for dinner? Isn't it interesting how easy it is for your mind to misremember things? I wonder if you can remember what shoes you wore last Tuesday." No, you can't. Think about that evening. Okay, well, let's see, last Tuesday, you went to the Young Democrat's fund raiser. You went home after work for about an hour, and you changed clothes and let's see, when you went in, it was so hot, what did you have on? They say, "Oh, yes, I wore such and such and with that I wore this pair of shoes."

Putting things into an appropriate context that is comfortable for the individual, lets them recognize the parts of that they can forget. When they put it in an integrated whole, they are able to remember. And I play a lot with the word "hole", spelled, "H-O-L-E" and "W-H-O-L-E", because when dealing with amnesia, you have to get rid of the "hole" in order to see the "whole". That kind of routing can be interesting for the person to play with any way they choose.

Mostly, I go from that kind of structure, setting it up to give them the opportunity to not tell me something. Sometimes, they just aren't sure they can trust me. That's straight out of Milton Erickson. He would demand that patients withhold something from him to prove that they could. Obviously, when they can withhold from someone else, they can also withhold something from themselves. That kind of practice is equally good.

We are talking a lot about forgetting. The process of learning how to forget and understanding about forgetting has its opposite and that opposite is the ability to remember and to remember how to remember. There's less threat in talking about how you forget, much less than there is in how to remember. But they mean the same thing. I will go about it from kind of that back door, in terms of opening doors. Sometimes, I put a whole bunch of doors in front of a person and have them opening different doors and talking about what's behind them. And finding out which door it is they don't want to open and then talking about when they might be willing to open the door.

Balance and Control

What I'm after is balance and control. That's what all these things lead to.

For example, I might use scuba diving if the person likes swimming. Scuba diving has this balance and this ability to turn slow motion somersaults under water and to have this *fine control*. To breathe in and to go up and to breathe out and go down, and to be able to get the perfect balance.

There was a lady with a lot of pain in her mouth and jaw from an implant. She sat there while I was teaching hypnosis and kept saying, "Is something supposed to be happening? I don't feel anything. Should I be doing something? Do you want me to close my eyes?"

I finally said, "I want you to sit there and listen. I don't care what you do. Just listen."

So she sat there and she listened. At the third appointment, I was ready to tear my hair out because nothing was happening and she didn't feel anything and never spoke the image because she couldn't. At the end of the third appointment I was talking about the bone forming cells, "Because bones are thicker after you have healed so you know the bone forming cells are always in your body." And I said, "I want you to picture those cells in your jaw."

When she came back, she said, "The pain went away for three days but it came back again." I thought, oh nasty word! And then she said, "But I knew if it went away, it could go away again." And I thought, "Bingo."

And then I asked, "What color is your pain?" She answered, "It doesn't have a color." I asked, "If it had a color, what color would it be?" She said, "Black."

"Fine!" I asked, "What shape is your pain?" She said, "It doesn't have a shape."

And this went on. I finally said, "Your assignment is to go home and draw me a picture of the pain."

And this woman came back with two marvelous paintings. There was a charcoal block and there were fragments with lightening chipping away at the pain. She didn't know what to do with the extra pieces, so she put them in a red river that was her bloodstream that was carrying them away. How could she create something like that? According to every scale of hypnotizability, she was a minus zero. We could have given up, but she had no other place to go. The other picture was of her jaw with her bone forming cells.

The bottom line was that she didn't get rid of all her pain but she got control over it. And that kept her from thinking she might as well kill herself. She could control it and eventually she began to relate the pain to other kinds of problems.

Question: What other metaphors was I using with her?

T: I used a sand bucket to prove something can happen on an unconscious level, but nothing happened. I spent 30 minutes and she finally said, "My arms are tired," and put her arms down.

And then I went into imagery and talked about looking in a mirror. Pain is something you can't see through, you can't see beyond the pain. You wash the window pane clear to see through to the other side. So much of the time, when you teach someone to get rid of pain, they don't know how their life can go on, because they've built their whole life around this pain. They have to have the expectation that it will be greener on the other side, that they'll have things they can do on the other side. You

250

kind of merge the wavy lines into a marriage of the past, present and future.

The last one I worked with was the music, symphony kind of thing, because there was an artist in the family. I kept trying to reach what I thought was inside of her. All of that was tied into this logic of these bone forming cells and the circulation carrying nutrients and oxygen and healing kinds of cells to that area.

It was all tied into: "It's your perfect right! You do not have to put up with what these doctors have condemned you to. You are not an automaton! You can choose. You can show every one of those [blank] people exactly what you think of them by proving you can do something about it, when they say you can't!"

Yeah, I get emotional.

When I work with someone who doesn't know about pain control, and isn't familiar with computers or switches, I would be likely to talk about the fact that when it is November, we have gone through an interesting phenomenon. One of the glories of the fall is watching the leaves change color. You watch the tree with all its leaves in the spring and in the summer with all this glorious color providing all the shade beneath. You watch the tree when fall comes and the tree gets kind of cold and the message is it needs to get itself geared up for the winter. So the sap, which has been providing the energy and growth for that tree all year, withdraws from the tree branches and the leaves fall off. You can see the limbs getting dry and bare and if you touch them you can feel how brittle they are.

All of the vitality and life-giving energy is being pulled back into the root system of the tree, into the foundation of that tree so it will be able to withstand that winter, all of the cold winds, all of the snow, and pain, and rain, and storms it has to go through. But the really neat thing when you feel the branches with their bareness and dryness, is the fact that the tree can withstand all of the storms it needs to. Because it knows next spring, when the sun comes out, it can stretch and feel that life-giving energy and vitality flowing up from that root system, moving out into the branches to start the new growth and development that is necessary for it to reach its full potential.

What we are about is the ability to withdraw into ourselves, to withstand life's storms and blizzards and attacks of any sort and to be able in the sun to grow again and to become strong and vital and move forward in that direction that we have the potential to be for ourselves. Anything less than that is really cutting yourself short and maybe breaking off one of those branches you may really need to use in the future.

Part V
Therapy with Pain

In his commentary "It's Okay to Let Go of the Pain", Alexander Levitan shares several vivid examples of Kay Thompson's inspiring teaching about therapy with pain.

The chapters in this section are an outstanding repository of Kay Thompson's experiential knowledge of, and expertise in, working with pain. Chapter Fifteen, "Patient Management and Pain Control", is an exceptional collection of most of Thompson's key teachings on pain. In this chapter, she thoughtfully examines basic components of the experience of pain, and demonstrates the necessity of working with most of them before dealing with the pure pain itself. Numerous poignant clinical vignettes illustrate her teaching. At the end of the chapter, Thompson discusses two fascinating surgical films which represent innovative clinical work with pain. Her masterful teaching is reflected in a systematic deconstruction of a variety of effective therapeutic interventions into simple, sensible and understandable segments.

In Chapter Sixteen, "Traumatic Situations", Thompson gives numerous demonstrations of how she talks with people in pain, and she shares many absorbing clinical vignettes and stories. Her spontaneous answers to a wide range of questions provide the reader with a fascinating array of clinical discussions. Several of her key ideas about pain, including the importance of belief, the effects of negative suggestions, and her thesis about what normal healing really is, are passionately presented.

Chapter Seventeen consists of selections from several panel discussions on pain control and contains a wealth of fascinating material. In most panel discussions, each panelist usually presents a brief summary of how they work with pain and then the panelists discuss a variety of subjects, through a question-and-answer format with the audience. These edited selections have been chosen from

Thompson's introductions and her comments and discussions, with the purpose of providing material not already available in the collected works. All transcribed excerpts are by Thompson. Entrancing hypnotic communications and stimulating question and answer segments on clinical work with a wide variety of medical problems are included.

Chapter Eighteen, "Creative Problem Solving", contains two sections. In the first, Thompson answers questions about helping chemotherapy patients with nausea and using time contraction and amnesia for pain control. The second section, "Therapeutic Uses of Language", opens with a presentation about working with chronic pain and includes several interesting discussions, including one about the conceptual pathways for hypnotic pain control.

It's Okay to Let Go of the Pain

Alexander Levitan

Kay Thompson was very gifted both in teaching and utilizing hypnosis. Even more importantly, she was a gift to the field of hypnosis. Her contribution to clinical hypnotherapy and to the therapy of pain was profound. In my own personal case, I modeled almost everything I did on what she had taught me, because it seemed so eminently sensible and easy to apply.

I recall the first time I saw her demonstrate pain control and physiologic control of bleeding, by inserting a sterile hypodermic needle through a fold in the skin of the back of the hand of a volunteer subject. She was able to convey with absolute certainty that there would be no pain, and that the subject had within his power the choice of which of the puncture sites, if any, would have a tiny drop of blood on the removal of the needle. There simply wasn't any room for doubt about the matter. And for good measure, she threw in the comment that healing would occur so rapidly that the puncture wound wouldn't even be visible in a few hours, which it wasn't.

Kay had proved to herself how effectively hypnosis worked for pain by undergoing two rhinoplasties (nasal reconstruction to open the breathing passages and improve the appearance of the nose) and a dermabrasion (polishing the skin of the face with a grater to remove acne and other scars) without the use of any anesthesia whatsoever. When I first saw her videotape of a woman having a surgeon pounding with a hammer and chisel in her nasal passages *and* shaving her facial skin, I wondered what kind of person would even consider undergoing such torture, until Kay identified herself as the patient on the tape!

I also recall her equally amazing demonstration of having a large hypodermic needle inserted into one of the large veins at the inside of her elbow, customarily used to draw blood, without a syringe attached, and then demonstrating that she could both decrease and increase the blood flow from the needle.

This demonstration gave me the courage to try the hand demonstration on a cancer patient who did so well, that I ultimately agreed to help her undergo an oophorectomy (surgical removal of both ovaries to diminish the supply of estrogen to her breast tumor) and operative hepatic catheter insertion, which prolonged her survival considerably. This patient was delighted with hypnosis because she could avoid the prolonged nausea and vomiting that she had always experienced with general anesthesia.

I also recall learning from Kay, a phrase that I subsequently employed whenever I was asked to see a chronic pain patient. It was a multilevel inquiry with an implied embedded command: "Has everything that should be done been done in regard to your pain? If so, then it's okay to let go of the pain." This question covered a multiplicity of topics, among them monetary compensation, diagnosis and therapy, revenge, secondary gain, need for control and need for permission to get well—which she always gave.

There was no nonsense about Kay. What you saw was what you got. In addition it was always for the benefit of the patient.

Kay realized that the mouth was an organ of exploration for both infants and adults. She was careful to see that the words that came out of hers were those that the patients most wanted and needed to hear. She was very gifted in neurolinguistics and applied this skill to verbal and nonverbal communication. Her posture was always relaxed as was her facial appearance. She utilized everything the patient provided and supplemented these with skills she simultaneously taught. She would gently press down on the shoulders of her patient with her forearms while working in the patient's mouth, thereby augmenting the patient's relaxation.

Her phraseology often had embedded hypnotic suggestions that pointed out the value of pain to us, but simultaneously advised the patient that they had powers they didn't even realize they had. She would encourage the patient to take the "hurt" out of the pain by pointing out that things which seemed very large to us as a child, such as a school desk, were now very small and no longer of use to us. She was not afraid to use command hypnosis and would occasionally forcefully say: "Stop that bleeding!"—and it would.

She knew that dentistry could not be performed without touching the patient and she endeavored to utilize everything that was available in the operatory. The aspirator became a babbling brook. The cautery noise was a buzzing bee. The splashing of the water from the drill was the contented play of two children splashing each other in a local watering hole. She would always attempt to understand what was occurring at each moment. One time when a patient appeared to be in satisfactory trance but was having pain from the drill, she discovered that he was so skilled that he chose to anesthetize the wrong half of his tooth, which was immediately corrected by Kay.

She taught because she felt it was not only her obligation but her privilege. She knew that most of us remember those who first taught us hypnosis with particular affection, since it has had such a profound effect on ourselves and our professional careers. She felt communication was at the foundation of every relationship and was thus able to relate to an extraordinary array of colleagues and patients. When a patient appeared anxious, she gave them permission to be as anxious as they needed to be and often suggested that it increase further, before gathering all the tension into a tight fist and discarding the contents onto the floor, so that "the procedure could proceed uneventfully and comfortably".

She would explain the physiology involved and then nonchalantly direct her hemophiliac patients to turn off their bleeding, while she extracted their teeth, knowing that it would work. She inspired many of us to expand her approach to our own fields. She taught me that it was not necessary to have my patients vomit whenever they encountered me in the supermarket, because they associated me with their chemotherapy. This also made the Super Value personnel much happier as well. I also became aware of the multiple messages I was sending my patients without even knowing it. I became more careful with my phraseology as well as with my body language.

She also set an example in her own personal life. She tolerated her malignancy with the same grace and self-control with which she interacted with her patients. She often asked for my advice but never questioned why she had to undergo the ordeal.

I have a personal belief that most of us are fortunate enough to have benevolent spirits looking after our welfare. I have always thought of Kay as being one of mine. Whenever a parking space becomes surprisingly available in the midst of heavy traffic, when a good medical result ensues for one of the people I have asked her to watch over, when my first grandchild is born exactly on my 35th wedding anniversary, which happens to be tomorrow, I thank Kay as well as all the other "angels" who look after me and my family. Interestingly, the more I thank them, the more good things seem to happen. Thank you, Kay, for everything!

Chapter Fifteen
Patient Management and Pain Control

Fear of Pain

You are not dealing with just the real pain alone. That part of it is just a tiny fraction of what is involved with pain. What you are dealing with is the *fear* of pain. When you deal with that, hypnosis can be very helpful. You are dealing first with the fear of behaving poorly. In our society particularly, one doesn't want to make a fool of oneself over pain. Therefore, you learn to go in and grit your teeth, hang on tight, and shove all of it into your stomach where you get that knot because you have to be an adult. You can't just fall apart and be hysterical. That would be behaving poorly because of the fear of pain.

Another part of the fear of pain is the fear of the unknown. If I tell you that a procedure I'm going to do is going to be painful, but it's going to take seven seconds, you say, "Okay, I can handle seven seconds, go ahead," because you *know* when it's going to be over. If I say, "Gee, we have to get that foreign body out of your arm and I can't use any anesthesia. I really don't know exactly where it is, so I can't tell you how long it's going to take, but you're just going to have to put up with it," then I have a feeling, by just changing it into the fear of the unknown about how long it will take and whether you are going to behave poorly, you are not going to stick your arm out and say, "Go ahead, I can deal with it."

And then we get down to the fear of the pure pain. The fear of the pure pain is really difficult to qualify and quantify because it's always surrounded by these other fears. The fear of losing our dignity regarding the pain and becoming hysterical is one of the bigger factors that we have to recognize. We have treatment for the physiological pain and the psychosomatic aspects of pain. But people still don't trust that they are going to be able to handle either the pure pain or the fear of the unknown or the hysterics and the falling apart, which might happen to them.

What happens with hypnosis? Hypnosis changes your tolerance for pain and changes your threshold for pain. We know from the clinical demonstration in which we relax the hand and pick up the skin on the back of the hand and make a fist and do the same thing, that tension increases the pain perception or what it is that you feel.

If the only thing that hypnosis did is teach the patient how to relax, that in and of itself would be helpful in dealing with pain. There are people who say, "Well, all hypnosis does is teach you how to relax." I look at them and say, "So! If that's all it did, that would be a very positive kind of thing." Relaxation enhances your pain tolerance and increases the pain threshold, so you are more comfortable and things do not hurt you as quickly as they otherwise would. When you are coiled tight like a spring, and somebody touches the right button, that spring expands and falls apart. When the spring is all loose and limp, no matter where you touch it, nothing is going to happen to it. It's going to be fine. So based on that, teaching hypnosis as a means of relaxation is an intervention for pain.

Perception

Hilgard[14] talks a lot about pain versus suffering and what we have to do in talking with the patient about these two aspects of pain. Most of you are old enough to remember the song "Anticipation". Anticipation is a great part of this intervention of pain versus suffering. When you anticipate, you look at something that is coming up and focus on it. You tend to magnify it out of all proportion to reality. I like to talk about the two words, *anticipation* and *anxiety*. Anxiety can be a very negative term while anticipation can be a very positive word, depending on the way you frame it. When you are anxious about something, the physiological response of your

---

[14] Ernest R. Hilgard, PhD, Emeritus Professor of Psychology at Stanford University. He and his wife were central figures in the field of modern scientific research about hypnosis.

body is that your heart beats faster, your circulation pounds, and you can't breathe quite as well and you get really concerned, uptight about what you are anxious about. So the physiological symptoms exist. When you are anticipating meeting somebody you really wanted to meet for a long time, the physiological symptoms that you have are similar. Your heart beats faster, and your circulation pounds, and you kind of flush and you get this knot in your stomach.

The physical symptoms for anticipation, which is good, and anxiety which is negative, are exactly the same. It's just the way you look at them psychologically that makes them different. So the relationship that the patient can then begin to understand is that the way they perceive what is going to happen, can have a positive or negative impact on their understanding of pain. When you deal with it that way, and they recognize that they can, simply by changing their attitude, decrease these physiological anxious kinds of symptoms about pain, the patient can be very much more relaxed, comfortable, and in control.

Control

Back to that fear of behaving poorly, of making a fool of oneself over pain. Hypnosis gives a sense of control so it impacts on that one fear that, most of the time we don't know how to deal with. When you are dealing with the idea of physical pain or psychological pain, you can use every means at your command to talk the patient into understanding that they have a great deal more control over their pain than they really anticipated.

There was an interesting experiment in dentistry where patients were given a machine, which they could use to stop whatever the dentist was doing with the drill. The patient would test this machine a couple of times and find out that it did in fact stop the dentist's drilling; it gave the patient absolute control. From that time on, they didn't have to turn on the machine. Simply knowing that they had the control meant that they didn't have to use it. They could relax because they had control. Much of what hypnosis does for the patient gives them that same sense of control.

One of my fun "play with words" is to say: "When you really have control, you don't need control because if you have control, you can get it back whenever you want it. It's only when you don't have control that you have to have it all the time, because if you lose control when you don't have it, you won't be able to get it back."

It's people like these researchers who give me the courage to make that statement because they demonstrate to me that it is in fact true. I work with a large number of agoraphobics because I'm the dentist they can go to. My standard reaction is, "Look, anytime you want me to stop, you raise your hand or say 'uugh', and I'll stop." They look at me and say, "Well, you can't. What if you are in the middle of extracting a tooth?" I say, "I can stop. It's going to feel kind of funny if your tooth is halfway out and you try to close your mouth. There isn't anything I do that I can't stop in the middle of." Just knowing that and testing me a couple of times gives them the recognition that they really have control. And that lets us do the dentistry. And that's a major part of it.

Language and Meaning of Pain

We're talking about language, verbal and nonverbal communication. It's our responsibility to give the message to our patient to make that patient more comfortable. That's what this is all about. It's a game and I have to outwit the patient by saying what they need to hear in order to be as comfortable as they want me to keep them.

I was fortunate enough to be taught by Leonard Monheim, a dentist and a member of the American Society of Anesthesiologists, who had written books about anesthesia. One of the things he said to me that really made an impression, was, "When you understand the patient, you have gone a long way toward understanding the pain." Hypnosis helps you understand the patient in a way you could not do otherwise. He understood about the doctor–patient relationship and the importance of evaluating the patient and understanding the value the patient places on the pain. If the patient places a high value on that pain, then you are going to have to work harder to change their understanding and perception.

You have physical pain, you have psychological pain, you have both and you have anticipation of either. When you are dealing with the patient, you have to recognize whether they place more value on the physical pain, or they really are uptight about the psychological pain or whether it's the combination or whether it's just they are scared about pain. Somebody who has a chronic disease or has a debilitating disease is more likely to be into the anticipation than they are into the actual right now kind of pain. I can deal with what's happening now but will I be able to deal with what is going to happen in the future?

One of the things that Erickson was most skilled at, and you often don't see in articles about him, was the ability he had to teach people amnesia for previous pain. Now the memory of past pain makes you anticipate future pain. So if you are having cancer pain, or intermittent pain, and you can learn to forget that previous pain experience that you had, then that eliminates the anticipation of the future pain. That gives you the satisfaction of enjoying the interval between pain without worrying about the next one. That sounds more complicated than it actually is.

The other thing that you tie into that is time distortion so that you condense the period when the patient is having pain. You make that period of time seem very, very short and help them to expand and enjoy the very long minutes when they are pain free in between these different attacks of pain. The obvious example would be in the time between contractions when a woman is giving birth, so you can expand the minutes between contractions and you can condense the length of time of the contraction, and it makes the patient go through the delivery process much more comfortably than she otherwise could.

And because there is a positive expectation in the future, it's easier to deal with because there is a limited amount of time that the delivery is going to take. Obstetricians can use hypnosis so well because they know what they are dealing with, they know within limits, how long it is going to take and they know that the positive result at the end will make it all worthwhile. We all know that the women who have had children forget the difficulty in delivery. The standard joke is that if women remembered how difficult it was to give birth, we would have far fewer children. So that amnesia effect isn't only created by hypnosis. It's created by the individual and by what they *get* out of what they go through.

People in Hollywood who go through plastic surgery, go through things that most people wouldn't consider doing, because it involves pain and a lot of suffering and a long period of recuperation. We say, "Hey, it's not worth it. Forget it!" But image is so important to those people. What they get out of it makes it worth the pain and suffering they go through, so they are able to go through plastic surgery repeated numbers of times.

So far as I'm concerned, we are talking about the reward they get for the pain and suffering they go through—the *value* that the patient places on the pain. When you make that determination, you have a much better idea of how to approach the patient hypnotically when you are dealing with pain.

What kinds of control of pain do we have? We have social, physical, physiological and psychological control. We have the cultural impact. There are the cultures in which we have stoic individuals whose ability to endure pain without showing it, without demonstrating it, is something to be rewarded, to be admired. There have been studies that demonstrate that Mediterranean people are far more emotional about pain and that the American Indian is taught to be very stoic and very impassive about pain, and all the examples you find in between. Some of the studies need to be redone in light of some of the information we are getting about pain.

Then you have the physical control of pain. When you break a leg, you put a cast on it. When you dislocate a hip, you put a brace on it. There are physical ways of controlling the pain, because the pain gets worse when you move it so you make the patient not able to move it. People go around in body casts for six months. I'm not sure if the pain of the body cast doesn't neutralize the pain of being in that cast, whatever it was that caused it.

You have the physiological kinds of ways. You give people medication that will zonk them out, that will take care of the pain. You give them pills, placebos, injections, some kind of internal thing to neutralize that pain pharmacologically. And you have the psychological control of pain, which is where hypnosis comes in. When we are dealing with hypnosis, however, we can impact on all those other aspects of pain—the physical, the physiological and the social.

We need to be aware, when someone comes into our office, of having an understanding of where they are in the sociocultural, in the physical, and in the physiological. Do they *really* like to take medicine? Is medicine something they expect, rely on, something that they know works? If it does, then that may be the easiest way to deal with it. If someone comes from a culture where they expect to have a lot of explosion and emotion and hysteria involved with the pain, and that makes them feel better, then help them feel better by letting them have that kind of emotional expression.

There are times when I think that people have a pressure cooker valve, which is a safety valve, and they kind of let off steam. You can let off steam about a lot of things. One of them involves letting off steam about pain. Pain may be involved with anger at having it or with guilt at having done this to yourself, and thinking how stupid you are and feeling you deserve to suffer. Then getting into that pressure cooker and letting off some of that steam through hypnosis and relaxation, if that's all the patient is willing to accept, will let it work a little more easily.

I said early on that hypnosis cannot really do any damage. Nobody has challenged me, so I'm going to challenge myself. One of the concerns that people express is about somebody who has a brain tumor and it's giving them headaches. When they go to a hypnotist and the hypnotist takes away the pain and that brain tumor gets worse, they are going to die because they didn't go to the neurosurgeon soon enough. My reaction to that is pretty clear: nonsense.

One of the things I think about is the idea about each cell in our body. The real amazement, I mentioned earlier, is that from one cell, we become two, become four and this trillion cell apparatus that we are. If that's true, then all the information in that first cell differentiates into all of us. Then every cell should have remnants of all of the information of all of the other cells. I don't understand it but it makes sense.

When you are dealing with pain, in the normal patient, not with the patient who is really psychologically impaired, their body *knows* what is going on. It is not going to *permit* that body to turn off a pain that it needs.

Turning Off Pain

I had a client with a back problem. He went to the orthopedic team and they decided it was too soon to do surgery. They suggested he use hypnosis to control the pain and he did that for a couple of years. Then they decided it was time to have a laminectomy. He had a really good result and he was fine and went back to work and the pain came back about three years later. He went back to the orthopedic team and they did the usual kinds of tests they had and couldn't find a thing. They finally told him, "Turn it off like what you did with hypnosis before." He said, "I can't. It's a different kind of pain."

They decided he was malingering because he had this great insurance program and he had been working pretty hard and wanted some time off. After they diagnosed the cancer of the spine, he was then able to turn off the pain in his back and keep it turned off until he died. He needed to understand where the pain was coming from. Once he knew the truth about the pain, he was able to deal with it. All of the people I have talked with who have had similar kinds of experiences have validated that patients cannot turn off pain which has not been appropriately diagnosed.

When I had a dental emergency on a plane, I couldn't turn off the pain. When the plane landed and as soon as I did the appropriate medical thing, then it was all right to turn off the pain. How many times do you hear stories about the patient who is in terrible pain and makes an appointment with the doctor and the instant he walks into the office, the pain goes away? Because the pain is needed to drive the patient to do whatever it is that is appropriate. Don't be misled by the fact that when the patient shows up, that the pain goes away. That is one of the diagnostic tools you have to utilize.

Comment: With self-hypnosis, I make an internal contract. I promise to go to get the care I need. As soon as I make that commitment,

I don't have any more pain. Sometimes, I renege and the pain comes back.

T: Our bodies are so much smarter than we are if we learn to listen to them. I remember when Bob Pearson told a story about a woman with back pain. She was at this party and her back was hurting, so she told herself, "I know you are miserable and I'm pushing it. If you will let up, I will make it up to you for this extra pain I'm putting you through tonight." The contract was fine. She kept her part of the bargain the next day. It sounds kind of funny. You negotiate with your body, you negotiate with your-self. When you learn to do that, it's kind of fun, the things that can happen. I do not believe that patients will ignore or mask a symptom that they need. I just don't believe that that's going to happen.

There are two sentences that are my philosophy about pain. I published them in 1967 and I have not changed my mind about those two sentences, which encompass all my philosophy about pain. They are so simplistic that people look at me with one eye-brow raised. Pain is a danger or a warning signal, period. When everything that can be done and should be done, has been done, there is no longer any reason to have the pain. That sounds really simple but when you take it apart, there's a great deal more understanding on the part of the patient.

We all understand and agree that pain is a danger or warning signal; it's a signal to drive us to do something, to get an answer. It's in the second sentence, when everything that can be done and should be done, has been done, where the diagnosis and treatment come in. Nowhere in that sentence do I say that the patient will get better. When everything that can be done, and should be done, has been done, the patient has the knowledge, the understanding, and control.

Having that kind of control gives them the ability to do with dig-nity the things that they otherwise would not be able to do. It gives them the ability to understand where the pain is coming from and, for example, to be able to take a radiating all encom-passing pain and reduce it to a much smaller, much more man-ageable size. When every test has been taken care of and the appropriate diagnosis is there, when it has been done and it's all that can be done, what good does pain do you? There's *no longer* any reason to have it. If pain is a danger signal, when everything encompassing that pain has been done, that can be done, it's self-defeating to continue to have the pain, because it interferes with your life. That's a very important facet of talking with patients about their pain.

Pain is kind of like a hysterical child. When a child gets started crying and gets really hysterical about it, even when the reason for the crying has been eliminated, the kid keeps on screaming. And you have to do something drastic to intervene, to interfere with that child's crying in order for them to realize that it's okay for them to stop because the reason for the crying has long since gone. And pain is kind of like that. It gets started, it builds up, and it gets hysterical, and even when everything that can be done and should been done, has been done, the pain keeps right on going.

That's what hypnosis lets you get a handle on. It lets you take hold of that hysterical pain and stop it, change it, reduce it, and remove it. Once you get rid of the hysteria surrounding the pain, the fear of behaving poorly and making a fool of yourself, and the fear of the unknown, it becomes much easier to deal with the pure pain that particular person is pursuing. That is what makes the difference in the way people who utilize hypnosis deal with pain.

Talking about Pain

How do I talk about pain? It depends on what I really want to say. I can make as good a case for pain stimulates healing as I can make for pain interferes with healing. And I can believe both of them, because it's important that I believe what I say.

Let's talk about the person who has been having pain, who has been hurting for a long time. I teach them a little about hypnosis. Then I'm going to say, "Actually, you are fortunate that you have had so much pain. The pain has identified for your body exactly where the injury is and is sending a signal to the rest of your body. You have all the cells already flowing and carrying the oxygen and you have increased the circulation to that part which is really good. And you need to recognize that the increase to that part carries the cells that carry the endorphins that carry the oxygen and the nutrients for healing. And they also carry away all of those waste products, so in that sense it's convenient that you've had enough pain as a warning to get your body all ready to encourage the healing process. And now that the healing process has started, it's okay for you to turn off the pain."

If it's someone for whom we are going to do surgery, I want to say, "You know, the only really nuisance thing about this is if you have pain after the surgery. Pain would interfere with the healing process. It takes energy to control pain, to turn off pain. All of that energy that you would be using to turn off the pain is energy you could use to heal. You don't want to have pain because you want to focus all your energy on healing. That's a really good response you can have. On the other hand, if you have pain and take a lot of pills for it, that takes a lot of energy too, because you are zonked out. The reason to turn off the pain is so you don't have to take pills and so you don't have to waste energy on pain. You can use all your intense alert energy for healing."

I'm taking two absolutely opposite positions on pain and I'm making both of them sound reasonable, because the body has the ability to respond in different ways when it needs to. The body has the ability to respond to pain that is post surgical in one way and to respond to the anticipation which is pre surgical in another way. Just because I'm taking two opposite positions, doesn't means that I am lying, or I don't believe what I'm saying or that what I'm saying isn't true. I make that point because people talk about trance logic as though it is cheating, as though these opposite ideas can't be in existence at the same time. That's not true. They really really can. *Two different things* with two different bases are both true.[15]

There are many, many routes, roads to get to there [your destination]. Some of them are very circuitous, some will have detours, and

---

[15] Note: Brief portion of program was not recorded. Ed.

some will be straight highways. Which roads you take depends on the negotiation you do with your patient, and it depends on the detours and roadblocks they throw up along the way as you drive to the destination. I don't care which road you take, because the bottom line is where the patient needs to go.

Dying with Dignity

Dealing with pain is one of the most significant things that hypnosis can do. Giving someone the understanding that they can have some control over the specter of pain, that sits in the back of most of our minds is one of the best services we can provide. Teaching people hypnoanesthesia may be included in the service that we provide, even though the patient may not need it at that particular point.

I really believe that all of us have this similar question, how are we going to come to our mortal end and how much pain is going to be involved with it and are we going to be able to do this with dignity? Hypnosis, oriental cultures and other different ways of approaching life systems are giving us a lot more of a handle over how to live life, knowing that the end of life is going to be able to be conducted with dignity and grace that we might not ordinarily have.

I generally resist working with patients who are terminal. I get into it a number of times with people who are very close with me, because I haven't been able to tolerate them having suffering that they would be unable to do something about. In many of these instances, I have watched these people make their own decision about when it is no longer worth being alive in the way that they are alive. They made the decision with the utilization of their body knowledge, with, "I have done everything I need to do, here and now, and there's no sense in dragging it out."

I think the hypnosis in all of those instances was a facilitator for the self-knowledge and the understanding and the control of pain. In all of these cases, the patients who were in the terminal state did not need pain medication because they had sufficient control over their bodies. I don't know whether they would have done that anyway or whether it was a result of the teaching we were doing. All I know is that it made it much easier for these people and that's what was important to me.

One particular friend of mine, who had developed lung cancer, eventually ran out of money and decided to stay at home and stop treatment. He stayed at home for a fairly long time. I was asked to come in and talk to him because he was on Demerol pretty frequently and was out of contact with his family. And I went in and we talked. I'm going to tell you what we talked about, because it impacts more on the psychological and the psychosomatic aspects of his pain than it did on the physical.

He had a wife and two children, and his mother-in-law lived with them. He had a really wonderful support group. His support group was just magnificent; it was my rock-climbing group of friends. They came in and sat with him and they said, "Don't worry about a thing. We recognize that this is terminal but it is going to be okay because we are really going to pull for you. We are going to teach your wife to drive. Just because you were such a jerk and never taught her to drive, that's okay, don't worry about it. We are going to teach your wife to drive.

"And don't worry about the fact that you don't have enough money to send your kids to college. We'll see to it that they get temporary jobs and we'll see to it and help them apply for loans and grants so they will be able to go to college. Even though you didn't provide for them to go to college, don't worry about that. We love you so much that we are going to do this for you. And don't worry about carrying on the mortgage on the home. We will make sure that your wife can get a job, so she'll be able to pay the mortgage and they'll be able go on living in your home".

Now obviously they weren't saying it quite in that way. They were saying, "We'll teach your wife to drive. We'll help your kids get jobs. We'll help your kids get loan applications." But what was he really hearing? He was hearing what a lousy husband and father and provider you have been. You are abandoning your family and they don't have anything. They aren't being taken care of. The depression that went with the pain was at least as serious as the pain itself.

So I went in one day and I sat down. I said, "You know, Bob must really envy you!" Bob was our friend. We talked about this idea of "Bob must really envy you." Of all the people in the world who would envy this man, he was the least likely.

So I sat there and rationalized why Bob envied him. I said, "He looks at you with your wife and your kids and he must really be envious of the love and support and what you have produced. And these kids are going to carry on your name and your grandchildren. That's really nice. Bob is never going to see that. He never had the opportunity to go to another country with his family and show them the wonders of other cultures. He never stays a long time and never gets any real knowledge of a place.

"You built this house and did all this remodeling yourself. Every time you walk into one of these rooms, your family is reminded of the work and effort you put into it. And it was so wonderful to have your mother-in-law move in with you. Your wife really, really appreciates the help that she's been." And you could almost see the expansion of his thoughts and his chest growing. And he began to recognize that his life had been worthwhile, by contrasting it with his friend whose closest relationship had been with an animal.

I said that, and we laughed about it, but it was *true*! It made the impact I needed it to make. It was unexpected, it was unorthodox, but boy, did it hit home! And from that point on, he didn't need any more Demerol. And that was what the message was there.

And the rest of that message was that a few months later, he was still looking fine. The day after his son's sixteenth birthday, he called in his mother-in-law and had this long chat with her about how nice that she had been around to help, and how much he liked her and appreciated her. And then he called in his younger son and gave him his instructions for life. And he called in his older son and explained what he was going to do after he died. And finally he called in his wife and had this chat about their life together. And then he said, "I bet you're sorry I'm sick? I bet you wish I weren't sick, don't you?" And she said, "Yeah, I really wish you weren't sick." And a half-hour later, he wasn't.

And the physician said, *"I don't understand why he died."* If anyone has had anything to do with lung cancer, it's really pretty bad. He kind of turned off his life because it was the appropriate time. And he didn't want to put his family through what he knew would come, if he didn't do that.

How do you explain that in physiological terms? You explain that in the knowledge and information in the cells in the body. Sometimes, just giving people permission to know that they know how to do the elegant things in life lets them do those things. I think that's really important. All of the other people I have been involved with have had similar kinds of experiences where the physicians said, "I don't know why they died. I don't know why they died." But they did when they decided it was time.

On her sixth visit to the hospital, one of my patients with cancer said, "If this is what it's going to be, I really don't want this. I think it's time." This was the night she died. This knowledge and information is hard for me to deal with.

Midbrain Stroke Patient: Eliciting Energy for Change

Sometimes it's necessary for us to be able to be uncomfortable in doing the things that the patient needs, in order to play the bad guy. I've worked with some midbrain stroke patients. A psychologist friend asked me to see this woman who had had her stroke three years ago and had been totally helpless since that time. She was very fortunate; she had a very close knit family. They really rallied around her. She spent her days in a recliner with her family doing everything for her. They were suctioning her because she couldn't swallow. Every time someone suctioned her, they would kiss her and tell her how much they loved her. They absolutely meant every single bit of this. She was having a problem biting through her lip. One of the sisters stood there, all day and all night, taking turns holding this woman's lip out so she wouldn't bite it.

I had no idea what my friend Arnie and I were going to do. I watched all of this love and I felt all this support in this room. I thought that I can't do anything that she isn't already getting.

273

I thought about Erickson and his German man somewhere in the deep recesses in my mind. I said to Arnie, "I really don't understand why you brought me here today. I don't think there's anything at all that I can do to help this woman." He looked at me. We hadn't talked about this before. I said, "I really think this is a waste of time." And he said, "What do you mean?"

I said, "Hypnosis is not going to do any good because you have to have motivation. She doesn't have any motivation to get better. Why on earth would she want to get better? She's lying here and has all of these people." I'm talking about her, doing one of the worst things that any therapist can ever do. "It's like she's a baby again. They love her, take care for her, take care of her every want and need. Let's face it. If she gets better, she's going to have to go back to work, she's not going to have people take care of her. She's going to have years of therapy before she can accomplish anything productive. Everyone's going to get bored with that. There's no way she's going to respond to anything we can do."

This poor, dear sweet psychologist was having a fit. This was not his persona, he couldn't understand this. I was pretty nasty for 5 or 10 minutes. "She just wouldn't want to do anything. I don't think there's a thing we can do." At the end of my tirade, this lady, who hadn't done anything for three years, raised her fist at me. I thought, "Whoopee!" I left. I left her angry, left her motivated, and I left her going to *show me*. We walked out and the psychologist said, "WHAAA?" I made an effort to explain to him. I went back four or five times before I quit being a bad guy.

That's really, really hard for me because I want everyone to love me. It was a very very difficult thing to do. But it was the unexpected. It was the thing that was going to get her off this, I can't do anything, but I don't need to do anything, because everyone is going to take care of my every want and need and the rest of my life is going to be spent like this. I can be depressed about it but I can't do anything about it. She found out that she could at least get mad enough to do something about it.

We went out three or four times and I finally backed off and eventually could be encouraging and supportive. The nice thing is that she did improve and I made an appliance for her mouth. She was eventually diagnosed with tardive diskinesthia and they changed the medication and we trimmed the appliance down. I used a bonding material and made a thing to hold her lip out there so her sisters didn't have to do it all day. She got to the point where she could sit up, she could use a fork and spoon, and could use a walker with the help of two people. That was probably one of the harder interventions I did. But looking back on it, it was interesting.

Question: How did the family react?

T: The family was so aghast the first time that they couldn't say anything. They were second generation Irish and very respectful of doctors and I was a doctor. Afterwards, I took the sister, who was the primary caretaker out and explained to her that I would probably keep it up for a while and it would have to be okay for me to do it. And because she saw the gesture, the raised fist, which was more than she had seen in three years, she obviously said, "Okay, nothing else has worked. Let's give this one a go."

Psychological Pain

I have had young patients, and on a couple of occasions I have aligned myself with the patient against the parent. That's kind of tricky. In one instance, this one man was a real hunk, big and muscular and a really neat guy. The father, who was in a wheelchair, resented and hated everything the son represented that the father could no longer do. He constantly belittled and berated and restricted his son from going anywhere. The son was polite and couldn't talk back to his father. What he did was clench his teeth and tongue thrust; it's a reverse swallow that pushes the teeth out. He had gone through orthodontics three times and it had failed within six months each time.

I didn't really talk to him about the fact that I thought he was sticking his tongue out at his father. As long as he saw me and we did some supportive hypnosis, he was able to control that and it was okay. If I had been in league with his parents, I wouldn't have been successful with the young man. Those of you who work with parental consent will have to work your own way around that. But it is tricky. You have to learn how to deal with it and figure out how to do it.

I tried to get him to go to a therapist the whole time I was working with him, and suggested to his mother that he might see a therapist when he went to college. In his second year of college, his mother called me and said, "He's ready now. Will you recommend a therapist?" He finally realized he would have to deal with these problems at some other level than sticking his tongue at Daddy. That was pain. That was definitely pain. It was a different kind of pain for him. It was something that was relatively important.

When you are dealing with pain, physical, psychological, psychosomatic, physiological, whatever, I think it draws on your own creativity. You look at the whole world of expectations about pain and what people have learned culturally. What they deal with is all of this other stuff. Once we can get rid of that with the hypnosis, dealing with what's left is so much smaller that it's worth spending the time to deal with the rest of it. You need to know something about the background of the patient, about his family, and be able to establish the kind of contracts you are going to get into in order to help.

Question: Could you talk about the story about Erickson and the German man who had a stroke?

T: A woman brought her husband in to see Erickson. Her husband had had a stroke, was in a wheelchair, and was not responding well to therapy. Erickson recognized that this man was very German and proud of it. He proceeded to say "Why should I help you? Look what the dirty Nazis did during World War II. You are a symbol. You are being paid back for all of the terrible things that the Nazis did to the Jews and to all of the other people in the war. This serves you right. You deserve everything that you get. There isn't anything I'd do for the likes of you. You are a dirty, dah, dah, uh dhah."

He kept it up until the man got up out of the wheelchair and ran out of the room, swearing he would never be back. When he came back the next day, he thanked Dr. Erickson. The idea there was that this man was imbued with self-pity and depression and the conviction that he was never going to walk, that this was going to be the rest of his life. Until you tap into the energy that the anger gave him, he wasn't going to respond to any other kind of treatment. Once he saw that he could get up and run out of the room, where do we go from there? We get better, don't we? That's what it took. That was what Erickson was willing to do, being uncomfortable yourself if that is what the patient needs.

I used to take myself by the scruff of my neck and go into a private room and talk myself into this. That's something I'd have to do to do something like this. It's tough to take that confrontational, Machiavellian relationship with someone who has come to you for help. They need the help. It doesn't matter if you are uncomfortable with it. If that's what they need, that's what you have an obligation to do. That was in the early 1960s. We weren't in the litigious society we are in now.

Acute Pain

Dealing with acute pain is easier than dealing with chronic pain. In dealing with an acute pain, you are dealing with a time-limited pain. For example, I had a friend who fell in a cave and dislocated his shoulder. I was the first person he called and I met him at the hospital. You know how a dislocated shoulder hurts? You don't want anybody to breathe on it, including yourself. He was sitting there about four hours, a half-day with this dislocated shoulder. Everybody said, "There, there, it's going to be all right, the doctor is going to be here in a minute, don't worry about it, the doctor will be here, you're okay. There, there."

What's the patient thinking? What the ____ *do you know* about this? It's my pain; it's not all right. Quit telling me that. Do something! Everybody kept patting him on the head verbally and saying, it's going to be all right. Enter the hypnotherapist or doctor. Recognize that there is not a word that comes out of my mouth that is spontaneous. It is all preplanned because I have this ultimate goal down the road and I want to get from here to there.

I walk in and look at the patient and say, "*Boy*! That must *really* hurt!" What happens? The patient says, "Thank God, someone understands." The immediate identification is established. Everybody else has been off the wall, way out there and didn't understand. I understand and say, "Oh! That must hurt from the top of your head to the tip of your toes!" At that point, he is ready to climb into my lap because he appreciates how well I understand. And then I say, "Now, I suspect it feels like it's been weeks and weeks. But how long has that been hurting." He says, "Four hours." I say, "I don't see how you *stand* it!" All I'm doing is exaggerating his pain. I haven't said anything about what I'm going to do or about hypnosis.

Now I'm going to say, "I *know* that really, really hurts. In order for me to help you, *help you*, I need some information." And the patient says, "Anything." I've said three sentences and I've established the communication with that person in order to get the response from him, so he can do what I know he can do, but he hasn't got permission to do before.

I say, "Okay, now, is it sharp, dull, throbbing; is it lancinating?" Every time I ask that question he answers me about each individual kind of pain. What's he doing? Every time I ask him about a type of pain, he has to think and make a distinction. Every time he thinks about it, he distances himself from the feeling of the pain. You can't think about and feel as intensely at the same time. I already know the answers to the questions. That's immaterial. What I want to know is can I get him to dissociate the emotion of the pain from the thinking about the pain? I can and so he answers all of these questions very nicely and obediently. I can see the pain level going down. While he's thinking about it, he ain't going to be feeling it.

At the end of that time, I'm going to say, "I recognize that it feels as though it hurts from the top of your head to the tip of your toes. But I need to be more specific about it. It doesn't really hurt here, does it?" And he says, "No." I say, "And it doesn't hurt here?" And he says, "Nooo," getting a little more suspicious. And I say, "And it's a little tender here." And he says, "Yeahhh." And I say, "And it *really* hurts right *here*," and he pulls back thinking, she wouldn't!

She would, and she does and she touches it!

And then I take my hand away and then I say, "And isn't it interesting that now that it is hurting only as much as it was hurting before, when you thought it couldn't hurt any worse, it really isn't hurting so bad."

I have a little tiny window of opportunity to do my intervention. In this case, it's enough time to get that shoulder back. In my case, it would be enough time to give an injection. In somebody else's case, it would be enough time to do this brief intervention. It might be enough time to simply continue with the hypnosis, if that's what you want to do.

There isn't a word that comes out of my mouth that is spontaneous. I have a goal. You start by identifying with the patient. You get them to distance themselves from the feeling of the pain. You bring back the pain intensely. You are showing them on an unconscious level that they can make the pain less and worse. You are giving them the element of control which they thought they did not have. And then you do what you know how to do. That kind of distinction or differentiation with acute pain is a really good way of getting the person involved and understand that they have some control over it.

Chronic Pain

With chronic pain, I think you have a different ambience. You are working with it in a different way. You are validating the pain they have and getting them to recognize, when everything that can be done and should be done, has been done. You have to take in account, all of this business of secondary gain, what they are getting, what they are crying about and communicating to you. They are communicating: "I don't want to be an invalid. What did I do that I am so guilty that I should be punished like this? This is terrible on my family. I don't want to do this to my family. My family really doesn't understand how bad I am and unless I have this terrible pain, they won't give the attention I want."

The hypnotherapy has to cover all of these issues of the chronic pain before you get down to dealing with just the sensation of pain. Each one of these is going to differ based on your understanding of the patient and their need for the pain. Back to Monheim (Leonard Monheim, professor of anesthesiology), when you understand the patient, you have gone a long way to understanding the pain.

Reinforcing Clients' Efforts

There is an interesting thing I find with people who have been in real agony over their pain. They come in and learn how to control their pain in their jaw, for example, with TMJ. They go home and their family says, "That's wonderful. That's amazing! How do you do it? Isn't that incredible? Okay, keep doing it. Come on, go back to what you were doing. Do the dishes, do the laundry. You're not showing us you have pain. We're not going to take care of everything anymore." They forget because the patient isn't exhibiting the pain, how much work and how much energy is going into controlling it. It is taking energy. This patient is working hard and feeling exhausted. Every once in a while, the patient needs to lie down and recharge his or her energy and the family says, "What's wrong with you? How come you are taking a nap? Get with it." You have to deal with that aspect too.

One way I do that is to get the patient to come back at regular intervals so I can reinforce them, so I can tell them how absolutely wonderful they are, that they are able to do these amazing things. Isn't it even more wonderful that they have been able to fool their entire family so they don't have to worry their family with having them know how much energy they are putting into this? "It's our secret how well you are doing. It can appear that you are functioning absolutely normally. Only you and I know how marvelous you are. What a super human being you are at doing this." They buy it. They just need somebody to really appreciate the work and effort they are putting into it.

Question: About a child in an emergency room. How do you deal with parents who say, "That's all right, this won't hurt."

T: I look at the parents and say, "How do you know?" It does two things; it says, "How do you know?" and it says to the kid, "Hey, this woman is really weird but she's taking on my parents and she's more likely to tell me the truth." So we have that kind of connection. Yeah, it alienates the parentsbut it gives me the opportunity to talk with the parents. Talking to the parent is generally not done openly hypnotically, but certainly utilizing calming and relaxation and explanation to the parents: "You know that Jimmy always knows when you are anxious at home. I'm sure you know how he responds when you have an argument and he gets really distressed and it's important for me to be able to deal with him without his having to calm you down. I wonder if it would be all right if you could get out of the room. That will be nice. The door will be open. There's no problem there. I don't want Jimmy to worry about you. I want him toconcentrate on what he and I have to do."

I will give you one instance with this 8-year-old boy who was doing the hysterical bit in my chair. "I want my mommy." I said, "Okay, Mommy can come in but you have to stop crying so we can communicate." And Mommy came in and the kid started crying again; while he was screaming, he was throwing glances to see what impact it was going to have on his mother. I said, "I told you, if you are going to cry, you are doing it for your mother and Mommy will have to leave." Mother went out again. The child started screaming bloody murder. I said, "No, this is my house and in my house you have to obey my rules. The agreement is that Mommy will come in only if you are not crying." He stopped crying and he looked at me and said, "When I cry, my mommy always comes! What he didn't know was that Mommy was sitting on the other side of the open door and said to my secretary, "You know, I have the feeling that Mommy may not always come so much anymore." So I hope that they all learn something from that one.

Hypnoanesthesia: Rhinoplasty and Dermabrasion [16]

First Film: Dental Surgery

These are surgical films. This is an X-rated film with subtitles, meaning it's not sound. This is a young man who is about to have some dental surgery and his hand is numb and anesthetic. And someone like me is saying, "When all of the anesthesia flows from your hand into your jaw, then your hand can go back down to your lap." So when his hand returns to his lap, we know that he is numb and anesthetic and we can go ahead with his surgery. This was his third appointment. The first one was to teach him hypnosis. The second was to decide whether he wanted to learn hypnosis for the surgery. Notice his eyes are open.

You can tell that there is no physical evidence of discomfort on his part. And in between procedures, he would sit up and talk to us and look at the bracket table which had an amazing array of instruments. This is saline solution rinsing out any pieces of bone that may have broken off in there. And a really good job of suturing, which was relatively important in this case. Up until now, this is kind of a normal procedure anesthesia for surgery. Except that this guy happens to be a less than 1% factor 8 type A hemophiliac who has had no factor and no concentrate before the surgical procedure.

This was the first time this was done within the catchment area in Pittsburgh. We have about 250 hemophiliacs in our area. The director of the clinic was *really* upset about the idea of doing this. She said, "Yes, you can do this without anesthetic but we are going to use factor." The oral surgeon said, "No, no, no, we know that he can do the anesthesia, we just want to demonstrate that he doesn't have to bleed." It took her a month before she broke down and said, "Okay!" with the, "*Uh*! I'll show you, he's going to bleed all over the place." I wouldn't be showing the film if he had, so.

---

[16] Note: Kay shows films to the group. Ed.

We chose the patient very carefully, folks. He tried very hard to live a normal life and not let the hemophilia interfere in any major way. He has some medical problems. You can tell he is perfectly comfortable during this procedure. He's not strong arming it through or denying the suffering that his physiological body is showing. He's sitting there letting us work.

Question: How specific were you in preparing him?

T: Very specific. I knew the entire procedure and talked about all the things that were going to be going on—the sounds, the feelings, and the instruments that were being used. And how it would sound when the root was moved and the compression of the bone in order to give the root the ability to move out of there. As far as being specific about telling him how he didn't have to bleed, not very, because he didn't understand the very technical aspects of it, so that part of it wasn't important.

We talked about the fact that his body knew how to not bleed and eventually he was always able to get the bleeding stopped. He could do this internally because his body had had a lot of experience by having these external factors put into it. His body had the experiences of knowing what happened as he went through the healing process. He would be able to do that himself, because the signals were there and he could accept and understand that he already knew how to do them.

He is comfortable and is not bleeding. The social worker who watched the process, told the director, "He had his teeth out and didn't bleed." The director said, "Well, that's nice but the third day is more significant." After the third day, the director said, "Well, that's nice but really the seventh day is more important." On the seventh day, she said, "The twelfth day is the really critical day." After 12 days when he didn't bleed, she finally said, "Well, maybe there's something to it." Now please understand that I understand that. If I had spent my life devoted to helping hemophiliacs survive and some jerk had come and said, "Well just tell them not to bleed," I would get a little bit upset.

We've done a number of patients with hemophilia. This is not an attempt to show you or tell you that hypnosis should be used in place of the regular things that hemophiliacs use. I do think that it should be taught as an adjunct. Everyone I have worked with has told me, "You are the first person who has told me that there is anything I could do to help myself." The helplessness that people with bleeding disorders feel, and to have some ability to control that and to have something that they can do, is very important. One of the things that happened with this patient, who was on a home program, was that his annual self-care bill went down from $36,000 to $8,000. Since I'm paying that bill, I would like all hemophiliacs to be able to learn to use the adjunct of hypnosis, because I think it would save us money, if nothing else.

Question: Why just an adjunct?

T: I don't want people to think that I'm saying that all hemophiliacs should turn off bleeding. I don't think that's practical or realistic. A great many are too narcissistic; they aren't going to do that.

Second Film: Rhinoplasty and Dermabrasion

This patient received no preop medication, no atropine, no sleeping pill the night before. Watch the assistance surgeon on the right side as the surgeon starts the procedure, because the assistant *really* didn't believe this. I have a friend who describes this initial procedure as "a knife up your nose". And the assistant surgeon says, "Oh! I really don't believe that!" The patient wasn't too sure about having whatever it was up her nose irritating it there. One of the things you do is sneeze to get rid of it. *Ahhchooo!* It didn't get rid of the knife so she had the good sense not to sneeze again.

They are using knives, files and chisels in there, to break the bone in the nose and open up the area so the patient can breathe better. (There is a lot of nervous laughter in the audience.) I don't think it's funny! The patient is lying flat and doesn't drown in her own blood. Since there's no suction used, she has to be doing something to not bleed. They are going right from the rhinoplasty into the dermabrasion—1500 RPMs is known as ultraslow speed. This is a very close shave. It is a round emery board taking all the skin off the face. The patient had X-ray treatment for acne during her teenage years that had left blue scars there. We've tried for years to get a clip of a standard dermabrasion and haven't been able to do it. I don't think they want to show the difference. Apparently, everything green in the room turns red from all the blood and skin that is suspended in the air. After watching this film, Jack Hilgard and Ted Barber both said, "You know, skin does really hurt. I don't understand how you can have it done without pain." Because there is pain and suffering. Once you make the incision into the abdomen, there are no pain sensors, they say. And they can't quite explain this one.

If you watch, the patient talks, so you understand that even in this relatively deep trance state, it's possible for the patient to talk, not scream, just talk. It's pretty clear, I think that there is no evidence of discomfort and distress.

Question: Was there anybody speaking with the patient?

T: With the hemophiliac patient, I was talking with him all the time. Mostly, I was talking with the oral surgeon, so he would have the courage to finish it. In the second film,, there wasn't anybody else doing the hypnosis. It was the first time it was done in Pittsburgh And there weren't many people comfortable with surgical procedures there.

This is saline solution, which is adding insult to injury.

Question: What kind of induction?

T: The induction happened. There was a rehearsal before the procedure. The physician went through the process and explained everything that was to be done so the patient knew what to expect. Patients in trance have a sense of humor, when something funny has been said. Even when they go through this kind of traumatic procedure, they can still laugh. There were no suggestions for amnesia. That was not even considered.

It normally takes three days for the seeping to dry up so the patient can look like that and 10 days for epithelialization. There had been no bleeding, no swelling, and no black eyes from the broken nose. The patient was smart enough to know that if you could go through this procedure without hurting, why would you have any pain afterwards, because that didn't make any sense.

So I didn't have any pain afterwards.

(Laughter.) "Oh my God!" (Applause!)

This is known as put your money where your face is. Believe me, the fact that I know I did this, means that I am not smarter than anybody in this room. If I can do this, everybody can do it. Motivation is the factor. When I say to my patients, *"I know you can do this,"* they believe me. I think that this is a major part of the process.

Chapter Sixteen
Traumatic Situations

I can and will say almost anything about pain. Let me give you a very brief introduction about where I come from in terms of dealing with pain. I'm glad you are all here. I hope you are all here. I firmly believe pain is a danger or a warning signal. When anything that can be done and should be done, has been done, there is no longer any reason to have pain. Period. End of story. I said that first in print about 1960 and have not changed my mind about it. I have had people make valiant efforts to back me into a corner so I would have to back down. I have not backed out of my position that I can deal with any kind of back pain without going backward on that statement.

What it really says is when anything that can be done about the pain has been done, that means everything that is appropriate and you know what the pain is all about. It doesn't matter if it is physical, psychological or physiological or a combination of all three. The phrase, "when everything that can be done and should be done", refers to treatment. In no way does this say the patient is going to get well.

The pain and the dealing with the pain is the issue. This stands up to working with terminal patients, chronic pain, as well as working with acute pain and traumatic situations. Then there is no longer any reason to have pain. That aspect says that pain interferes and it interferes with the quality of the things that go on. That is the important point that we can achieve in discussing this with our patients whether we have two minutes or two hours. When you are dealing with traumatic acute kinds of pain, I deal in a more authoritative, interventional way. When it is someone with a chronic pain and they are told that they have to learn to live with it, I deal with that in my approach in a more time oriented way.

I feel I need to give my patients some understanding of what's involved in their pain. I walk in and I take charge!. That's what they want in that situation. I ask, "What kind of pain is it? When did it start? Where is it worse?" That indicates that there are places where it's not so bad. If I ask, where doesn't it hurt, they can't deal with that. Where is it worse? They have to circumscribe it.

It's back to the Erickson philosophy of sometimes the way to teach people to lose weight is to teach them to gain weight. Because any gain can be a positive loss when you realize that you can only gain by losing. There are some people in here who listen very well to that statement. You take very practical realistic statements in terms of where the person is. You disrupt their conviction that any reality is fact by changing around any facts they thought could not be changed. You affect a paradigm shift. Put aside your assumption that you know the way the world works. Consider that it can work differently and then show them that it can.

If a client has pain in a traumatic situation where the pain has just been introduced, I want to say, "You don't want to hurt, because pain interferes with healing." If I don't get to them for three days, I say, "Boy, you are really lucky, pain really stimulates healing, you are well onto healing, let me tell you about it." They think, this has got to be crazy, but she's offered to talk about it so I'm willing to listen. There is an advantage to being able to be willing to have them think that I'm crazy. Because all the other people they are dealing with have been normal, rational, unconcerned people. I kind of wade in with both feet and say, "Let's do something about this, it's silly to hurt like that!" I *want* their attention. Once I get that, I will take my chances.

The one thing we talk about is teaching people to handle pain with dignity and die with dignity, to do all these things with control. We don't know how to give them that control without zonking them with medication. The alternative to that is hypnosis. When you are dealing with pain and you have those other factors involved, recognize the power that you have when you say to someone, "I can teach you to control ..." You don't even have to finish the sentence after the word control, because it's all of the above. That control is something that they need to be given an understanding about because they are going to say, "But, this pain is real!" I'll say, "I know it, all pain is real. But the pain is interfering with your getting better. The pain is interfering with your enjoying your family." The pain is interfering with whatever I can come up with that the pain is interfering with. The pain interferes with healing with the immediate traumatized patient.

I believe that the reason people who utilize hypnosis heal faster is not because they heal faster than normal, but because they heal at the normal rate, and that pain itself slows down healing. This is the premise I present to my patients. I had all these broken bones after an accident; I had a couple of broken legs. And I had this orthopedist who did not believe in hypnosis. When he took the first X- ray he couldn't see the break. He wouldn't let me see the X-ray, which I found absolutely fascinating I went and had my own taken. I tend to be ornery and am not threatened by all the physicians who don't know anything about hypnosis.. I didn't want to be off my legs for the 12 weeks he told me it was going to take. I was lecturing in Vermont in seven weeks, without a cane, without crutches.

I needed to focus all my energy on healing. My unconscious was selective. I only had my left leg in a cast. I was going from the hospital bed to the wheelchair. It was kind of curious that my unconscious made the decision to heal the left leg faster. I was able to demonstrate to my physician that I could get out of the cast and use that leg and at least use crutches. At that point I was able to focus on healing in my right leg. There was this absolute understanding because I was getting these hot flashes in my left leg. I finally realized I was sending the nutrients and energy to that area in order to speed up the healing and it wasn't happening in my right leg. And when he said I could use my left leg, then all of a sudden it got transferred to my right leg. I kind of scratched my head and said, apparently my unconscious knows what it is doing. Later, the only thing my physician said, is that, "You know she really does heal remarkably rapidly."

You can hear the conviction in my voice when I say this. So I can say to my patients, "If I can do this, you can do it too." So get busy. You can be as miserable as you need to be, but you don't have to be painful about it.

Question: What do I tell patients who are very inquisitive and want to know why pain interferes with the healing process?

T: They are told that the circulation is directly related to the healing process. When I was healing I took gelatin and drank gallons of cranberry juice. I explain that part and I explain the part that rest plays in the healing process and in the repair of cells. I explain the process of the repair of the broken bone. I talk about the energy that it takes. And then I tell them how they can control pain by explaining to them about tension, which is a culturally acquired phenomenon in our society. I ask them to deliberately make themselves tense all over their body for a while and hold their breath and relax. And I ask them to do that for a second time. And I ask them to watch what happens to their hands. They get a warm flush in their hands. That flush is the increase in circulation that carries the healing nutrients into the area. When you are tense, you restrict the circulation which interferes with the healing process.

Question: In a stress reaction, does pain automatically increase healing?

T: When I feel the patient has been in that situation, I say that pain stimulates healing. The first time I used that reasoning was with a patient who had all her teeth removed for preparation for a denture. She had two dry sockets and a sinus perforation and had not been out of pain for three days and nights, and her physician had prescribed medication that didn't work and she was in severe pain. (Chapter Seventeen, panel discussion). And I said, "Why not try this?" I was still using the word "try" because she was my third or fourth patient. She went into a deep trance in 20 seconds because she was highly motivated.

I said, "You have really been pretty lucky. You have been in pain and focused your attention to that part. You have really been aware of the increased circulation, and the heat, the inflammation which has been caused by that pain and you felt the discomfort. You have been constantly aware of that area of your body. Those were precisely the things you needed to do to in order to have all the nutrients and all of the healing cells and all of the circulation carried in there,that were necessary. I wouldn't be surprised if you would just heal so rapidly there that we would be *amazed*." She was out of pain.

She called the next day and she was still out of pain. What literally blew me away at our follow-up visit was that the right side, where she had the dry sockets was more healed than the left side. That scared me. It really did. I hadn't seen anything like this. I didn't have any concept of what was going on. I didn't tell her that it scared me. I told her how marvelous and wonderful it was that all these things came true. She had no further problems with it.

There are people who say, "You are cheating, you are deceiving the patient. You are saying these crazy things."All I am doing is changing the way they look at what is happening. I am giving them a quasilogical explanation to tie in with whatever they need to know. If they need to know that pain interferes with healing in order to prevent the pain from starting, I can use the circulation to justify that. If they need to understand that the pain they have been in for three or four days can be utilized to stimulate healing, I explain that. I can't give you the physiological reason why these things happen. My justification is as good as anyone else's. I'm giving them more options to look at what's happening and other ways to look at things. We get in these ruts.

You haven't done any intervention that can possibly hurt the patient, if you do this in a matter of fact way. I had a patient who had a root canal, and he didn't know it was supposed to be terribly traumatic. And my patient went to work and his boss said, "You had a root canal, do you want to go home for the afternoon?" And he called me and said, "Did I really have a root canal, because everybody thinks I should be in such pain?"

If I say, "Yes, you had a root canal," and he listens to the other people, he can develop pain because they expect him to. If I insulate him and say, "Yes, you had a root canal but those other people don't know what they are talking about," then he goes back and is able to withstand them. We haven't really changed what he had done; all we've done is changed the way he looks at it. I'm offering patients the option of looking at things differently.

I'm not going to say, "You will have no pain." I say, "You will be pleasantly surprised at how very comfortable you will be, as long as normal healing is progressing." What is the opposite? If normal healing is not progressing, you will have pain. They may have the degree of feeling that they choose to have. I risk nothing when I talk to them about this because I tend to start my talking with, "You know one of the really neat things about this is that you can learn so much." I don't say, "You have to" or "I want you to" or "You must." I say, "One of the neat things you can learn."

I talk to them about it in a direct pain, nutrients, healing, trauma fashion. I go into a metaphor, "You know, it's kind of like," and I give my analogy and then say, "I suspect you can be pleasantly surprised at how very comfortable you can be." There is no risk, with the patient saying, "That did not work."

In the chronic pain situation, I use a slightly different approach. With a burn patient who is nauseous and in pain, I like to use this kind of intervention. Pain control is a matter of degree. The degree of control that individual has is related to the fact that all feeling need not be painful. They can *feel* other things without having to feel pain or they can feel the degree of pain with which they are comfortable. Except in the trauma situation, I tend to be open ended, to offer a lot of options and opportunities.

How many people in this room would have the guts to walk up to someone with an open wound who was bleeding like crazy and say, "Stop bleeding!" and expect the person to do it? Every dentist in the room would say, "Yes." The only reason that we are so hesitant is that we were taught that we have to bleed, and that bleeding can be a very painful procedure and is a danger signal. And that is only true until whatever can and should be done has been done. As soon as everything that needs to be done, has been done, then there is no reason to bleed either. Patients need to have permission by God in the person of the doctor, particularly in the acute or terminal phase of pain to do what they have the potential to do. Nobody has ever told them they don't have to hurt, they don't have to bleed, until someone gives them permission to not bleed or to not hurt.

I talk about the two verbs, can and will, the "in-trance-ative" verbs. I believe that every individual *can* go into trance. That's where my confidence comes from. I do not believe every patient *will*. That's negotiable. When I communicate with them I believe you can Mr. Patient! Whether you will or not, we will talk about it. I am not confident that every patient will turn off all their pain, because I don't have the right to say that. I am confident that they can.

And I can teach them so they will turn off enough to be really comfortable. Does that help? I can be confident about this. I maintain that every physician should have one operation a year, every dentist one root canal a year, every nurse should spend a week in the hospital, and every therapist should have at least one trauma every year. You forget how it feels to be on the receiving end. And I think we need to try it.

Question: How much of my success rate do I attribute to my non specific expectation that people can do these things?

T: Ninety-nine percent. My expectation has a great deal to do with it and they tell me that. I have worked with people who have failed to learn with other people. They say, "The difference is I know you believe." That may be corny. That's where Milton Erickson taught me to come from. This nonsense about remaining objective; remaining objective does not mean you do not care. There are those people who can remain objective and still be compassionate. And I think that's important.

Question: What would I say for bleeding?

T: Pretend you are 13 and I'm about to take out four first bicuspids. I haven't given you Novocain, because you are not going to have an anesthetic and doing this is a real fun kind of thing because look what it's going to do for your future. I say, "You know, the only really nuisance thing is if you bleed after I get the teeth out, because that gets in the way. What I'd like you to do after I get the teeth out, is put your head back, let your sockets fill to the top and turn off the bleeding." I do the same thing with older patients. They look at me and say, "What! Are you crazy or something?"

I look at them with my wide-eyed, sincere look and say, "Well, all you have to do is control your circulation and you control your circulation all the time. If you think back to when you were a little kid, and remember when you were out playing and it was really hot, and when you stopped running your mouth was so dry it hurt underneath your tongue. You could feel every blood vessel in your body open up and the blood racing through to cool you off and you could even feel yourself turn pink. And remember in the wintertime, when you played out in the snow and stayed out too long, and when you finally went in, your fingers were so stiff they wouldn't bend, and your feet felt like you were walking on stilts, because you turned off your circulation to keep it here where you needed it in your tummy?

"You already know how to control your circulation. Don't worry about how to do it. Just close your eyes and let it happen." That's the end of the instruction. I say that whether or not those people were in a trance that I recognized happening. The stress situation of surgery is enough to produce spontaneous trance. Our whole orientation is negative toward bleeding and toward hurting. I have the right to give them the opportunity to have the best things happen.

Question: I worked with a patient who was going to have an abortion and our hypnotic work didn't help her from experiencing pain. I wondered afterwards if she needed to feel the pain as punishment. Is there any way around that?

T: I don't know if there was any way around it with that particular patient. My general response would involve dealing with the physical, physiological and psychological and the recognition that real pain can be very painful, but that feeling pain need not be a real kind of feeling. I would do that kind of teaching. It's all right to recognize that there are different ways to work it out.

In a very real sense, a caring kind of recognition that one has the right when one feels one has made a mistake to do whatever is necessary to correct that mistake. When one looks forward to the consequences of having to live with the mistake and recognize that in balance, this is so much and this is so much, and having given the appropriate amount of thought to it, it is so much better to feel the necessary degree of remorse and guilt at this time than to have to deal with it in the future.

Question: About dealing with individuals who have terminal pain.

T: They really are only, in many instances, reassured that they are alive by having the pain. There is this idea that when the pain stops, they are going to be stopped as well. You are going to have to live with that, is what many are condemned to because the alternative is not preferred. They are told they are expected to live with pain in order to live. They have the ability to enjoy the quality of life. I get into a number with terminal pain and chronic pain, "It is your right and you owe." It's your right to do what you need to do, but you owe your family the opportunity to let you know how much they love you and care about you. They want to help you and support you and let you know that. Regarding the quality of life, I've worked with a large number of terminal patients and many have chosen their time to bow out.

I'm working with a man who has cancer of the lymph glands and has metastases with the lower jaw. He's in the VA hospital, has no relatives or friends. Why bother living? He's in pain all the time. His therapist asked me to see him and I taught him relaxation because he was so uptight and gave him some exercises to do for relaxation. I was desperate the next time to make his life worthwhile. That's what I'm looking for. My life was worth living. We should not have lived in vain.

As I was fishing around, it turned out he was a fisherman and had gone to Italy when he was in his 40s, and this was the highlight of his life. He was able to stand on the shore, watch the fishing boats and the sunrise and watch the fish brought in by the nets. And we did this real imagery and that wasn't enough.

And I said, "Isn't it too bad, that there are so many people who will never have the opportunity in all their lives to see the beauty you have seen there? And there are so many people, even in this hospital who haven't had that opportunity. I wonder whether you would be willing to share this marvelous private memory that you have with these poor individuals who will never have a chance to see anything that beautiful?" And I knew he had been in the art room and said, "Would you be willing to do a painting to let them share in this beauty that you have seen?" And he said, "Yes." And I quit. When you get that kind of commitment, that means that there is something worthwhile there. And we have something for him to do that says, I am special, I have something some others don't have. I can share this with them in the time I have left and it means that my time is really worth while.

Question: About using the word terminal.

T: We are all terminal in this room. The medical community is telling them that they are on the fast track toward dying. I don't make any presumption. Everything I say is positive. They make the choice about what they are going to do with this. You have a limited life expectancy and they have a lot to do with determining the use of those limits. Patients hear the medical terminology. I am dealing with a woman who has ovarian cancer and I believe we are going to beat this one. The doctors have said that your odds are not very good, this is terminal cancer. My first job is to give her the ability to be insulated from those kinds of negative attitudes.

One of the things I have been asked about is that I have the reputation and I'm so good because everyone refers to me, and I'm confident and sure it's going to work. How do the beginning people, who are quaking in their boots, manage to do this? Every time that I walk into the OR where there's a hemophiliac about to have surgery, and he and I have the contract that I'm going to teach him that he doesn't have to bleed, I am *terrified*. Every time I pick up a scalpel and start in on somebody, my hand is shaking inside almost as much as my stomach. Every time I go in for surgery myself and the doctor picks up the knife and sets in, I think, "I wonder if it will work this time?" When I am waiting for them to do whatever they are going to do, I think, "You have got to be out of your mind, you can't do this. Why don't you run down the hall? You are screaming inside, how can you look so calm?"

When I work with patients who are going to undergo some traumatic situation, when I am going to be involved in being a party to inflicting this, I say, "I understand that your conscious mind isn't really sure about this and it is perfectly all right to wonder whether this is going to work. Recognize that this is on a conscious level and you have been raised culturally to expect that you cannot do this. If your unconscious is concerned, it will let us know. If you can let me start, it's because your unconscious tells me when you are ready and it will be fine." I have had patients who could not let me start, and so I don't.

When one of my patients who was good at demonstration hypnosis was waiting for me to begin, his heart was beating so hard that the bib was thumping. I said, "I know how you feel." And he grinned, because he knew that I knew. I said, "When your unconscious is ready, you will discover that your mouth will open." He got this strange expression because his mouth opened against his will. He said, "I didn't think I was ready." It's okay to have this conscious level of wondering and concern, it's your unconscious that we need to be dealing with.

Every time it works, I say, "Thank You." Culturally, I still have this fear. On an unconscious level, I go ahead and don't let it stop me. It's okay to be afraid as long as you don't let it interfere and learn that you can go ahead anyway. It requires something we are all taught to not do. It requires trust in the patient or the client. It requires the guts to say to the person, "Tell me when you are ready." And when they tell you, to believe them. And I still get scared, but I go ahead and do it anyway.

I never cease to be amazed and delighted and thrilled at the *marvelous* things that people can do. And the fact that so many of them do them because I ask them to do them is the most humbling experience that I can imagine. You don't hear, in a lot of the talking about Milton Erickson, the gentleness and the respect for the individual. You hear about the technique, the manipulation, the Machiavellian approach where he is authoritative and abrasive. What they don't tell you that is underneath all of this is the infinite respect and love for the human being just because he is a human being.

Every person has the right to that respect. I think the patience we exhibit with those patients who have pain is one of the ways we show that respect. Any time I think I am scared I have to remember how much more scared they have to be. My neck is not on the line. I can walk away and they can't. I have to work harder because of that.

I believe in their unconscious as much as I believe and trust in my own. Even though I'm scared, I'm going to go ahead. I'm going to give them the opportunity to do these things.

Chapter Seventeen
Pain Control
Selections from Panel Discussions

In this historically important clinical meeting of the Society for Clinical and Experimental Hypnosis in 1972, Dr. Kay Thompson showed a film of both rhinoplasty and dermabrasion surgery, which she underwent using hypnosis as the only form of anesthesia, and discussed the important implications for the field of hypnosis.

T: I guess I didn't know how it was supposed to feel before I went into surgery or I might not have done it. It was a dentist who came up with the idea of anesthetics around the 1840s. I think that dentists work with a field that hurts more people, more casually, more of the time than most people will admit. Granted, that there are both individual and cultural differences. At the time, when these people were having surgery done before anesthesia, there were also people who believed that the only way that hypnosis worked was if the patient went into a convulsion. So convulsions were expected and so was pain during surgery.

I feel that there are many things other than skin that hurts. If I may go back then to dentistry again, anyone who has had what is commonly called a dry socket knows that it isn't skin. It is one of the most excruciating pains which goes on for about 10 days with all the kinds of treatment that we can use short of hypnosis. Hypnosis can alleviate the pain. The dry socket occurs when a tooth is removed and a normal blood clot doesn't form. There are exposed nerve endings sitting down in that hole in your jaw, and every time when your heart beats, that tooth thumps. It is extremely painful. I suppose that this is one of the reasons I'm so interested in hypnosis and feel so strongly about it.

What I expected was when we went into it (my surgery), the surgeon and I would discuss what was happening. I was not distracted and I was not asked to imagine other things. We did talk about what he was doing, how long it was taking, the changes that were taking place, and things he expected of me. We didn't talk about pain, because that was my job. My job was to keep the pain turned off. As far as anxiety is concerned, I think that probably few people were more anxious than I when I went into that surgery, maybe not more than most people are when they go into surgery, I had not had anything done before. I had been an experimental or demonstration subject. I had my neck stuck out very far. There was that kind of motivation. I was extremely anxious.

I stayed outside the OR about an hour and half on the cart. By the time I went into the operating room, I was probably ready to chicken out. My conscious reaction when he started in with the scalpel was to say, frantically, "What the Hell do I do if this doesn't work?" I was as afraid of pain as most patients are. The relief I felt after the incision was the glee of, I guess it worked! Something I can't describe for other people. But the recognition that there was no pain, I'm sure was very reinforcing for me.

This is the reason I object to the rationale that you feel the pain but you deny it. You say, I can feel what is happening but it just doesn't bother me or just doesn't hurt. I think I heard an explanation for this in a talk today, when the speaker said something that appealed to me. I'll paraphrase how I understood his comments: "If I only deny the pain, then I should have the tissue damage that people normally expect as a result of abuse of the tissues." In this specific example, there was no tissue damage, there was none of the swollenness or the injury you would expect with this kind of surgery, as evidenced by the fact that the healing took place in half the usual time.

I go back to my own practice, when I was convinced of this when we had a control case that was unexpected. A patient had all her posterior teeth removed at the same time. She had two dry sockets which I had previously described and a sinus perforation. She was extremely unhappy and she was very miserable. Three or four days went by and her dentist and physician weren't able to help her. And obviously if I wasn't able to help her with hypnosis I wouldn't be telling this story. The pain went away in 20 seconds when she went into trance because she was highly motivated. This didn't bother me because I expected she would be able to do that.

The thing that shook me up was that the healing had been delayed and interfered with on that side and she was very poor as far as circulation and inflammation, everything that you don't want. She went home with suggestions for healing and sleep and proper nourishment. At the follow-up visit the next day, the side that had been traumatized and in pain was further healed than the side that had been healing normally. I make no pretense about explaining this. But I do feel that this has to do with the actual removal of the pain, so healing can proceed at the normal rate. If somebody would start to investigate healing and tissue damage they might come up with a few more ideas on this question of pain.

(Spontaneous applause.)

Moderator: I'd rather hoped that we would have a little more controversy!

T: The surgeon who did this had never used hypnosis before. And he used hypnosis on the next seven rhinoplasties that he did and the next four facelifts that he did without any other anesthetic and with no additional training. I thought this was very interesting because he didn't discriminate. He just took every patient who came in. Granted that the people who were having this done may have had certain variables in common. I still think that was a pretty impressive statistic too.

T: Never let men have the last word. I agree that research needs to be explored. I presume that the only way that kind of definition of pain (experimental pain) can be valid would be if it was from the same person. It would take somebody like me, who has had that kind of surgery done going into the laboratory and letting you pound my finger, to describe whether the pain for me is any different. I think the motivation is very different. Obviously, when I had the surgery done, you can see that we chatted back and forth and that I wasn't too unhappy. It took a lot of the normal kinds of anxiety away from it.

The demonstration kinds of things that other people, as well as myself do, indicate to me that it is a different kind of perception. The stimulus, the motivation, and need are very different. When

I put needles through my hands or let other people do this, there is a different kind of internal response than there is when I am having surgery. Everyone who has ever had rhinoplasty has said they would never have this done again. I had this one done twice. The surgeon was not happy with the first result. I still wasn't able to breathe. So I went back in and had it done a second time.

So far as motivation is concerned, the dermabrasion was his idea. I did not want to have it done. I went along with it. So I had very little real internal self-image kind of need for that particular part of it. I wasn't real hot about the whole idea unless we could have it done my way, which was with hypnosis. Laboratory kinds of pain, I feel from my own experience, are a different kind of perception. (Thompson, 1972.)

Pain Control

Introduction

I'm Kay Thompson and I'm a dentist and I induce pain. (*Laughter.*) And you laugh, but how many of you like to go to the dentist? So where I come from in my work with pain has a slightly different significance, because I'm dealing not only with the fact of acute pain and the anxiety surrounding that, but I'm also dealing with where I come from with hypnosis, which is all those years with Milton Erickson. And just about the time when I get comfortable talking with patients about their pain, I get a patient who is going to use anesthesia for pain control. And, frequently, I am the one doing the surgery and that demands a different level of intensity of hypnosis on both my part and on part of the patient, and a different understanding of pain. It's immediate, it's urgent and it's intense.

I was listening to the convocation with Betty [Erickson]'s remarks and was impressed that she brought up that Erickson was a physician and how he never forgot the physical body of the patient. We have the physical, the psychological and the physiological. Pain is a warning signal. It's not only a warning or danger signal. When everything that can be done and should be done, has been done, there is no longer any reason to have the pain. I published that first in 1967. And I will defend those sentences against anyone who cares to take me on.

How do you spell pain? Yeah, you can spell it a-n-x-i-e-t-y and other ways. You can also spell it p-a-n-e. You can teach people to see through that pane to the other side. So what they're looking at gives them a different perspective depending on how they choose to see through it. The work takes physical symptoms and lets people interpret them. And one of the symptoms is that the physiology involved in anxiety is the same as involved in anticipation. If people can be taught to reframe their anxiety into anticipation, then you are dealing with the pain without actually having to confront it. I have tried a number of times in my practice to remove pain, knowing that everything that could be done and should be done, had been done. I want to tell you. I failed beautifully. Because it was not my pain to remove, it was the patient's pain.

One case was a root canal with subsequent recurring pain. We did what a friend calls E-T-K-T-M, every test known to man. She was referred from me to her physician first who said, "Ah, it was obviously a tooth. It's not my problem!" She was referred to the oral surgeon and then to the radiologist who referred her to a neurologist who wanted to refer her to a psychiatrist. And at that point, this 17-year-old girl said, "Dr. Kay, I'm not crazy." And we started around with a different group of people. I did some investigation and discovered that her family had a history of neuralgia. And I called the physician and got a little irate because even though it appeared to be a tooth, it might not really be. When she was treated for the neuralgia, the pain in the tooth went away. In the meantime, I had done everything I knew how. She was a really good trance person, she was able to go into trance, could produce anesthesia, amnesia, hallucinate, and do all this stuff we would like to have. But after the first three hours she couldn't turn off the pain.

Because we weren't addressing where the pain was coming from. I've had that happen numerous times. I think we could remove it for a little while. And as Phillip said (Phillip Baretta told a story of someone whose undiagnosed serious cardiac problem manifested in physical pain), if he could have removed that pain for a little while, that little while would have been too long. We need to look at all the aspects of pain. My soapbox is primarily my clinical work with acute pain. Yeah, I do some other things. But we need to remember that that aspect can be very impactful on the patient's life. It takes a different kind of work with hypnosis to work with that different kind of pain.

Question: About being stuck with how to help a client remove her pain. The client had been a refugee in World War II and had recently revisited her home in Europe.

T: I tend to take a particularly simplistic stand. How dare you remove her pain? Excuse me! Certainly, she would say no; she has a right to that pain, she deserves that pain, it's hers for very valid reasons. What I would be interested in knowing is whether she can remember back to the traumatic events and remember how traumatic they seemed?

Remembering back to some of the places that she was, and some of the homes she was in, and some of the places she may have been hiding. And how overwhelming they were and how big everything seemed. And she was so little and helpless. And you said that she went back, and I'm wondering if she saw any of the places she had been when she was a little girl? I'm wondering if she was able to understand that the rooms weren't so big and overwhelming and the places she hid in weren't nearly as threatening. And obviously the places hadn't changed. It was the perspective she was using that had changed. Maybe since she had changed her perspective in the size of those things, she could also change in the emotional value of them and begin to recognize that there were a lot of other things she had changed in her life since that time. And she needed, and not you getting off being stuck, she needs to get off being stuck where she is in that perspective. And grow up with that along with all those other things she had been able to change since then. And see if she can put that in some other kind of perspective in her life.

Because they have a right to their memories. It's just that they need to recognize that their memories aren't exactly as accurate as they might have thought they were.

Question: About a man whose pain would move to a new location in his body whenever he learned to control his pain in the previous location; it is currently in his knee. Through therapy, he had finally been able to set boundaries at work with his coworkers for slacking off.

T: It's kind of interesting if you think about that for a few minutes. There's no reason for the pain. It may be that we don't *know* the reason for the pain. The fact that one finally steps aside and decides to look inside rather than outside. And recognize that when in your life you really have to take sides, that you can separate things into the front side, the backside, the upside, and downside. And that the working side of what he has been doing has permitted him to keep inside all the things that he really should be putting aside. And when he puts them aside he can go inside and deal with whatever the downside of the things that are causing the pain may be. Changing the side of himself that looks back as a little child into the side of him that is now grown up. And that this knee jerk reaction that he has to wanting to kick out in anger at all of the people that are slacking off on that other side, certainly has a lot to do with his recognition and understanding of the things that he himself is dealing with on the side.

(Spontaneous applause.)

Panel member comment: That's a hard side to follow!

Question: How do you use metaphor with pain?

T: I tend to be very nonmetaphorical when I am talking about acute pain in my office. And I can take a position very easily that the patient needs to hear. I can do diametrically opposed statements. Pain interferes with healing. Pain stimulates healing. If the patient has been having pain, then pain stimulates healing. If I want the patient to not have pain, then pain interferes with healing. And I think that you will be absolutely amazed that this is going to heal faster than the other side where you haven't been having pain. And I do use the word pain. And I don't avoid calling a pain, pain. I don't use discomfort or euphemisms. This is not the only way I use it. This is one of the ways it can be done.

Question: I'm interested in what you are talking about in terms of anticipation and meaning of pain. I had a root canal and it was one of the most significantly painful events in my life. Recently I was told that I need another root canal. I'm having a lot of difficulty with anticipating this surgery.

T: I've had 12 root canals in my mouth; I have not had an anesthetic for the last four. On the upper right first molar, there are three nerves, two on the outside and one on the inside on the roof of the mouth. I was on a plane going down to Grand Cayman for a continuing education program when that particular tooth blew. I happened to have my root canal instruments in my purse.

(Spontaneous laughter.)

I was with a plane load of dentists. And I couldn't turn off the pain while we were on the plane. I'm sitting there knowing that cold will stop the expansion of the gas that creates the pressure that creates the pain. I was chewing ice. And I get off the plane saying, "You are supposed to be smart enough to turn this off. This doesn't have to hurt!"

And I chose my dentist from this plane load. And we made a reservation with the only dentist on the island, to use his office. The instant we got the reservation, the pain stopped, because I knew I was going to do what needed to be done.

And I told the dentist he could use a local if he wanted to. And he didn't have an aspirating syringe, and he said, "You are going to have to do this yourself." And he was drilling away and I was fine and he found the inside canal and the outside backside canal. And he couldn't find the front canal. And I had visions of all this tooth structure disappearing. And I said "*Uuuh!*" And he stopped. And I said, "Let me turn off the anesthesia and then I can guide you to where the canal is by the way it becomes more sensitive. And when you get into the canal, I can turn the anesthesia back on again." And we did that. And I said, "Uhuh, uh huh … Uuuuuh huhhh," and I went back into trance.

And that was fascinating to me, that my body could do this. It just was a major revelation. My conviction is what comes across to my patients when I am talking to them. Your apprehension needs to be converted into that anticipation that you can do the same kind of thing. And that needs to come from reframing. And that you have the confidence and trust in the person you are going to. And that person is willing to let you use your autohypnosis. And how do you get them to do this? I say, what do you have to lose? I can only help you, there's no downside. If it doesn't work, you can do what you would have done.

You program yourself by reframing that experience into the positive experience that you know it can be. You need to understand that at the base of the root of the tooth, where the apex is, that everything narrows and it comes into a narrow canal and into the rest of the bone. If you turn it off right there, they can clean it out and not have any problem doing it. It's your attitude that needs to utilize the same kind of reframing that you use with your own patients to do that with yourself.

It Does Not Need to Hurt. I believe that and you can get yourself to believe that as well. I would get to know a little bit about your background. And I would take experiences where you have had things that have hurt or bothered you and at a later time you have been able to do them without letting them bother you. And other experiences when you have changed the way you looked at things. Like the house you grew up in, kind of thing. And because it's not fair to let something that has hurt your back then influence where you are today. I think it's a really important issue. I use, "It's not fair!" all the time. "Take turns and play fair." We learn that as babies. When something happens to us that we don't like, we say, "It's not fair." That has been instilled in us. It's still in us. We need to recognize and understand and utilize that. It's not fair for you to let something that happened a long time ago in a different circumstance and in a different situation influence the response that you are going to have today or tomorrow. *It's not fair!* (Thompson, 1994.)

Panel on Pain Control

In this panel discussion, Dr. Thompson shares some of her favorite brief and effective hypnotic inductions and presents several seminal ideas, including the importance of confusing the client's concept of what pain is and helping terminally ill patients acknowledge the value of their lives.

Introduction

So far as I am concerned, hypnosis is the ultimate in self-control. And now that I know that I know hypnosis I never have to be afraid of pain again. I know that it works for acute pain, anticipated pain, chronic pain, and unexpected pain such as an automobile accident. I'm dealing a lot with the anticipation of pain, now that I am seeing many TMJ pain patients. This is in the same chronic realm as arthritis and other conditions like that. I am helping patients deal with the worry they may behave poorly over the pain, helping them deal with the aspect of the unknown part of the pain, and I'm helping them deal with the pure pain and how much they need to suffer from the pain that they are having. That says that I want them to restructure their attitude toward and their need for the pain response they have

It's up to me to do an intervention by confusing their concept of what pain is. In order to do that I have to identify with them very, very clearly. The hypnotic intervention starts as soon as I see that particular individual. Eventually, I can get around to having some gut level feeling about what it is I need to say to the patient. I have certain kinds of statements that are accurate facts but they tend to be a little bit difficult to follow. In as far as I have already identified with the patient, I'm giving them information that seems to be very appropriate for them.

I might say, "The pain of discovering that it really is a pain, is much less than working with it to do something else about it, that you didn't know what to do before you knew about the pain."

Or I say, "And you can become so entranced with really knowing all there is that you need to know, about how to make the experience of that pain change into something that it wasn't when it first began, only because you hadn't thought about it as being what you didn't think it was."

That's a pretty rapid trance induction. I'm not belittling the pain. I'm getting the patient to recognize that they have options and that we can progress from that kind of interaction to utilize the options which I'm going to be able to teach them. My conviction is that everybody can learn to do something about their pain without even necessarily sharing with me where that particular pain comes from, the physical, psychological or the physiological. That may not be any of my business. But we can still teach them to deal with the pain.

Question: How to work with people whose sleep is disturbed by pain?

T: It happens all the time with TMJ patients. It's one of the kinds of pain they have. It isn't a matter of interrupting their sleep so much as learning pain control-teaching them self-control and autohypnosis and identifying the kinds of things which contribute to and go into pain. It has been my learning that once they learn they can control the pain, they learn it doesn't have to interfere with their sleep.

Question: About self-blame in chronic pain.

T: I think that those comments (from another panel member about incorporating how to treat depression when it is a part of the pain problem) are important. We aren't teaching you how to use hypnosis in the absence of all the other appropriate behaviors. We are assuming that you are going to do those and that you then understand when hypnosis is an appropriate intervention.

Question: About using hypnosis with a client with skin pain, cholinergic urticaria. Whenever he is stressed or the temperature is raised, he has a repeating acute knife-like pain all over his body and it is incapacitating.

T: My feeling about that is that the individual has to break out somehow. I wonder how much they need and what other behaviors they can learn and what surface they need to have involved. There are a tremendous number of multiple meaning words that can go with that kind of skin lesion. The Erickson philosophy of how big a patch of this do you really need would be the effort I would make to teach that individual—to let them jump out of their skin in only a small part of it, while you were looking for whatever else might be involved in it.

Question: What techniques would you use with acute pain such as postsurgical pain?

T: Postsurgically, I treat the body with great respect. It has every right to be angry and insulted at the assault on the body. But to deal with pain takes energy. And that energy takes away from the time that you could be spending healing. Everything that can be done and should be done has been done, therefore there's no longer any reason to have pain. Let's take the energy you are wasting controlling the pain, by teaching you how to turn off the pain. Glove anesthesia and switches is my particular favorite and then spend that energy on healing.

Instead of just leaving a void there, I am going to give them positive things to do rather than taking away just negatives. I'm going to say, "Instead of spending all this time on pain, these are the things that your body needs to do to heal itself—circulation, oxygen and nutrients." Give them metaphors for enhancing their body's own natural healing responses and make them so busy doing positive things, that it's easier for them to not have to concentrate on the negative things.

Question: How might you work hypnotically helping a person move to a realistically hopeful future orientation, since there are often so many blocks and so much grief work?

T: The position that I've been taking this morning has been kind of pragmatic and coming on pretty strong. I tend to do the same thing with patients in surgical situations and terminal situations. I make a very, very strong, very serious, very committed acknowledgment of the fact that their life has been very worthwhile. That's one of the first things that I think is necessary. Everybody else, in this sense of helplessness, wants to take over and do everything for them. They begin to think that they are not capable of anything.

My effort is to validate their existence by helping them understand that their life is really very valuable. In that sense, in order to be able to continue the value of that life, these are the things that you can do. "After you go home, gee, you know for the first week it is going to be important to spend x number of hours per day just paying attention to your body's needs. But after that first week these are the things you are going to notice." Incrementally, I start giving them homework assignments that automatically say, "Oh! She isn't really worried about whether I'm going to come through this operation, because she wouldn't be talking so much about a month down the road." It is kind of an automatic reassurance for them. So that I'm comfortable that they have the understanding that my life and I as a person am real and valid and I can begin to deal with this.

The other thing is my absolute all out belief that these people can do it. If I can do this, then they can do it. I am no smarter than they are. And they *know* that I believe that. They can't let me down! I'm quite willing to put it on those terms. Do it for *me* if you won't do it for yourself. *You are not supposed to do that but I do.* (Thompson, 1988.)

Intermediate Language Workshop

Recovery from Anesthesia

Question: Do you have any suggestions about recovering from anesthesia?

T: I think that giving the patient control is one of the issues there. Talking about the wearing off of anesthesia is important. It's important to get a little bit of feedback from the anesthesiologist in terms of the kind of anesthetic and how fast it's going to wear off. When I had my total knee done, I had an epidural because my orthopedist wouldn't consider doing surgery without it. I knew my anesthesiologist because he had taken my course.

I get back to my recovery room and, of course, it's supposed to be two hours before you're supposed to move your legs. I'm moving my legs in less then 10 minutes. The nurse in the recovery room got really upset, because I wasn't supposed to do that. And she runs over to him: "Oh, Doctor! She's moving, dada-dadada." And the doctor said, "Oh, she just wants to get out of here. Send her back to her room."

I was doing whatever I needed to do to neutralize the anesthetic. You can talk to the patient about their ability to increase circulation so that they can carry away the effects of the anesthetic. And talk about the positive aspects of waking up with curiosity about how soon they are going to be fed, how soon they are able to drink and empty their bladder. You are going to survive this by giving them all these other things to do. Their unconscious has less time to focus on, "Oh my God, I've just had surgery, I'm going to be sick." Yeah, some people get sick, there's no question about it, but there are all these other things you need to do in order to heal and you're not going to have time for that. (Thompson, 1997).

References

Thompson, K. (1972). Pain panel, Society for Clinical and Experimental Hypnosis Meeting, Boston, MA.

Thompson, K. (1988). Panel on pain control, Fourth Erickson Congress, Brief Therapy Conference, Phoenix, AZ.

Thompson, K. (1994). Panel discussion on pain control, Sixth Erickson Congress, Tracking Ericksonian Methods, Phoenix, AZ.

Thompson, K. (1997). Intermediate language workshop, Seminar on Erickson Methods, Phoenix, AZ.

Chapter Eighteen
Creative Problem Solving

Question: About how to help chemotherapy patients with nausea.

T: A psychologist I know does a lot of work with chemotherapy patients and talks about this whole process and how it makes them sick. Starting with the symbolism, I would say, "There are a great number of valid reasons for this to make you sick. When you were a little kid ..." then give some of the reasons why the child got sick. Either someone tried to force you to eat some food you didn't like or a doctor stuck a tongue depressor down your throat. So you learned how to be nauseous, you learned how to throw up, and you learned how to respond in a negative fashion so they would understand that.

That became kind of a body language for you. Right now you are in a situation where you are having to have something done that you really, really don't like. And there is no question, it has every right to make you sick. And you can be really sick of it. But that is not the time. And then tie in the relationship to the early learning and adapt and modify, so they can see that they have learned to deal with other things.

In addition to giving them that, give them the kind of positive things. Not being nauseous can be very positive for them in terms of their nutrition, in terms of their overall health, and in terms of their feeling of fullness and well-being. The feeling of fullness is another one to play with because frequently the feeling of fullness and nausea go together. You can tie that all in with salivation. When something happens that scares you, you tend to salivate a lot. When a good steak comes near you, you also tend to salivate a lot.

One of the things you have to do is learn to discriminate when it is appropriate to salivate when something good is happening or when it is just a fear response of salivation, because salivation goes with nausea. You teach them how they do not have to increase their salivation. With chemo, you frequently don't have a lot of saliva. You can use the salivation as a signal. When they feel the salivation starting, that will be a signal to put all these other things to play, because they will not have to dadadadada.

Question: You were talking about working with a cancer patient, getting them to forget or ignore the original pain. Could you give some approaches for getting that going with a patient?

T: Memory. If you think about a nice day, like it is outside. You go down to an outside mall and you run into a friend. You stand there and talk to a friend and all of a sudden, you look at your watch, and 30 minutes have gone by, and it seems like it was only 5 minutes. In January when you are in exactly the same place at this mall and waiting for a friend to meet you, and they are 3 minutes late, and the wind is blowing, and it is cold and it's miserable and sleeting, it feels like it is 30 minutes, instead of only 3 minutes. And it is the way you look at it that makes the time expand or contract. And you've had that kind of experience in your life and then you would tap into those kinds of experiences.

One of the word phrases that Bob Pearson and I played with a lot at the ASCH workshops was "remember to forget" and "forget to remember". It means the same thing both ways but can be interpreted differently. Talk to the patient about the ability to remember how to do this time expansion and contraction. When they actually go back and regress and remember something in the past, then anything that happened in the future cannot yet have happened, because they are back there in the past.

When the patient truly regresses, nothing that has happened after that time has truly occurred. So they can remember how they felt before the nausea or how they can remember how they felt before the pain, and they can talk about that and communicate that to you, and they can feel that. While they are back in that time frame, none of these other things have happened. They can then bring back the memory of that and put it into today's time frame and let the kind of in between time disappear.

Erickson would say, "I really thought the Pirates were going to win that game with Colorado last night. The final score ended up, it was three to four." And then he would say, "*What I really would like you to do is go into this nice comfortable trance.*" He might do it a bit more elegantly than I did. And the person would go into their trance and do their work. And when he was finished working with the person, he would say, "It was actually that Colorado three run homer in the last of the ninth that really sealed it for Colorado and the Pirates really didn't do very good at all."

He finished the sentence that he had started back here and the patient is amnesic for everything that happened in the intervening time. That was one of his favorite methods for teaching somebody amnesia and, of course, time distortion. The intervening time could have been 45 minutes and the patient looks at the clock and says, "Hmm, what happened?" Trance went on in that interval. Memory is the thing that is most useful in getting people involved in those sorts of things.

The patient understands with the stream metaphor (see Chapter Twenty-four) that they are a closed circulatory system and that they are the stream. I don't have to say, "Your body, your circulation is the stream I was talking about, and the flood is where the surgery is done." They figure this out for themselves. They are really, really pretty good at that. How long does it take? It's a reasonable story, it's the kind of story you can sell to your patients. Then you sit back and wait and the nicest things happen.

I didn't used to say the current was picking up the waste products and carrying it off. You know what happened? My clients got swelling. I finally figured out that I was sending all this blood into this area to heal and it was sitting there. I was smart enough to put in the "current carrying away the waste products". It was like magic, it really was. Because the explanation was incomplete and they needed to understand all of it. It was a really, really useful kind of thing. There are lots of other fancy things you can do with circulation and with healing. That's one of the ones I use over and over, every time I get a chance and that's really an important thing for those people.

Why do people heal in half the usual time? Please note I said half the usual time, not the normal time. I believe that healing with hypnosis is true normal healing. Any other healing is not normal healing. If you have pain, that interferes with healing, so it's not normal. If you are zonked out with drugs, that interferes with healing, that isn't normal. The only normal healing is the healing we do with hypnosis.

If you have broken a bone, and you have an X-ray of it after it has healed, you can always tell where the bone was broken, because it over heals. Instead of being in these nice straight lines, there are all these bubbles of extra bone there. You always have the bone forming cells in your body, they are always active, aren't they?

I say to my patients, "What I'd like you to do is recognize that you can figure out where the bone forming cells are in your bloodstream. And you can really focus and send those bone forming cells ..." And if you have someone who knows what they are, you call them what they are, but most people understand bone forming cells. I continue, "You can send those bone forming cells, along with the oxygen, along with the nutrients into that part. *You can be absolutely amazed* how really, really quickly that part is going to heal up and heal together." Just telling them that they can do that because nobody ever told them is important.

Why do people stop bleeding? Because I tell them to. Nobody ever told them before. When you were a kid and stepped on a can or stepped on a nail or something that your parents didn't think might be really good, what did your parents say to you? Your parents said, "Oh, it has to bleed. It's good to bleed and clean it out." Did they ever tell you how much to bleed? No, they didn't. Did they ever tell you when to stop bleeding? No, they didn't. I see myself as completing that suggestion when I tell them to stop. This is for grownups as well as children.

I say, "When you were a kid, you were told that bleeding was really good, and it is." And if I really want to be nasty, I say, "You know bleeding always stops." And I wait and they figure it out and say, "Oh!" I say, "Nobody ever told you how much to bleed. What I'm doing now is telling you to let that socket fill with blood and stop bleeding." They look at me and say: "I can't do that," or "You're crazy!" or "What are you talking about?" I say, "Everybody knows how to control bleeding," and go off into one of these metaphors.

When the patient understands that I believe they can stop bleeding, they put their head back and do it.

It's partly because I believe that they can do it. They *feel* that conviction, not necessarily that they will, but that they can. That's all I ask, that you give patients the benefit of the doubt. That they *can* do something. Whether they will or not is the negotiable item. You have a responsibility to do that, to offer that to your patients. What's the worst thing that can happen? They bleed like they would have anyway.

Give them the option to do these wonderful wonderful things that their body has the ability to do. Give them your conviction that it is possible. When you communicate to them that they can do this, there is a much, much greater possibility that they are going to do it. (Thompson, 1995.)

Therapeutic Uses of Language

In these excerpts, Thompson discusses several very important topics, including how she works with chronic pain and the conceptual (versus neural pathway) model for hypnoanesthesia.

Chronic Pain

The first thing if we are dealing with a chronic pain is to talk with the individual about whether or not they are able to make the pain worse. Everyone else talks to them about making the pain better. I go back to the Erickson idea. If you can alter the pain in either direction, that in itself is the foundation for change. When we are dealing with pain, people are so used to having a lot of effort invested in that pain, that it is a much safer, much easier way to get a perspective on the pain. When we get that perspective on the pain we do it by asking if they would be willing to make it worse.

317

I don't use scales a lot; I will with people with chronic pain. I ask, "On a scale of 1–10 what is your pain now?" They may answer, "Four." I say, "What is the worse it has ever been?" "Nine." Then I ask, "What do you have to do to make it worse?" Everybody else wants to know what you do to make it better. When is it better? You may ask about when it is most intense, but that's different, because they have to back off and look at the pain. When you ask them, what they have to do to make it worse, they have to feel the pain. They have to think about it in a way that gives them the experience of the pain.

I say, "Make it worse." They say, "I can't." I say, "Yes, you can. What kinds of things make it more intense?" They say, "It seems to get more intense when I'm busy."

I ask, "Is that because you move around a lot?" They say, "Yeah, or I concentrate a lot." I say, "Do whatever you need to do to make the pain worse. Do it now." They'll sit for a few minutes. "Okay, what's your pain now?" They respond, "Six." When it is six, they have succeeded in making the pain worse. Did you hear what I said? They have succeeded in making it worse. That's not a failure. It's a success. That's a way they have not been taught to look at their pain.

Once the patient is able to make it worse, then we teach them the physical symptoms that they recognize in order to make it worse. Obviously, when they have taken it from a four to a six, and I say, "Okay, now let it go back down again," the way I say it, is not, "let it go to a four again", it's "let it go back down again". In many instances they learn to let it go down to a three, instead of a four. When it is a six, what they always do is tense their body, increase their circulation, enhance all the awareness. When they release that, sometimes just because of the reaction to that release, the pain will lower.

The analogy is one of the ways that I teach people to go into trance, when they think they are uptight. I say, "You think you are uptight. If you want to be tense, let's teach you how to be really tense, because you are not doing a really good job of it." And they get very indignant. I say, "I can't teach you how to relax unless you first have an understanding of tension. What I want you to do, is when you are ready, I want you to take a really deep breath and hold it. And when you hold it, have your entire body very tense, hold it as tight as you can." And I show them.

I say, "When you are ready." They'll take the breath, and, at the top of the breath, I say, "Now hold it." You hear the change in my voice. I want the authoritarian to come out in my voice. "1-2-3-4-5, let go of your breath and the tension. That was reasonable but it wasn't really very good. Next time, see if you can do it better. I want you to hold your breath so hard, you can feel it in your ears." Do you know when you hold your breath very hard, you can feel it in your ears?

I watch them. The second time they really tense up. The second time when they do it, because I told them they've done a lousy job, they really tense up. The second time, when they let go, I'll say, "Watch what happens with your hands and arms." I count slower so they are holding their breath longer. When they let go, and they watch and feel what is happening, they feel a rush of circulation, this warmth, and a real lethargy. Part of it may be the response to the circulation, part of it may be they are getting into the lactic acid, part of it may be that they are learning.

Whatever it is, I say, "Fine! Now, that is so much better than you did before. You are beginning to understand that you are walking around with a medium level of tension all the time. Your body gets so used to this and used to creating the lactic acid. Until you learn how to make yourself more tense so you can understand the opposite of that which is relaxation, you don't really have much chance of dealing with the factors that go into controlling the pain."

They look at me as if I'm off the wall, but that's all right. I have proven so far everything that I have said to them. When you take some simple physiological steps that you know will work and bring them to the attention of the patient, then you have started to build the foundation of trust that you need. Then you can talk to them about the pain and about the tension.

I get into the pain is a danger and warning signal. You talk to the patient then about the fact that you are really impressed that their body is so tuned in and so aware. "But you know what? Pain is really kind of funny." I talk to them about how pain is kind of like a hysterical child and how when it gets started, it doesn't know it is safe to stop. What we are doing here is teaching it that it is now safe to stop. I say, "Now, if you continue to have that pain, you are actually detracting from the diagnostic purpose that that pain can serve. You need to turn off the pain, while the medication, chemotherapy or healing process is going on so that if there is any change in your body, that your therapist or doctor should be aware of, then you will have the pain back. So that you will know that something has changed. You need to understand how to use this marvelous tool of pain."

When you present pain as a marvelous tool, rather than something to be afraid of, something to dread or something to anticipate, you have the patient changing their perspective about it.

For example, I put migraine in this category. It is a recurrent pain. It is an anticipated pain. It is a pain that they expect they are going to have again. There are factors of chronicity in any recurrent pain. I don't think chronic pain has to be steady. The threat of that pain is what makes it chronic. You have as much of a threat with migraine or a cluster (headache) as you have in terminal cancer. It is going to come back. You have some of the fear of the unknown. I only know it is going to happen. I don't know when it is going to happen. You have that anticipatory fear.

Sometimes it is actually a relief when that pain comes, because you know what to expect then. You know how long it is going to last and you know when it is going to go away. You live in dread that the pain is going to happen at a time that will be very important to you, when it is very inconvenient for you. That's a great deal of the consistency of chronic pain. You are sitting there and wondering when it is going to happen next, not whether it's going to happen, but when it's going to happen next. That puts it in the category of chronic pain.

Oncology Patients in Experimental Situations

I am as straightforward as I can be with oncology patients who are in experimental situations. I have a patient who has been fighting cancer for years. If we could bottle her attitude, I could retire now from the royalties from selling that bottle. My patients have no problem with the "everything that can be done" aspect of it. I say, "Your body has to heal itself. We are giving your body the raw materials. Now we are going to talk about how the immune system functions so you can enhance what your body is doing."

Question: Regarding double-blind situations when the patient may not be receiving the experimental drug, so everything that can be done has not been done.

T: I say, "I'm sure you have read a lot about placebos and I want to give you the statistics about how often placebos are at least as effective. It is my belief that the placebo is effective, because it frees your body to do the things your body knows how to do, without the interference with having to worry." Basically, I have to be honest. I will bend my statements as much as I can. But I'm not going to tell them something that might not be true. I say, "I have so much data about the placebo effect and how important it is. And data that says that the individual, then can do whatever it is necessary to do, and we are going to free your body to do everything possible to make sure that it can help itself."

Reinforcement

With these kinds of patients, I think they need the reinforcement. In those instances, my voice, and they don't listen to it, they turn the tape on and there's this background music, and they go do what it is they need to do. But it's the fact that I'm there, that I'm in contact with them through the tape. It's the "somebody believes in me" reassurance. It's the exercise that I demand that they listen to the tape. They are forced to do the introspection that they might otherwise avoid doing.

I have a generic ending, "Bringing back with you all the good feelings and the knowledge you are using there, no matter what it is you are doing now." So they can use it in the morning before work or evening before going to sleep. I don't make it specific that they have to come out of the trance. I am a firm believer in making a smorgasbord of tapes. I have a number of different tapes and I believe people know which tape they need to hear. And there will be different foci on the tape, so they have the option, if they are tired and want to be more energetic, if they are wired and want to go to sleep, or if they need to focus on the circulatory system or on the immune system.

Dissociation: Out-of-Body Experience

If that person is somebody who can't deal well with pain, maybe that's the person who needs to experience pain in the other room, so they can *leave*. I knew a woman who had a life-threatening illness that they had not been able to diagnose. I think I'm probably still the only person who knows this. When she was in the hospital, she was so sick, that one of the doctors said she wouldn't make it through the night and she heard him say that.

What she did was dissociate, have an out-of-body experience. She dissociated her body up to a corner of the room and stayed up there and she watched the pain, and the illness and fever drip out of her hands and her feet onto the floor. She heard what the doctors said with that body that was having that happen. After about three hours, she came back into her body and she was okay. She wouldn't talk to anybody about that because they'd say she was crazy. But that was all right, I was already crazy and she could talk to me about that.

Hypnoanesthesia and Neural Pathways

One of my clients wanted to learn hypnoanesthesia. I was working on a cavity preparation on the front of her tooth. I was drilling away and it was a deep cavity preparation. I started in the back of the tooth for the preparation, and she said, "That hurts." I said, "Hmmm," and tried again, and she said, "That hurts!" I said, "Okay." I went into the front, and she said, "Soooo," and then the back and she said, "I don't know what you are doing but that hurts."

I am scratching my head. I finally decided that she was being so literal, that when I had explained to her that the cavity was in the front of the tooth, she turned off only one half of that tooth, because

322

that was all that I was working on. I said, "Please turn off the back half of the tooth, too, so your filling won't fall out." She said, "Is that what I'm doing?" and promptly turned off the back half of the tooth.

"You can't do that. It's one nerve, come on."

When I told her to turn off the back half of the tooth, she did and I did the preparation and I did the filling, and I went away and wondered what had I learned that time?

Knowing that hypnoanesthesia doesn't follow neural pathways is why you can do checkerboard kinds of things. It's really absolutely wonderful what people can do with hypnoanesthesia. But that's also what disturbs a great many of the physiologists, because those people who work in surgical situations and who work with pain patients assume that the pain relief, if it's utilizing hypnosis, must follow the neurological pathways. That is not a valid assumption. So that, when you are doing this, you have to be aware that hypnosis violates some of the physiological and neurological kinds of expectations. That's all right. That's what hypnosis is so good for.

Once you do, what I call, a paradigm shift, which means you set aside your assumption that you know how the world works, then it opens a great many things to you as a person, in order to believe in the things that other people can do—*belief*, as well as motivation. (Thompson, 1987.)

References

Thompson, K. (1987). Workshop on Therapeutic Uses of Language, sponsored by the New York Society for Ericksonian Psychotherapy and Hypnosis (NYSEPH), New York.

Thompson, K. (1995). "Creative problem solving", paper presented at a workshop during the 24th Annual Advanced Workshops in Clinical Hypnosis, cosponsored by the Minnesota Society of Clinical Hypnosis, the Behavioral Pediatrics Program, Department of Pediatrics, Medical School, and Department of Continuing Medical Education, University of Minnesota, St. Paul, Minnesota.

Part VI
A Holistic Approach to Dentistry

In "A Lasting Impact on Dentistry", Harold Golan succinctly outlines Dr. Thompson's profound contributions to the field of dentistry. Peo Wikstrom describes Dr. Thompson's significant influence on dentistry and hypnosis in Europe in "A Master to Remember".

In Chapter Nineteen, "The Oral Cavity: The Emotional Learning Center of the Body", Kay Thompson presents one of her most passionate teaching themes, the psychological importance of the oral cavity. She vividly evokes how the child learns to relate to the world through the mouth and explores multilevel meanings which the oral cavity can represent for the individual. As a result, dentistry, which requires an invasion of this space, can elicit deep psychological responses, and it is vital that dentists understand the psychodynamics involved, according to Thompson.

Through presenting a detailed discussion of clinical examples, she educates the reader about the psychological complexity with which many dentists work on a daily basis and proves that the dentist is, in fact, a therapist too!

Dr. Thompson opens chapter twenty, "Hypnosis in Dentistry", with an excellent general introduction to hypnosis and gives a systematic evaluation of the many different medical and dental conditions with which hypnosis is effective. She then thoroughly explores the utilization of hypnosis in dentistry, with multiple examples of hypnotic communications about habits (gagging, bruxism, thumb sucking), pain control and managing physiological issues such as bleeding.

A Lasting Impact on Dentistry

Harold P. Golan

I heartily acquiesced to writing a chapter introduction for the collected works because I have had extensive professional dealings with Kay over many years. Our interactions varied over time, sometimes full, other times sparse; but I was always aware of Kay's presence, as the smiling, laughing pupil of Milton Erickson, as poet, teacher, executive, friend and woman of principle. Her teaching about the psychological importance of the oral cavity and linking of hypnosis with dentistry had an enormous impact on dentistry in the United States. She was clearly ahead of any other woman whom I have known in my many years of professional practice.

Her influence was widespread. I vividly remember when we were teaching together at Oswego Lake, New York, in the early 1970s. Milton Erickson, as senior faculty, looked to a handful of us, including Bertha Rodgers, Kay, Larry Staples and myself, to provide key lectures for the symposium. I can still recall Bertha and Kay walking along the lake, seriously discussing some aspect of hypnosis.

Kay's influence and teaching spread beyond the United States as she accepted invitations to teach hypnosis throughout the world. At the annual meeting of the Society for Clinical and Experimental Hypnosis (SCEH) at the University of Glasgow, Scotland, in 1980, Kay was the chairman of the advanced dental group, while I was head of the basic dental group. We had a splendid collection of students from all over the world.

The most intensive professional interaction I had with Kay, was having her as a role model during the many years when I served as the executive officer of the American Board of Hypnosis in Dentistry (ABHD) and she served as a diplomatic presence on the Board. We frequently discussed problem patients in dentistry, some of whom were mistreated due to lack of basic psychodynamic teaching on the part of the dentist, which was such an important part of Kay's protocol in treating patients.

It is difficult enough for a dentist to learn graphically and mechanically everything he needs to know about the head, neck and cavity.

That Kay also recognized the psychodynamics of these areas is one of her great gifts to the profession. Through Kay's holistic approach to patients, the symbiosis of both psychodynamic treatment and mechanical ability led to new and effective ways to treat a large range of serious and difficult dental problems.

How fortunate we are to have had Kay's presence and influence on our profession.

A Master to Remember

Peo Wikstrom

My close friend and colleague Kay Thompson was truly a master to remember. I feel she is still among us. When I look back over 30 years of our life together in hypnosis and therapy, I remember so clearly why and when it started. It definitely was a serendipitous happening at the International Society of Hypnosis (ISH) Congress in Uppsala, Sweden, in 1973, when I was the rather inexperienced secretary. In fact the job had been thrust upon me due to the unexpected illness of the overworked secretary. It was left to me to arrange the program on induction methods for a panel with six discussants, including Josephine Hilgard, Erika Fromm, Bob Pearson and Kay Thompson from the United States, and John Hartland from Europe.

When someone proposed a sixth American panelist, Erika and Kay loudly protested, "*No! No!* No more Amer-i-c-a-ns!" They wanted another European panelist, and Kay said, pointing to me, "You'll take it." I accepted with fear in my heart. As the chair, she later introduced me, "Peo has chosen time distortion, and if he can cover this huge issue within his allotted 10 minutes, he really needs time distortion!"

Next morning, I approached Kay while she was sitting on a bench in the University park. "You are the President of ASCH. Would you accept me as a member of your society?" I asked. "Certainly," Kay replied. In a way this opened a gate to my personal growth and

327

development, and perhaps also was a contribution to the European history of hypnosis and therapy.

Kay was a master of the language of the unconscious and a true follower of Milton H. Erickson, becoming my mentor and therein also an example for many dentists in Scandinavia using clinical hypnosis. I invited her to come to Sweden and teach some of the courses I had organized for the Swedish Dental Association (SDA). Kay was a rich source of stimulation for my own interest in music, art, and human behavior, especially body language and diversity of verbal expressions. Kay invited me to assist her in workshops in the United States during the 1970s and 1980s.

During my years with Kay, I tried to improve my American English, so I asked Kay, "If you are a true friend, please correct me when I make mistakes." She agreed but after a while gave up that mission. She explained, "I don´t want to correct you any longer. Sometimes, you say wonderful double-meanings without knowing it. And I don't want to miss them."

Kay was a master of language, and having a refined mind, she played with words in a calm, relaxed, and witty manner. She was especially marvelous with stiff and anxious patients.

Because of Kay's influence, Ericksonian hypnosis was fully accepted in Scandinavia, as well as in the European Societies for Hypnosis (ESH) in Switzerland and Germany where she also taught. In our courses we used her teachings on dental hypnosis and her techniques for gagging, pain, and anesthesia problems. One of her major contributions is her development of the importance of motivation in hypnosis. Many practioners in my field have enhanced their effectiveness by using motivation as Kay suggested.

Kay deserves to be remembered for her unique position in dental hypnosis and therapy and as a model for dentists worldwide.

Chapter Nineteen
The Oral Cavity
The Emotional Learning Center
of the Body—The Dentist is a
Therapist Too![17]

The Mouth as Transition

I'm into puzzles and word games as most of you know now.

(Note: Kay asked the audience to answer each verbal puzzle; her question is to the left and the answer follows. Ed.)

Shakespeare's real estate? Bard's yards.

Whitman's pepper? Walt's salt.

Poet's Sylvia's fury? Plath's rath.

Lewis's postscript? C. S.'s P. S.

Opponent of the man who wrote the Raven? Poe's foe.

Man who wrote *The Return of the Native* is late for school? Hardy's tardy.

Man who wrote *Stopping by the Woods on a Snowy Evening* is missing? Frost's lost.

Sailboat's steerer belongs to playwright of *The Crucible?* Miller's tiller.

---

[17] This paper is from Kay Thompson's private prepared notes, with the addition of a few question-and-answer segments from the actual plenary address presentation.

Alternatives for the writer of *Ulysses?* Joyce's choices.

George Bernard's rules? Shaw's laws.

This is to get you in the right mood so when I get you all riled up you won't mind.

It's interesting how difficult it is for a dentist to be recognized as one who might also be competent with the utilization of hypnosis and maybe even have a little understanding of psychodynamics. This presentation posits the premise that, "the dentist is a therapist".

It really has always confused me that people feel a need to apologize and explain away the fact that I'm "good with hypnosis, even though I'm only a dentist". I hear that a lot- it has even been called my "first career", assuming that I could not do what I do and know what I know by being "only" a dentist.

So far as the *psychology of dentistry* is concerned, years ago Milton Erickson taught me and others that the psychological dental therapy has to be within the realm of the dentist and should be done by the dentist. He also was adamant about the teaching of hypnosis being best done in mixed degree professional groups—physicians, dentists and therapists, because people all learned more respect for the different professions and more knowledge about those professions.

When I think about that, I'm reminded of the courses that we had in Pittsburgh when we did advanced clinical work in dentistry. How fascinated I was by the fact that all of the physicians and the therapists tended to cancel their sessions, so that they could come and watch us do honest to goodness physiological work, because they were so fascinated by it.

An attitude is extant to regard the profession of dentistry as that of a mechanical profession. And if I asked for a show of hands I'm sure that most of you think that it is a mechanical profession. Because of that, it's outside the realm of "real" doctor or "real" therapy. Yeah, parts of our field are mechanical, there's no question about that. I have to know more than you do, I have to know the therapy and the mechanics. But it is also true that unless we have the skill to get the patient to sit down in the chair and open his or her mouth, it doesn't make a bit of difference how good I am with my hands. I could have, as they say in the profession, the best hands, but if the patient isn't going to let me use them, then the mechanical skill makes no difference.

By the nature of my profession I am forced to do difficult and sometimes potentially painful procedures to repair the mess of a mouth that makes its way to me. It is necessary for me to give the owner of that mouth as much support as possible and to explain about the essential repairs on the basis of how the mouth had or had not been cared for in the past, particularly when you are seeing someone who has not been to the dentist for 25 or 30 years. To tell them what kind of repair is necessary and what necessary maintenance is needed to keep it in repair, approaches it from a mechanical viewpoint, as though it were a car.

But, frequently, the owner of that mouth has severe concerns about my working on that part of the body because it is a body part and that specific body part of the mouth, and not a car that will undergo restoration.

It is not that people have teeth, it is that *teeth have people*! A very slight difference but very significant. So let's take a look back in time to see how that relationship and that concern developed in that oral, linguistic region. The dentist deals daily with the psychological significance of the oral cavity, which goes beyond the momentary "treatment" and focuses on the oral cavity as crucial for the lifetime development of the individual. Dentists can provide insight into, and have a powerful influence on, the psychological homeostasis of the individual. Now, how did that relationship develop with that oral linguistic organ? I believe that the reason that many of you in this room don't like to go to the dentist is because it invades the mouth, which is the *emotional learning center* of the body. And I'm going to defend that particular position because I firmly believe it.

I don't care whether you believe the Freudian concept of oral, anal, and genital development; this is physiologically the way the body develops. From the physical development of the baby and beyond, to the acquisition and mastery of language skills, the oral cavity is a primary focus and the source of nutrition, frustration, satisfaction, learning and communication and power.

When the child is born, the immediate focus on the oral cavity begins. It might even begin before that, because pictures of babies in utero show them sucking their thumb and responding to music as well. They are listening, they are hearing. When a baby is born, the first thing it does is take a breath and cry through its mouth.

When the baby is hungry it cries through its mouth and somebody comes and feeds it through its mouth. When it is wet, it cries a different kind of cry, and the adults around figure that cry out and somebody comes and changes it. When it is unhappy or afraid, it cries yet another kind of cry, and somebody comes and nurtures it and helps it not to be unhappy and afraid.

When it is happy, everybody else is happy too. It coos and goos and gets reinforced for that. I think it is normal and natural that the mouth becomes a focus of *power* for the baby, where all its wants and needs are made known and taken care of.

Then what happens? The baby begins to crawl and explore. And when it finds something on the floor, does it do what an adult has done? Pick the object up and examine it, feel it, look at it? Naah! It goes into the mouth. So that object teaches that baby hard, soft, hot, cold, heat, texture. And the pain of teething may be the primary pain the child experiences, even though it may not be able to localize it in the mouth. So again, *learning* power and learning *power* are concentrated in the mouth.

Everybody comes into this with the ability to learn power through their mouth and to use power that they learned in their mouth.

Continued learning and reliance on the oral cavity comes with the development of language, which is another oral skill, but one which has more encompassing significance for us. This oral skill "trance-lates" early into individual lasting learning. The psychodynamics of the doctor–patient relationship can be influenced by early learning patterns for language, when words first became symbols for meaning.

Words are symbols for meaning and experience. We know what symbols mean long before we put words to them.

As a child moves around and learns, what is he doing? The child crawls around and he knows it's a floor long before he knows it is called "floor", and he knows what you are sitting on holds you up long before he knows it is a chair. So very soon when the adults say the word *floor*, the child sees the symbol for floor. When the adult says the word *chair* the child sees the symbol for the chair. We learn to associate the "image" with the word. This is the way we learn much of our associative words. Today, when your mind is searching for an elusive word or phrase, we deliberately run through words in our brain? No, we run through images in our brain, looking for a clue that will tap into the right word.

Next, what happens? The child learns to put strings of words together, by babbling Dadada, Bababa, Mamama, and what happens? Mama gets reinforced. "He said Mama! He said Daddya!" From that point on, they become individual words. We start to play word games with children. We do repetition, we do riddles, we do tongue twisters and we do stories, all of which help us unknowingly develop our vocabularies and our minds. Anything that is fun is not perceived as learning, is it? "Joyce's choices" was not perceived as learning. It was just fun because you were playing word games. Anything that is fun doesn't have to be a lesson, unless it is painless and permanent, until somebody displaces it with something else.

So children learn, "She sells seashells by the seashore," and "A skunk sat on a stump. The stump thunk the skunk stunk and the skunk thunk the stump stunk." That's one of the harder ones I had to learn.

Where do you go from that? What are you learning? You are learning words, you are learning symbols. You are leaning fun. You are expanding your feelings and vocabulary, your emotional learning center at the same time. And then you go to school. What happens in school? You get these codes. You can scramble words or unscramble words, so you have messages that you can give to other friends of yours so nobody else can figure them out. One of the stories I have told is about the habitual drunk who went to church on Sunday morning and saw a woman sitting in a pew that was to be occupied by someone else. He walked up to her and said, "Marden me padam, this pie is occupewed, mollow fe and I'll sew you to a sheet."

People think that this is absolutely hilarious and they develop alternative languages and they are learning through all of this. One of the research things that is coming out now is absolutely fascinating and I want to learn more about it. When people learn a second language simultaneously with their first, it is learned in the same area of the brain, but when they learn a second language when they are adults and they already know the first, it develops in two distinct regions. So there is a different system for learning that second language, when you are an adult learning it than when you are a child when you learn both of them together. That might have some significance for some of the things that we do.

Along the way, if we are lucky, we have loving families who tell us bedtime and other time stories. The stories, a lot of the time, are often about good and bad, right and wrong; good guys wear white hats, and everyone lives happily ever after the storybook ending. How much do you suspect that the child who is listening to the story listens for the moral in the story? Now why is she telling me that story? What am I supposed to be learning? How should I resist this effort at making me understand the difference between good and evil? Nahh! They are there getting this kind of feeling from the words that are being said to them. It makes them *feel* good. They like it. They don't listen for the moral in the story. We aren't suspicious of why that particular story is told. All we want to do is to get the story. That's all that is important to us.

We pay very close attention to verbal and nonverbal communication. We talk about them and we pay homage to them. But we also must acknowledge the persistence of the unconscious mind and its determination, its persistence. The potential for trance may gradually diminish as other communication skills develop, but I believe the internal language association stimulus remains. That internal language stimulus is what we tap into when we are working with hypnosis and words.

Rossi explains that on the basis of state-dependent learning and talks about memory being explanations for behavior and trance. Candace Pert says, every peptide can be found with its receptor in the hippocampus, which is where memory is consolidated. By accessing a certain series of memories through a peptide substance, you get an emotional state. And the learning that takes place in that state is best remembered in that same state. When we tap into that kind of emotional state, we can go back to it anytime and recreate it for ourselves. It can be positive learning and can be negative learning. When we as doctors or therapists work with that, it's helpful if we know where that emotional state person is coming from.

Negative learning in this manner also can be insidious, in the same way that bedtime morals can be insidious. Sometimes we learn the bad things and sometimes we learn that we are bad. And sometimes we are lucky enough, through hypnosis and therapy, to transform that to learning what not to do ourselves, by experiencing other people doing it.

So, all of what I have been saying is that much of our early learning is sensed in our mouth, and kind of like a hidden snapping turtle, swims up to bite us at a later time when we least expect it. Chewing on a mouthful of that combination of aggression and vulnerability lets us taste a new reality.

Look at how many of our body language words revolve around the oral cavity. At the same time that the individual is learning language, they are learning vulnerability. The power of the cry gets diminished. The parents say, "Oh, let him cry, he's got to learn." The cry, then becomes one of helplessness.

This is the cry for help that is in effect when the patient or client comes to us. They would not *be* there, if there were not something out of phase that they are powerless to fix. And frequently it is related to all of these words that they have been hearing.

In their vulnerability there is a regression to a simpler time, when words were more eloquent and went straight to the meaning. A low key discussion gives you an insight into the patient's past. It is simple enough to request a regression during that recounting without any need for formal trance. "If you think back": those four words request a regression. If you think back to where you had lunch today, you see the place where you had lunch. If you think back to what you ate, you see what it was you ate. You get the image before you can give the words, when I say, "What did you have for lunch?" But you do it so fast, and you do it so much, you don't know how you do it, until you slow down and bring it to your attention. When you remember when you so enjoyed a particular favorite movie, or a special trance state, you regress to that state in order to do that. And this state dependent memory can help to reframe inappropriate responses.

People talk to me about the fact that I come on pretty strong. Yeah! I do! In my profession, where I have a very limited time to work with people, that's something that becomes necessary, because the patient wants to depend on the knowledge and the integrity of the doctor. When you take your car to the mechanic, you want to trust that the mechanic knows what he is doing. You, as the doctor-healer must serve as the authority figure. It doesn't matter what mode that car comes into you, whether it's sullen, fearful, subservient, frightened, hostile or hopeful, it's up to you not to take it personally. And to help, by earning the trust of the patient, so you can respect the development of these behaviors and the baggage that can result.

And that baggage is carried with our luggage of learned emotional language. To be opened at some later time and place, possibly in a most unexpected way, maybe in my office, with everything inside that luggage all jumbled together, because nobody is keeping it in its individual place. And it may be that when your patient goes to the dentist, that dentist gets that mess of luggage.

When do you go to the dentist? When a child is about 2½ or 3 and there is still a need for resolution about these feelings connected with the power of the oral cavity. If the dentist invades the oral cavity with no respect for psychological trauma, the child can be imprinted with a fear that will last for a lifetime, and generalize unless and until someone is able to defuse that memory and that behavior.

If the patient-client is lucky enough to have a relationship with a doctor who is psychodynamically oriented, even though she is only a dentist, it can be one of trust, vulnerability, learning and the comfort of self-control. Then we can proceed to change their perspective to a present-day reality.

Why, then, is it "only a dentist" and not "only a gynecologist" or "only a cardiologist" or only an "allergist or a therapist"? They too have a limited scope of practice. Is one's worth measured only by one's degree? And is the dental degree purely a mechanical one?

O. Spurgeon English,[18] many, many years ago said, in one of his teaching lectures in the hypnosis seminars, that there are some people in all walks of life who have the ability to handle other people, and there are some who, no matter how many books they read, will never master that skill.

Why do we make dentistry such an alien part of health care? Is it that the oral cavity has so much psychological significance that it is to be avoided? Many phobic patients have had unforgettably frightening dental visits, but in other cases, the negative experience might not have anything to do with dentistry, but generalizes to the oral cavity. For those patients, any situation that compromises their personal space is going to create a difficulty with coping with dentistry. It is not the fear of pain for anyone of you going to the dentist, it is the fear of loss of control and of making a fool of oneself over the pain.

And dentists more than most other people, routinely develop a relationship with the patient, but when we do it we invade their personal space. If we do it with respect and permission, that's one thing. If we walk in and bounce into the mouth without a by-your-leave, we deserve to be bitten!

---

[18] O. Spurgeoon English, MD, professor and department chair of psychiatry at Temple University Medical School from 1933 to 1964. English's textbooks dominated the field of psychiatry in the mid-20th century. He was the founder of psychosomatic medicine.

There is very little recognition of the value and psychological importance of the oral cavity, but you know what, there is obsessive attention paid to all the *other* cavities. Everyone understands the focus on the anal and genital phases of development, but pays lip service, a belittling phrase in itself, to the oral phase of development.

Look at all the emotions which are easily accepted as psychological manifestations of symptoms when they are expressed through the oral cavity. People often *say*, in these ways that are so important symbolically, what they cannot say verbally too. Why are bulimia and anorexia demonstrated through the oral cavity? Is it so difficult to interpret the nontraditional communication from the oral cavity as speaking through the oral cavity?

Let's consider this from the purely clinical perspective. Can you perceive the need for a psychodynamic understanding behind the situations I am going to give you? They are routine clinical proce-dures done by dentists every day, but which would never be attempted by physicians and therapists who judge the dentist's therapy credentials.

I will present the circumstances and you decide whether there could be any psychological implications in any of them. Please remember to add to each of these the apprehension that patients feel because they are anticipating pain.

1. *HIV/AIDS patients.* There are no psychological problems when you are working with HIV/AIDS patients. They just come in and open their mouths. That's all there is to it. Sure!
2. *Hemophilia.* What about doing surgery on a hemophiliac? Particularly without anesthesia other than the hypnosis and especially without using any concentrate or Factor 3. That's routine dentistry? Yeah, it really is, but there are all these psychological factors connected with it.
3. *Hepatitis.* What about working on active hepatitis patients and the concerns they have and the concerns I have as the dentist?
4. *Homosexuals.* We've gotten a little better at dealing with homo-sexual patients but some of the homosexual patients still have a lot of trouble going to the dentist. That was one of the first psy-

chologically oriented patients that I had. They are not so sure about the dentists' comfort with them.

5. *Bulimia and anorexia.* We have the eating disorders. Bulimics destroy their mouths. The acid when they vomit just takes all of the enamel off the inside of their teeth. They feel very guilty about it. They don't want to tell us. They have to share that secret with us even if it's unwillingly. Let me ask you. What are the ethics and the psychotherapeutic obligation with the knowledge, if I'm the only person who knows that person is a bulimic, and they don't want me to tell? What do I do?

They are destroying themselves and their mouths and I'm not allowed to tell anyone. Anorexics are very good at disguising their problem. Dentists are better in many ways at determining an anorexic than other people. Do we deal with it directly? Do we tell somebody? Because we are getting into the ethics and the psychotherapy obligations at this point, again. What do we do folks?

6. *PTSD.* How many of you saw *Marathon Man?* How many of you were upset with the dental scenes in *Marathon Man?* Making it a little more close to home, PTSD is something that dentistry deals with. It has significant dental impact on the torture victim whose teeth/mouth were the focus of the torture. And that happens oftener than it seems to. And we need to be aware of that. The survivors of those kinds of torture get toothaches and have to go to the dentist. I had one patient who wanted a general anesthetic and all of his teeth removed and dentures, because he couldn't face going to the dentist. He was a Dutch individual who was tortured in World War II by having his teeth extracted without any anesthetic. I probably wouldn't want to go back to the dentist if that had happened to me.

7. *Gagging.* Everyday we see patients with these potential problems. You all know how frequent sexual abuse is. And the dentist deals with it all the time. Because people who have been sexually abused get toothaches too, and they need their mouths taken care of routinely. How many of you want to deal with the gagging "habit" with a patient who was abused but has repressed the memory? I talked about that baggage all jumbled up and tumbling out; that's one of the times when it sometimes comes tumbling out, when you try to take an impression and

someone vomits all the baggage all over you and you have to deal with that.

8. *Phobia.* Or how do we complete restoration of the mouths of people who have been abused orally and have developed a phobia about dental work? How do you deal with that phobia without in some way, at least implying that they can get over the relationship of the abuse?

9. *Involuntary deviate sexual intercourse.* We get the rape victim who has to go to the dentist, but hasn't dealt with her fears. What do I do with that? Do I address it psychodynamically or am I just a mechanic? If I am just a mechanic, I ain't going be able to do anything.

10. *Smoking.* Then of course we have the routine work with smokers and their addiction. Those are the kinds of things we just shrug and say, "This is another one."

11. *Sleep disorders.* Lately I've been seeing ordinary sleep disorders, from sleep apnea to plain old snoring. We are supposed to have dental mechanical aids that are going to deal with this.

12. *Bruxism.* And then I had the therapist who called me and asked me what bruxism was, because he had a patient he was working with. I had a little bit of a problem with that. Had he done or was he capable of doing the physiological evaluation necessary to rule out physical origins for the bruxing? Or was he just believing that it was all psychosomatic? Because if you have one tooth that is a little bit high, unconsciously you work on that tooth to try and grind it down. And that ain't psychosomatic, it's physiological.

    I work with bruxism that manifests itself in TMJ pain. Does anyone here know what that is? TMJ is temporomandibular joint. If it is bad, you would gladly cut off your head at the neck, if it would stop the pain. But sometimes it's really a psychosomatic disease. Am I going to send that patient to the psychiatrist who doesn't understand what bruxism is in order to treat it? He doesn't know the meaning of the word, let alone the psychodynamics involved or the physiological diagnoses involved to rule out disc and joint disease. You are learning more about dentistry than you may want to know.

13. *Thumb sucking.* Sure it can be a habit. They do it in utero. But it can also be a way of expressing a great deal of frustration and dissatisfaction with one's family or something else. There are a lot of adults who are thumb suckers. That is something we also

have to deal with very, very carefully. They don't like being told that this may have a psychological significance.

14. *Surgery.* If the procedures we perform within the oral cavity were done anywhere else on the body, you would have a general anesthetic unless you are really, really good with hypnosis. We do them routinely in our offices. This takes a skill in preparing the patient to tolerate the process, at least partly because you have all these sharp instruments under your nose and you see what is going on. And it puts you at a distinct disadvantage unless you have the trust of the patient and have the nonverbal communication that says, everything is great. When the root of the tooth accidentally cracks during surgery, it makes this God awful crack, and you hear it all over the place. A dentist told me that when that happens, he says, "Finally!" As if he had wanted it to happen all along. Hey it works! I use it now.

15. *Cavities.* How many of you consider a cavity or restoration as a very simple thing? How many of you look at it as taking away a part of your body? Therapists agree about the need to mourn and grieve for loss of a body part, but they don't generally do it appropriately for tooth loss. They are very blasé about it. Where did the tooth fairy come from and why? Is it to ease the concern about the loss of a part and make it less scary?

Finally, how many of you like to go to the dentist? If you don't like to, why don't you? Might that influence your own attitude toward the oral cavity therapy? Or are you happy going to "just a mechanic"?

What I learned from Dr. Erickson was that it was not the induction of trance that was important, it was the utilization. And the utilization regarding dentistry demands an understanding of psychodynamics and psychotherapy to help the patient. To complicate our work with hypnosis and therapy in dentistry, it has to be accomplished along with our "mechanical" aspects, and most of the time we can't address the problem directly, because the patient does not want to discuss the reasons for their difficult behavior, which includes resistance to our work. And we not only have to work around their psychotherapeutic resistance, we have to work around their resistance to dentistry. All of this must be done as "brief therapy" since we have a limited number of appointments to fix the patient and fix the teeth.

Some patients come to our offices knowing they are receiving therapy, and that's okay, because they can deny it to their friends, because they are "only going to the dentist". I have a number of those. If it is so simple to demonstrate a need for the use of and understanding of psychotherapy and psychodynamics in dentistry, why is that role still ignored? Because "real" doctors think the body is all that is important, and the mouth isn't part of the body. They discount this communication organ and all it can tell them. And because therapists don't want to accept the responsibility and the obligation they have to deal with the oral implications of the patients they treat. And they don't know dentists who can.

Because therapists think only of "deep" emotional response and the mouth is too superficial. They ignore what they perceive is superficial. But the "deep" unconscious is very close to the surface in the oral cavity because you listen to your own unconscious and understand what is going on. And long ago, memories, every once in a while come up with a jolt and hit you. And you wonder where they came from. Maybe they came from that time way back, when you were learning power and learning power was focused in your mouth.

You become so entranced with really knowing all there is you need to know about how to make the memory of this experience change into something that it wasn't when it began, only because you hadn't thought about it as being what you didn't think it was.

And I've said that so often that some of you now don't have to go into trance, to stay out of the trance that I'm asking you to go into, and you can really hear the message that is in there. Because you are able to transcend the mundane into the magic of the mosaic of the many marvelous memories that you prefer, to the kind of things I'm asking you to think about that may not be as comfortable.

People aren't usually aware of their dominant assumptions, until they are challenged. And I'm challenging. The language of hypnosis challenges them. We speak of a paradigm shift. But the new paradigm has to function with the availability of new facts not available to the old.

Progress is not a steady curve. It is a series of events that create the information available in that new paradigm to make new connections possible. In the paradigm of change we spark the energy that oscillates within us. We link in series the transformers that recharge our storage batteries with direct rather than alternating current. This conduction of positive polarity discharges the negative current and the resistance is impeded. But we are galvanized as we remember to ground the voltage charge so the meters register only commutation values and we are safe.

Part of us is always working toward our emotional best. I'm putting this forth as a wake-up call to physicians, therapists and dentists to recognize and accept the dentist's responsibility to the whole patient and ability to provide appropriate psychological support to our patients and help them through the trauma of oral care. It is also a wake-up call to physicians and therapists to take the psychological significance of the oral cavity into serious consideration when tapping into that vast linguistic resource we all utilize to work with people—the Mouth! Thank you.

Okay, if anybody has any challenges or questions?

Question: Question about giving doctors/dentists a list of suggestions to give patients during surgery.

T: Which is very nice when you have a dentist who is willing to do this. Slow the bleeding down is different than stop it, and sometimes I want the patient to stop it, so I am very careful about the words I use. I was talking this morning about a nurse anesthesiologist who was given a list of statements to say during general anesthesia and the patient responded to those suggestions. We hear on an unconscious level at a much earlier age than we have culturally learned to respond.

Question: What helps you make a decision about reporting ethical obligations?

T: It depends a lot on the person. If that person is in therapy, I can go to the therapist and talk to them. If it is a young child, I am obligated by my license to talk to the family. In many instances I will talk directly. If it is an 18- or 19-year-old I will talk directly and I will confront that person. Physicians don't have an ongoing relationship with their patients. Therapists see patients when there is a problem. But a dentist sees a family on an ongoing basis and becomes a part of their lives. And the trust relationship that we develop will frequently permit that individual to talk to us when they can't talk to anybody else. But we'd better know how to talk and that's the hard part. I did a presentation to the Yankee dental congress a few years ago and the whole day was about language.

Question: How do you work with sound in dentistry?

T: You can use negative auditory hallucination [not hearing a sound that is present] or reframe sounds during surgery. That isn't hard to do. You can have a selection of music from hard rock or classical in your office and when the patient comes in, he can put the headphones on and listen to the music. Automatically, when they listen to the music, they go somewhere else and they don't pay attention. And I have to yell at them to get them to listen to me.

Chapter Twenty
Hypnosis in Dentistry

Dentistry and its techniques have improved greatly in recent years, but among the problems yet to be solved is a very fundamental one: how to get people to come into the dental office, sit in the chair, and submit to dental treatment. Estimates vary, but the National Institutes of Health (NIH) reports that only about 40% of our population seeks dental care and that a majority of those who avoid the dentist do so because of apprehension and fear.

Hypnosis offers one method for making dentistry more tolerable for the frightened patient. The patient can be taught to go into the trance state with the understanding that he will then be able to handle the dental situation with comfort, dignity and control. Hypnosis actually occurs spontaneously every day at the dental chair as a result of the stress of the situation and the special interpersonal relationship that exists between the dentist and the patient. Patients respond to suggestions from the doctor because of the rapport developed between them, and suggestion is the foundation for hypnosis.

The scientific basis for the dental application of hypnosis and suggestion is the proven relationship between tension and lowered pain threshold: the greater the tension, the lower the pain threshold, and the greater the pain realization factor. The person who comes to the office tense and frightened, but who looks with confidence to the practitioner for help, can learn to concentrate and relax and go into a useful trance state. The relaxation raises the patient's tolerance level and pain threshold, and this may be all he needs to get through the dental procedure with comfort. When the patient is comfortable and cooperative, the doctor is more relaxed and able to work more rapidly and surely.

Much of the delay in the acceptance of hypnosis in all the health professions has been due to a lack of understanding of the hypnotic situation. Before hypnosis can be utilized effectively, practitioners must understand something of its dynamics. It is, however, a difficult subject to study scientifically because the hypnotic situation is not a constant. It fluctuates with the needs of the patient and the doctor. Also, the reputation of hypnosis continues to be influenced by our past cultural tenets and the historical perspective in which it is viewed.

History[19]

Some knowledge of the long and complex history of hypnosis is helpful in understanding the phases through which it has passed to reach its current tentative position in the health professions. For the reader interested in more detail, many current references are available (Kroger, 1977).

The British Medical Association, in April 1955, approved the use of hypnosis for certain medical situations. In 1958, the Council on Mental Health of the American Medical Association recommended that instruction in hypnosis be included in medical school curricula. Two professional organizations, the American Society of Clinical Hypnosis and the Society for Clinical and Experimental Hypnosis, have established component sections in many countries to encourage high ethical and teaching standards.

Hypnosis finally is being accepted as a valuable adjunctive tool for the medical practitioner. It is recognized by many scientists, and data are being collected that should increase our knowledge of the nature of hypnosis. These contributions will eventually permit hypnosis to be both understood and accepted.

Myths and Misconceptions

Unlike most other disciplines of the healing arts, hypnosis has not been modernized over the past 50 years. Many practitioners,

---

[19] See Chapter One for history of hypnosis.

consequently, assume that the cultural qualities attributed to it during Freud's time are still valid. A more realistic approach is needed to correct some of the misconceptions. Although there are many interpretations of hypnosis, it is generally agreed that it is an altered state of consciousness. This state is somewhat related to what happens when an individual is reading and does not hear or respond when another person speaks. Beyond this, the agreement ends.

It may be easier to understand what hypnosis is by first recognizing what it is not. First of all, hypnosis is not a state of unconsciousness, accompanied by loss of autonomy and total amnesia. Neither is hypnosis something that someone does to another person; all hypnosis is self-hypnosis. The doctor simply facilitates the learning of the trance state and then helps the patient to utilize it, and the patient will also remember afterwards anything that is important to remember.

Theories of Hypnosis

There have been many theories regarding hypnosis. A few of the more current ones will be considered here. Theories of hypnosis and its phenomena are generally developed from observations of behavior. Since behavior itself is not yet well understood, hypnosis then becomes even more difficult to explain. Often the theories of hypnosis have been postulated in attempts to explain either the induction procedure or the phenomena, but in so doing the reasons for how and why hypnosis occurs have not been considered. Portions of each theory do not hold up under close experimental examination.

A belief held principally by a number of analytically trained individuals has been that hypnosis is a "regression in the service of the ego", in which the person experiences an infantile regression and elevates the therapist (doctor) to the role of parent. Numerous variations on that theory have been elaborated, all including some type of parentlike dominance and childlike submission. In experimental research, however, the submissive individual is not better at hypnosis, nor are patients more responsive to male authority figures. Transference theories have been another outgrowth of the psychoanalytic interpretation, but today it is generally accepted that transference is incidental to the trance, and no more common than in any other therapeutic modality.

Hypersuggestibility has also been frequently used to explain hypnosis. It does not, however, explain the process by which trance is achieved, nor does it account for the occurrence of spontaneous phenomena that have not been suggested. For a while a "dissociation theory" was promoted. This theory was based on the patient's ability to separate his awareness of an event from his emotional response to it. However, it does not adequately explain the presence of hyperacuity rather than the expected amnesia. Then, too, it is easily demonstrated that many other states exhibit this dissociative process.

Hilgard (Hilgard and Hilgard, 1976, page 185) has postulated a neodissociation theory of hypnosis. According to this theory, the normal ego controls our everyday behavior but coexists with some "outside consciousness" behaviors, that are capable of functioning simultaneously with the normal ego controls. This theory is a more tenable explanation of the variety of responses of which the patient in trance is capable.

For many years, T. X. Barber maintained that hypnosis was not a state at all, but simply the individual's recognition that he has the capacity to produce the phenomena commonly attributed to hypnosis without needing a "trance" (Barber, Spanos and Chaves, 1974). The many surgical procedures performed without anesthesia make it difficult to accept this theory. Recently, Barber has adopted a new theory of hypnosis that adapts to the natural trance utilization theory developed by Erickson that most clinicians advocate.

Orne and others have demonstrated experimentally that hypnosis is a "state" that can be produced and manipulated (Orne, 1972). The acceptance of incompatible occurrences as logical is one of the phenomena that can be replicated in this state, thereby distinguishing it from role-playing or simulating. Research into the theory of hypnosis continues today throughout the world. Possibly sometime in the future a theory that provides an adequate explanation for all of the ramifications of hypnosis will be developed.

Current Clinical Concepts of Hypnosis

Most clinicians accept hypnosis as an altered state of consciousness, similar to, and yet different from, many of the meditative states. If it is a natural capacity found in every normal individual, then it is something that can be learned to varying degrees in the proper circumstances. It is the focusing and concentration that result in the trance and permit the achievement of the desired phenomena. In this altered state of awareness there is an increase in concentration and an acceptance of appropriate (although sometimes seemingly illogical) suggestions. As a result, sensory and motor capacities are enhanced. Many doctors regard this ability as one of heightened awareness, or hyperacuity. In fact, some people are motivated to learn hypnosis because it promises a higher degree of self-control.

There are recognized "mechanics" that can help to establish the hypnotic situation. Motivation is probably the single most important factor. Beyond this, there must be concentration on the goal to be achieved. Both patient and doctor must believe that something good can be accomplished.

Much of the effectiveness of trance as used in the clinical situation is based on the motivational factors involved. This motivation is influenced by the verbal and nonverbal communication of the doctor as he uses both direct and indirect suggestions. The patient heeds the doctor's suggestions more carefully and accepts statements more literally than he would if he were not in a trance.

Hypnosis Utilization

Hypnosis is generally used for one of two basic reasons: to enhance control and to improve memory recall. Increased control may involve behavioral as well as physiological responses. When hypnosis is used to improve recall, it enables the psychotherapist to enhance recovery of memories and thus help an individual gain an understanding of a problem and its potential correction.

Hypnosis is not magic, nor is it a cure-all. It should never be used as a substitute for other necessary treatment, but it can be a very useful *adjunct* that enhances the effectiveness of the chosen treatment. It must be used within the doctor's own field of competence. It is extremely important that the doctor not attempt anything with hypnosis that he is not qualified to do without it. Just as a dentist who can administer general anesthetics does not have the right to take out an appendix, neither does he have the right to treat the patient's nondental problems by the administration of hypnotic principles. It must be remembered that the induction of trance does not accomplish the therapeutic goal. It is the utilization of the trance as a means to an end that is helpful. Simply learning to go into trance will not achieve anything.

Hypnosis can be used to some extent in all branches of medicine. It was accepted early on in obstetrics and gynecology. In addition to being helpful during the delivery, it is useful in eliminating hyperemesis gravidarum and in preventing spontaneous abortions. Most of the possible gynecologic symptoms respond to treatment using hypnosis.

Dermatology is another field that quickly accepted hypnosis because it influences the psychosomatic factors inherent in skin disease. Hypnosis has been used to reduce or eliminate reactions to allergens and histamines. Warts also have responded to direct symptom removal suggestions.

In some of the other fields of medicine the acceptance of hypnosis is still slow. Orthopedists have been very reluctant to work with hypnosis, despite the fact that when it has been used, the results have been gratifying, especially with back and joint pain. Genitourinary problems, such as urine retention, chronic bladder irritation and those necessitating treatment with hemodialysis, can be alleviated. Sexual dysfunction: hypnosis is used in this specialty as well as in psychiatry. Clinicians treating head and neck disorders use hypnosis for a wide variety of problems such as detection and alleviation of psychosomatic symptoms, adjustment to contact lenses, and throat spasms.

Hypnosis is very valuable in pediatrics because children respond well and quickly to imagery and other trance-inducing techniques.

It can be helpful in the treatment of many children's problems, from enuresis to dyslexia, from stuttering to learning disorders.

Internal medicine uses hypnosis in a wide variety of applications. It can be extremely helpful in treatment of various cardiovascular disorders such as essential hypertension and coronary disease. The psychosomatic aspects of many illnesses respond to the hypnotic approach. For example, it has proved helpful for migraine, ulcerative colitis, anorexia nervosa, and asthma. Severely burned patients also respond amazingly well to hypnosis.

The uses of hypnosis in anesthesia and surgery are probably the most commonly recognized. Total hypnoanesthesia is utilized for only a small number of patients. It is generally restricted to patients for whom other types of anesthesia are contraindicated because of particular health problems or other reasons. Hypnoanesthesia used in conjunction with chemoanesthesia is becoming more widely accepted. Hypnosis has many uses with respect to surgery. Preoperatively it is useful in alleviating fear and encouraging cooperation. It has been used during surgery to decrease bleeding and to achieve complete muscle relaxation. Finally, suggestions for postoperative comfort have proved useful, including good bladder and bowel function, healthy appetite and rapid pain-free healing.

Hypnosis and suggestion have been well received in oncology. Too often they were used as a last resort, but now a variety of approaches are being employed in conjunction with other methods of treatment. In addition to controlling pain, hypnosis can minimize the side-effects of radiation and chemotherapy, and stabilize the patient's emotional state. It has even been suggested that the change in attitude affected by positive hypnotic suggestion can increase resistance to the malignancy by somehow influencing the body's immune system and natural defense mechanisms.

Psychotherapists, whether psychiatrists or psychologists, can use hypnosis for any aspect of the therapeutic relationship. Therapists work with many psychopathologic states and must determine the advisability of teaching the patient to use hypnosis. It has proved valuable in a wide variety of applications in general therapy. It can be taught for pain control. In counseling psychology it is used in the treatment of anxiety, chronic stress and depression, and in working with habits such as excessive smoking and obesity. It also has applications in marital and family counseling and in the treatment of sexual dysfunction and severely disturbed patients. Hypnosis has proved effective in dealing with fears and phobias and in enhancing study habits and concentration. It can help achieve overall restructuring of a patient's attitudes and behaviors.

After such an exhaustive list it must be stressed that hypnosis is not applicable to all patients and that failures are a distinct possibility. The value system of the patient, the secondary gain from the symptom, and the motivation to use hypnosis and to get well must enter into the treatment modality. Hypnosis is not a panacea. If this is remembered, its use can be appropriately and effectively channeled.

Learning Hypnosis

For clinical purposes, hypnosis is an extension of the interpersonal relationship between the doctor and the patient. It is a natural skill that all normal individuals possess, but one that they have frequently either forgotten or do not recognize. Formalized and somewhat ritualistic induction techniques are therefore useful because they provide the opportunity for both dentist and patient to observe that something different is happening. This realization permits the trance state to be established and used in the treatment process.

There are more than 100 induction techniques that have been identified by name, including progressive relaxation, sand bucket, eye fixation and arm levitation. All of these techniques are designed to provide feedback to help the doctor and the patient know when the hypnotic trance state is achieved. Most doctors use these techniques in a permissive manner, enhanced by the use of the imagination. Some doctors, because of their own personality or the immediate needs of the patient, prefer to use an authoritarian approach. Whatever the technique, once it has been learned, it becomes possible for the patient to reenter the trance more quickly and easily on subsequent occasions.

For trance induction, the patient is asked to follow a series of graduated suggestions that use the principles of concentration and motivation. Frequently the patient is asked to imagine something and attach a strong emotional component to it. The emotional component makes the suggested imagery more effective.

After the basic induction procedure, additional suggestions are used to encourage a deeper trance state and thus ensure the desired response. Depth of trance is defined experimentally by the patient's ability to demonstrate certain phenomena, with the more difficult phenomena indicating a more profound trance. Phenomena evident in the light trance include relaxation, eye closure and slowing of muscular control and activity. In the medium trance, there is the beginning of some autonomic control, resulting in analgesia and catalepsy (rigidity of limbs). There is also some time distortion. All of these phenomena permit the patient to sit comfortably for long procedures with minimal chemical anesthetia. The deep trance permits the patient to remain in trance without closing the eyes, to achieve total anesthesia and control of bleeding, and to follow posthypnotic suggestions, thereby retaining unconscious control after the procedures are completed. As with any generalization, it should be remembered that these designations are only approximations, since clinical trance varies according to the patient's motivation and interpretation of the situation.

After the trance induction, the utilization phase begins. At this time the dentist-facilitator gives the patient appropriate suggestions regarding his dental needs. Because the patient in trance is less critical than he might otherwise be and will have few reservations about accepting the dentist's instructions, it is extremely important that the dentist realize the effects that such direct and indirect suggestions may have. Verbalizations must be positive, and nonverbal communications must match them. If the dentist tells the patient, "This will be a very simple procedure," but frowns and shakes his head, the patient will not be inclined to accept the statement. Similarly, a statement that "you have so much saliva in here I can't see what I'm doing" will increase the patient's apprehension. As a more positive alternative, the patient could be asked directly to "turn off your salivation" or be given an indirect instruction such as, "You know, it would help me to do this procedure more rapidly if you could get your mouth to become drier, so I could see more clearly."

Positive suggestions for the postoperative period are also given while the patient is in trance. If the dentist briefly outlines the expected progress, the patient will understand what to expect and have fewer questions regarding such feelings as thermal response, soreness, and increased circulation. Positive suggestions that promote rapid, uneventful healing can also be given. The dentist must realize that the interpersonal and intrapersonal relationship is constantly changing with the situation, the time, the motivation and the personalities involved. This is analogous to the use of drugs. A standardized dose is only an approximation, to be modified by the doctor's recognition of patient factors. Further, both patient and doctor understand that the results of the drug will not be immediate. It must be realized that hypnosis is a type of subtle handling of the patient in which the "standard dose" is varied to suit the patient, and one must be willing to wait for the results.

As the doctor-facilitator becomes more skilled in observation, he will easily recognize the patient's spontaneous readiness for trance and can bypass formal induction techniques. An approach that I have found very successful, and that is readily recognized by those involved in behavior modification, is the use of analogy and metaphor. Some examples of this will be given in the discussion of dental uses of hypnosis. One way to prepare individuals to accept change is to initiate confusion and get a shift in attention. This can be done by telling stories. The patient will not need to raise defenses against a story. Instead, he can listen to it as he did as a child, wondering not only what the story is about, but also why it was chosen. At the same time, the unconscious mind, activated by the trance state, listens to the multilevel messages in the story. It picks up nonverbal cues and persuades the conscious mind that this is, after all, only a story, but possibly one with a moral to be remembered and used.

With the patient's understanding that the trance is his own, termination of trance then becomes simply a matter of recognizing that the reason for the trance has been accomplished and that it is no longer necessary to remain in the trance. Trance termination is as individualized as the methods for entering the trance. It may be slow or rapid, may follow a set pattern or may simply end. Once the formal trance is terminated, any necessary posthypnotic behavior can begin. Examples of such behavior include maintenance of anesthesia for pain relief and reduction of circulation to a wart so that it will fall off from lack of nourishment. This is the method for generating long-term benefits from utilization of trance.

Utilization of Hypnosis in Dentistry

Much of the dental application of hypnosis overlaps with the basic principles used in medicine and psychology. As previously mentioned, the interpersonal relationship is an important facet of the communication effort. When there is good rapport between individuals, trust and curiosity will make teaching and learning the hypnotic trance a rewarding experience. The doctor, as facilitator, must constantly observe, work, reformulate and practice to be able to offer the patient appropriate suggestions. Utilization of trance requires that the facilitator listen to what the patient is really saying on all levels, since the chief complaint is often not the real reason the patient sees the dentist.

Although most practitioners automatically learn to listen, they do not deliberately make use of this skill. A dentist might begin to get training in induction techniques by taking a recognized course on hypnosis as taught by practitioners. The next step would be to practice the techniques and get constructive feedback. It is probably advisable for the dentist to begin with patients or office staff who are also friends and who like and respect him. Working with children can be a great help because they are naturally expert at hypnosis.

It is reassuring to recognize that hypnosis cannot do any damage to the patient. It is not an all-or-nothing procedure. If the patient simply learns to relax, that is beneficial. If nothing happens, the practitioner has done nothing irreversible and is just where he would have been without hypnosis.

It must be remembered also that there are some people who, for reasons of their own, do not want to be helped. For example, there are individuals who have enough secondary gain from their symptoms or difficulties that they might prefer to keep them. Recognizing this will make it easier for the dentist to accept the limited help he can provide.

Fear and Apprehension

Among the primary reasons patients do not seek dental care are fear and anxiety. Dentistry must deal with these problems if it is to offer a total service to patients. It is true that the dental profession is getting better at treating patients, but many patients do not seem to be getting better at receiving dental treatment. Part of dentists' responsibility is to perceive the factors involved in the motivation of each patient and use them.

Most patients are capable of integrating their fears quite well if they are given the opportunity to do so. The utilization of simple positive suggestion combined with appropriate hypnotic techniques enables the dentist to offer help. Often careful semantics, gentle operating techniques, and simple explanation of the necessary procedures are all the patient needs.

Most of a dental patient's anxiety is the result of a previous bad experience combined with fear of the unknown. When a patient is relaxed and in a trance, it may be necessary for the dentist to point out that the learned anxiety can be changed if the patient redirects his thoughts and emotions toward more desirable goals. An explanation of what should be expected can reduce the fear of the unknown but only if the patient is trusting and comfortable enough to listen to suggestions in a way that results in a new and better perspective.

There are a number of ways to approach a patient who is tense and frightened. The dentist might elicit an acknowledgment of the fearful, uptight behavior and suggest that the patient can be shown how to relax. As a first step, the patient can be given a simple demonstration of how tension increases pain. The patient should be asked to completely relax the hand so that it has no tension. The dentist can then press lightly on the back of the hand with an explorer. Next, the patient is asked to make a very tight fist, and the dentist again presses with the explorer. When the patient realizes how much more sensitive the hand was when made into a fist, the dentist can extend this example to explain total body response to tension. The dentist who is concerned about helping the patient can then show the patient some simple deep breathing exercises that aid relaxation. Progressive relaxation can be used to encourage still more involvement in the phenomenon of hypnosis, if that is desired.

Another useful approach to the tense patient is to give him more control over the dental situation. This is accomplished by establishing appropriate guidelines. If the patient thinks that sitting immobile in the chair until something hurts is the expected behavior, the dentist should say something like, "If you think this might be going to bother you, raise your hand, and I will stop so we can discuss it." The patient may test this statement once or twice, but then will develop enough trust in the effectiveness of the procedure to relax and accept it.

The patient will find it increasingly easier to relax as he learns to trust the dentist. As relaxation is increased, the pain threshold is raised. It becomes more difficult for the dentist to hurt the patient, and the patient is thus encouraged to relax even further. At this point, good dentistry can be accomplished with full cooperation on the part of the patient, and both dentist and patient can be well pleased with the results.

Habit Control

Many oral habits do not respond well to the dental approaches currently used. Hypnosis alone cannot treat these problems, but it can reinforce treatment aimed at eliminating them. The dentist should first know how to treat the dental problem without hypnosis. The only thing that is then necessary is that the dentist make careful use of semantics and logic, so that the patient in the trance state can accept even semilogical statements as making sense and all multiple-level messages as being positive. The effectiveness lies in the patient's recognition that the unconscious can listen to and hear meanings that promote change, giving him more motivation to give up the habit than to retain it.

Thumb Sucking

Intervention is appropriate only if the thumb sucking is interfering with the oral growth and development of the child, not if it is just something that bothers the parents. It is not necessary to institute a formal trance, but for those unfamiliar with working with children and hypnosis, it might be well to do so. As is the case with all dental hypnosis, the main skill involves knowing what to say to the patient once the trance is established. One possible approach is to get the child to agree that adults do not suck their thumbs, and that it will be only a matter of time until he will give it up. The dentist might raise some question in the child's mind regarding the possibility that the thumb is actually in control of the child's behavior and then question why it is that particular thumb (or finger) that is the problem. A discussion with the child can bring out suggestions from both patient and dentist regarding ways to change the habit and to test their effectiveness. These suggestions can be put into a behavior modification framework that includes home exercises to reinforce the change and signals to remind the patient to make the change. The child's family is asked to refrain from negative comments about thumb sucking and to encourage and support the new program. When this outline is presented while the patient is in trance, the prospects for change are excellent. A reward after a prescribed period of "no thumb sucking" (i.e. 30 days), is also part of the treatment. This is usually something the child has wanted and that he has tried unsuccessfully to earn before.

Tongue Thrust (Deviate Swallowing Pattern)

The deviate swallow responds well to hypnosis, which is usually attempted after numerous orthodontic corrections have failed to hold the teeth in position. The child is taught how to go into and remain in an active trance and is involved in exercises to correct the habit. In my practice, I utilize variations of the Garliner myofanctional therapy approach (1976, page 435). I explain to the child that he learned to swallow incorrectly and that there are exercises that can help. The exercises are then explained and assigned on a gradual 1 or 2 per week basis. We agree that the child will go home and twice a day will go into trance, go to his special place in the trance, and practice the exercises the agreed-upon number of times. The change in swallowing quickly becomes more automatic. The parents observe the child's eating and drinking behavior, as well as the resting swallow pattern. Continued observations should reveal that the swallowing pattern has been successfully changed.

Bruxism

The pain–dysfunction syndrome frequently associated with bruxism responds rapidly to control of the habit through hypnosis. For this reason it is one of the few oral habits for which the technique of symptom substitution is justified.

The patient is first taught how to go into trance, and during that trance is taught how to use autohypnosis. The instructions include an explanation that treats bruxism as an energy source. The patient is shown how to change the negative energy that is destroying his teeth and underlying structures into a positive type of energy that can be used to build up more appropriate muscles such as the wrist grip for tennis. The patient is instructed to hold a rubber ball or a piece of foam rubber in his hand when he goes to sleep. During sleep, each time he has the impulse to grind, he will instead increase his grip on the ball until the spasm passes.

This approach permits the dentist to regard bruxism as a habit rather than a symptom of a more serious psychological problem. If the bruxism does not respond to this type of symptom substitution, any further psychotherapy is outside the province of most dentists. It might then be appropriate to recommend that the patient have a consultation with a therapist to determine if there is something of more psychological significance to the habit. This approach to bruxism is to be used only after all other appropriate dental treatment, such as night guards and occlusal adjustment, has been completed.

Gagging

Gagging is one problem that frequently can be helped only through the appropriate utilization of hypnosis. Hypnosis is usually a last resort for the patient, who has exhausted all usual methods of treatment. There is a consistent pattern in my own approach to the gagging patient, particularly the denture wearer.

A semilogical approach utilizing an ego-strengthening attitude is helpful. This permits an assumption that the patient learned to gag to avoid or get rid of something unpleasant, and that the gagging subsequently became a way of rejecting anything distasteful. It is the responsibility of the patient to learn how to utilize hypnosis to permit the unconscious mind to unlearn this generalized response.

The treatment begins with a very thorough history taking, at which time the dentist listens for clues regarding the attitude of the patient, his family, and his friends toward the problem. This provides information regarding the patient's motivation to eliminate the inappropriate gag reflex. It also gives the dentist an opportunity to explain that since the gagging has developed over a long period of time, it may take a while to get over it. The history taking is followed by a brief discussion of dental hypnosis and a demonstration. The patient is shown examples of tension and given an explanation of the way in which this type of stress affects the entire body. He is then taught autohypnosis as a means to learn progressive relaxation, which he is expected to practice at home at agreed-upon times.

At the second appointment, the patient is generally taught a breathing technique to correct the gag reflex. In addition, the dentist discusses with the patient the advantages of eliminating the habit. Again, the patient goes home to practice the correct breathing technique, which provides a tangible reason to get over the gag reflex, rather than requiring that the change be all psychological. At the next appointment all the behaviors learned during the first two appointments are reinforced, and preliminary impressions are taken to demonstrate that the patient has successfully overcome the difficulty.

For the patient who is not edentulous or the patient who already has dentures but cannot wear them, the approach still involves ego-strengthening and quasi-logic offered during the trance state. The positive benefits are developed gradually in many instances but are of long-lasting benefit to the patient.

Many types of dental pain respond to the control offered by learning hypnosis. It is important to remember that hypnosis may not be effective for many patients, and that some patients prefer to keep their pain. Hypnosis is, however, one of the possible approaches to the handling of the patient's problems that possesses special and highly significant values at both the psychological and physiological levels.

When patients are under stress and expect to feel or undergo pain, the doctor automatically becomes a facilitator; hence his comments may be taken as specific suggestions. If the doctor pays close attention to positive semantics and provides both a logical explanation and optional responses, the patient can become more involved in discerning the type of feeling occurring rather than in responding to the feeling of pain. A conscious effort should then be made to avoid negatively charged words such as *needle, hurt, burn* and *pain*. The description offered should be designed to confuse the patient, causing him to wonder what it is that he will feel, rather than how much pain will be felt.

A method of administering a local anesthetic provides an example of this confusion approach. When the topical anesthetic has taken effect, the doctor should say something strongly incongruous to the patient just as the injection is given. A sample statement might be: "Now, just wiggle your left ear for me, please!" After the injection is completed, the dentist can explain the effectiveness of the distraction so that future injections can be completed more naturally because the patient understands that it need not hurt.

Hypnoanesthesia can be utilized as an occasional substitute for chemical anesthetics if the patient's motivation is sufficiently strong. The patient can be taught to turn off the pain sensation in the area involved. This can be achieved by teaching the patient glove anesthesia (imagining the hand is placed in ice water so that all feeling leaves it), by turning off the sensations that carry pain impulses to the brain, or by "taking a trip" so that the patient's mind is not paying attention during the procedure but is somewhere else more desirable. All types of dental procedures can be performed utilizing hypnosis as the sole anesthetic in appropriate situations.

The control of the autonomic nervous system that is made possible through hypnosis can enhance relief of pain arising from tumors, the temporomandibular joint pain–dysfunction syndrome, and facial pain from other sources. The types of control offered the patient can be direct (such as muscle relaxation) or indirect (dissociative). The patient accepts responsibility for control of his symptomatology. Hypnosis enables the patient to re-examine his attitude toward the pain and restructure his adaptive response to it. There is a great deal of satisfaction in teaching patients with severe chronic pain how to gain sufficient control over it to function in a comfortable manner.

Physiological Controls

In many of the articles on hypnosis, there are references to regulation and cessation of the circulation of blood to an area, as well as to increased speed of tissue healing after injury. This indicates that the trance state permits the patient to control the physiological processes of the body through the automatic nervous system.

Patients seem to be able to control bleeding with much less effort than one would expect. Recognition of a patient's stress during surgical procedures lets the doctor offer a verbalization something like this, given in an assured, self-confident manner: "After these teeth are removed, it will be helpful for both of us if you will not bleed excessively. Please let the sockets fill to the top and then turn off the bleeding." Although the patient may not believe such a statement, the dentist must be convincing in the presentation. The patient then recognizes that other people apparently can and do stop bleeding when asked, or the request would not have been made. If the patient asks for an explanation, a brief analogy will suffice. The automatic control that occurs when one blushes or when one uses a cold shower to close off the blood vessels are useful illustrations. In addition, the patient is told not to worry about how to do it, but simply to relax and let it happen.

This approach works well with hypnoanesthesia, which can be used in conjunction with either local anesthesia or conscious sedation. Additional motivation may come from explaining that bleeding control permits the dentist to complete the procedure more quickly. A surprising number of patients stop the bleeding completely, while others reduce it dramatically. Salivation control is achieved in a similar fashion. A comment that the dentist can do the job more efficiently if the patient will turn off the salivation can be very effective.

Recently, I have had rewarding results in working with hemophiliacs, using hypnosis to control bleeding. Without the use of fraction or of concentrate, Type A hemophiliacs with less than 1% Factor 8 have been able to control bleeding during surgery and postsurgically with hypnosis. This alone should encourage many more health professionals to investigate the potential of hypnosis. Just as patients are able to control bleeding and salivation, they also seem to heal more rapidly through use of hypnosis. Hospitalized patients who use hypnosis for comfort are discharged from the hospital more quickly than those who do not use it. There are fewer complaints from patients, and tissue repair is much faster than it is for those who are not using hypnosis.

References

Barber, T. X., Spanos, N. P., and Chaves, J. F. (1974). *Hypnotism: Imagination and Human Potentialities*, Elmsford, UK: Pergamon Press.

Erickson, M. H. (1958). "Naturalistic techniques of hypnosis", *American Journal of Clinical Hypnosis*, 1, 3.

Garliner, D. (1976). *Myofunctional Therapy*, Philadelphia: W. B. Saunders.

Gill, M. M. and Brenman, M. (1959). *Hypnosis and Related State: Psychoanalytic Studies in Regression*, New York: International Universities Press.

Haley, J. (ed) (1967). *Advanced Techniques of Hypnosis and Therapy: Selected papers of Milton H. Erickson, M.D.*, New York: Grune & Stratton.

Hilgard, E. R. and Hilgard, J. R. (1976). *Hypnosis in the Relief of Pain*. Los Altos, CA: William Kaufmann.

Kroger, W. (1977). *Clinical and Experimental Hypnosis*, Philadelphia: J. B. Lippincott.

Orne, M. T. (1972). On the simulating subjects as a quasi-control group in hypnosis research: "What, why and how", in E. Fromm and R .E. Shore (eds), *Hypnosis: Research, Development and Perspectives*, Chicago: Aldine-Atherton.

Pierce, J. M. and Thompson, K. F. (1980). *Hypnoanesthesia and Control of Bleeding During Oral Surgery on a Hemophiliac*, (Film), Shadyside Hospital, Pittsburgh.

Part VII
Clinical Demonstrations

This section opens with an insightful commentary by Sidney Rosen, "The Evocative Power of Language".

These masterful clinical demonstrations are our only glimpses into Kay Thompson's clinical work. She refused to do therapy in public because she felt it compromised the confidentiality of the volunteers, and she shared that "any therapy that was done during these demonstrations, was purposely kept outside of the awareness of the audience" as Erickson, her mentor, had done. In these demonstrations, we listen to the weave of her magical, entrancing language into suggestion, motivation, changing perspectives and word permutations, which expand any fixed idea about a symptom or reality. New options and realities are presented in metaphor, stories and convincing reasoning, which completely absorb the listener's attention.

Dr. Thompson was unusually intuitive and had an exceptional ability to develop rapport with a broad range of clients. Being perceptive, she taught, was partially the result of years of observing patients with meticulous attention and accessing interpersonal communication on multiple levels of consciousness. She once suggested that if we reviewed her clinical demonstrations, she could explain every one of her interventions by noting her studied observations of the client.

These demonstrations and clinical discussions explore her therapeutic communications, clinical goals and engagement with clients and provide a unique and profound learning opportunity for the reader.

Chapter Twenty-one, "Conversational Inductions with Utilization of Spontaneous Trance", contains two delightful conversational inductions. The first demonstration is a wonderful example of ego strengthening messages given within a metaphor about playing music. In the second, Thompson plays with sailing and control.

In Chapter Twenty-two, "Strategies of Hypnotic Utilization", Thompson directly addresses therapeutic issues in two outstanding clinical demonstrations. This is a rare opportunity for the reader to observe Thompson doing therapy and to hear her define themes, discuss her clinical interventions and explain utilization. In the first demonstration, Thompson utilizes hiking up a mountain as her surface metaphor for therapeutic communication. Several of her favorite metaphors are threaded through this absorbing journey. In the second demonstration, Thompson teaches the client a great deal about physiological control within a series of fascinating metaphors.

In Chapter Twenty-three, "Pain Control and Healing Enhancement", Thompson gives an impressive demonstration of her work with pain. Following a trance induction through a formal structured technique, Thompson first convinces her client that there is no longer any reason for her pain and then redirects the client's energy toward soothing and healing her injured area. Detailed physiological instructions are an important part of Thompson's absorbing communications.

In chapter Twenty-four, "Clinical Posthypnotic Suggestions", Thompson ingeniously incorporates numerous posthypnotic suggestions in two elegant clinical demonstrations. These captivating examples are an important display of the possibilities of therapeutic language.

The Evocative Power of Language

Sidney Rosen

While conducting therapy or teaching, Kay Thompson would say, "Not a word passes my lips before I have thought of it first." When I heard this statement in a workshop I found it hard to understand. I knew that she did not mean that she was obsessing on or even consciously naming each word that she spoke. That would have slowed her verbalizations almost to a halt. I realized that the "thinking" must occur on an unconscious level. After reading instructions to her musician friend in Chapter Twenty-two it was clear to me that she utilized time distortion in the same way that she instructed him to do.

Kay frequently taught that, "I believe that everything that I say, once the patient walks in that door into my office, is leading toward the ultimate goal." So we have evidence that Kay was methodically/meticulously processing her language on multiple levels. One was incorporating orientation toward the goal, sometimes including preplanning exactly what she was going to say, as in her work with patients in acute pain situations. At the same time, she was utilizing trance in several ways. She openly described developing an intense interpersonal trance for accessing her and her client's unconscious process. And she utilized time distortion during her communication, to scan what she was saying prior to speaking.

In general, Kay's approach to therapy and to teaching (she tended to equate them) was relatively simple—even as it was hidden and decorated through her brilliant and creative use of words, images and nonverbal communications. It is mostly an injunctive approach. She prepares her patients and students by directing their attention toward their own "knowing and power" even as she presents examples, images, and metaphors to "jump start" their inner searching so that they can find resources to apply to their concerns and needs. She suggests, "So you already know everything you need to know about how to increase your circulation to carry the oxygen and nutrients to heal the parts of your body that need to heal." Then, just to make sure that he knows, she repeats previous suggestions: "You know how to make that happen by thinking warm to carry that flush ... to carry oxygen into that area ... to carry away waste products."

Unlike Erickson, who almost always answered questions with another story or metaphor, Kay often explains her interventions in relatively simple terms. In Chapter Twenty-two, for example, she points out that she used metaphors of climbing, the growth of a flower and the utilization of "pebbles", or blockages on the path to augment growth and mastery. She notes that she induced relaxation with the imagery of a swimming pool and the warming sun.

The depth of searching was tied to getting into the water with the recurring question, "How deep do I want to go?"

As Erickson did in his story, "Dry Beds" (Rosen, 1982), Kay adds directives for reinforcement. Erickson had instructed, "You can practice starting and stopping, starting and stopping." Kay says, "When you practice relaxation, practice imagining taking a walk to the swimming pool or taking a walk beside the river. You can tune in to the ability to relax and produce your own endorphins and enkephalins, your own interferon." She might preface an injunction with a phrase intended to bring the communication down to the level of a child. For example, she explains (Chapter Twenty-two) that she introduced more complex language after "protecting it" by saying "it *really doesn't matter* whether the front of your mind hears it". Erickson might have appealed to the child by inducing regression and talking as an adult to a child, telling corny jokes or speaking in simple language.

It is obvious that Kay and Milton shared some very common elements in their work—the use of metaphors, reframing and post-hypnotic suggestions. However, they were quite different in their content and delivery. For example, Erickson's stories tended to be at least a step removed from him, referring, for example, to anthropo-logical facts, experiences with previous patients, and most closely to family tales, all presented with mild amusement. In fact, tape recordings of his last years are punctuated by repeated laughter, which caused him to cough frequently. On the other hand, Kay's stories are more likely to refer to her own interests and experiences and they tend to be presented seriously, often using poetic language.

Instead of directly ordering or even suggesting certain skills, Kay will gently, almost casually, suggest them, as in Chapter Twenty-two: "You need to get in touch with the fact that you now can learn to use the switches that carry the feeling pain to that part of you body that you want to control." She then presents the example of a rheostat "to know whether it's safe to turn it all the way off".

In her treatment of temporomandibular pain Kay clearly illustrates her practice of turning destructive into constructive and perpetua-ting the result with posthypnotic suggestions. First, she has her subject transfer tension into a clenched fist. Then she says, "Every time yours jaws come together ... there's going to be an automatic signal ... electric current ... into your hands ... clench your fist." She has previously pointed out that while clenching the jaws is destructive, clenching the fist builds up forearm muscles for swimming or playing tennis. Finally, she suggests, "When that stress is coming back, you can use ... the same clenched fist and tightness."

In Chapter Twenty-four, Kay's word play is extensive and especially rich (e.g. "that void that you have avoided filling"). In this chapter, as in the other chapters on clinical demonstrations, her conversational inductions and trances include innumerable "interspersed suggestions". They are so continuous that "interspersed" is an inaccurate term. Everything that Kay says in these sessions, including her questions, constitutes suggestions regarding multiple subjects, including trusting yourself, distorting time perceptions to suit your needs, to living today and to taking and letting go of control. And she adds, "It was all posthypnotic suggestion work from my frame of reference." Her unique way of delivering suggestions is marked by her obvious joy in playing with words and her open eyed enthusiasm and expectation that her subjects can do the things she asks.

There is so much to be learned from these chapters, not only about how to do therapy, but, on a deeper level, about how to conduct one's life. As expressed in Chapter Twenty-four, Kay's comment about control was especially meaningful to me. "It's only the people who don't have control who have to have it all the time to be sure they don't lose it. When you are sure you really have it, you don't need it because you can get it anytime you want it."

Like Kay, I often look at life as moving from one kind of "trance" to another. As she indicates in Chapter Twenty-four, therapy can help a patient "to come out of the trance he was in, in order to have the opportunity to go into another trance".

It is impossible to summarize the artistry of Kay's therapeutic communications, unique style, and her ways of maximizing the evocative power of words. Reading and rereading the transcripts in this section will help people to get a feeling for Kay's special style and creativity and the variety of ways she utilizes the power of language. Readers will undoubtedly try to imitate her at first, adapting her examples to their own work.

But in order to truly emulate Kay Thompson, and indirectly, Erickson, I believe that we need to enter into a "therapizing" or a "teaching trance", in which we focus on the needs of our patient or student, ask ourselves what the situation calls for and trust our unconscious mind to guide us in guiding and encouraging his or her growth and healing. When we do this we can tap into and utilize appropriate material from our life experiences and from the rigorous practice and training Kay so consistently emphasized as necessary to feed our unconscious. Like Kay, we must always be aware of the evocative power of words, because hypnotherapy is fundamentally a process of healing with language.

Reference

Rosen, S. (ed.) (1982). *"My Voice Will Go With You": The teaching tales of Milton Erickson*, New York: Norton.

Chapter Twenty-one
Conversational Inductions with Utilization of Spontaneous Trance

Two Clinical Demonstrations with Volunteers

First Demonstration: Playing Music [20]

T: That part of you which says, "Hey, what is in this that I can use later?" You don't even have to worry about it, because you are busy absorbing it, so that thinking about it isn't necessary. What do you do when playing the guitar that is kind of like the same thing?

V: A friend says that my emotions come out when I play guitar. My experience is that I shift into an entirely different experience of myself and that things take on a depth and meaning that I don't allow in an ordinary state.

T: So you move into that kind of movement in order that the motion can let you deal with the emotion that mentally you might not be motivated to use otherwise? It's really kind of nice to have a safe place like that to go. I think that you are doing the same thing with hiking. Did you ever do the campfire bit? End of the day and the really nice tired.

V: I did one on a rafting trip in the Grand Canyon. Extraordinary.

T: How many people on your trip?

---

[20] Note: There was a problem with the recording, so the beginning of this tape starts in the middle of the conversation between Dr Thompson and the first volunteer. Ed.

V: Some good friends and acquaintances.

T: Did you do the whole trip?

V: We went halfway to the ranch and hiked out.

T: Very good. It's a really nice feeling when you have been through that for the day and you have kind of tested your resources. The nature part of that is so overwhelming and yet it's nice because it isn't overwhelming, because you can just sort of accept it and absorb it. And then you pay it back that night with your music, because that's what you do when you've had dinner and you're tired and sit around and everybody gets into that mood which is so appreciative of everything that happens. The music that comes out is more than just music. It's really a way of saying the most marvelous things.

I think a lot of times that's one of the things that we are all kind of jealous about learning. We know it's in there somewhere— that ability to reach for it and to access it whenever we want to and whenever it's appropriate. Part of that pride of being able to give back and share is one of the things enough of us don't really pay attention to. We're too into the competitive aspect of living without realizing that the only person who counts in that competition is yourself. Being able to enjoy with friends and to work with them and compete to get that boat to do the things it really needs to do to get through the rapids. The absolute thrill when you come through a really tough one and you know that the water had the ability to take that boat and flip it anytime it wanted to.

It's the ability you have and the skill of working and doing what you are asked to do and told to do sometimes in a hurry. It's really different because it's competing against yourself and not with somebody else. When you're through, you can sit back and do something we very rarely have a chance to do. You can say, Hey, I did a good job today. I deserve to be really proud of how I handled myself and the way I functioned. I need to sit here and let that combination of absolute reverence for the outdoors and for the water and the moon and the weather work together. And the fact is that you are a real part of that and you can have within that a kind of exhilaration, that nobody can ever take away. Because when you tap into it, it's the ability to say that no one, no one understands that kind of thing unless they've been there. Once they've been there, there's no way, anyone can even chip away at a little bit of that.

When you get enough of those kind of experiences, it's almost as though you could build on those and you could have the kind of stepping stones you need to climb any hurdle that has been put in front of you. You have enough satisfaction and absolute conviction that you are doing what you need to do. And it's so very, very special. And the neat part of it is that when you do that, you can choose the people that you bring along with you. You can choose the people who really hear what you are saying and feel the kinds of emotion you feel.

And when you play that music, you reach out with your song. And your voice, when it does that, isn't really yours. It's a combination of all the voices that have ever done that, because you have joined a community of people who understand a great many things that most of the people in this world will never have a chance for. And I think what you get from that is a need and a real desire to share that. You have the skill through the knowledge that you have used this, through the ability with the guitar and playing around with the piano and your singing, and there's a way of reaching out to a lot of people through your music.

And you find you can take what nature has given you and you can take the nature parts that you have learned to coordinate and to capture. And really make them do what you want them to do in order to let you understand that you are a part of this. And the rhythm in that kind of response really deals with what is way down inside of you that you want to give back. That music that's inside you can create, I was going to say,a symphony, but it really can be a ballad, because it has words that reach people in ways that a symphony can't. You can feel music and you can enjoy it, but there are still people who need the words, who need the picture painted for them. Anyone who can sing of that kind of response can do so much more than the person who just talks about it.

And you can let your voice and your knowledge and your ability go with you through so much of the memories you have, because those kinds of memories let you do whatever it is that you really want to do, and that you need to do. And if you think back and remember all of those kinds of good feelings, each one of them being a stepping stone toward that place that you are going to go. You realize, *that's better*, that the competition of having had to remember melts, dissolves, and just fades away in the satisfaction of feeling the knowledge, the security, the skill as you let yourself enjoy knowing how to believe in yourself.

It doesn't really matter that we all believe in you. The only thing that matters is that you know yourself and your potential. And any time you really need to, you can use that music as a path, a path you have traveled so many times before. And when you first start walking on a path, you have to watch, you have to pick your steps pretty carefully. Very soon you get the rhythm, you get the flow, just like the music. When that happens, you don't have to watch the ground any more. You can start to look around and you can feel the sounds and as you hear the real softness of the circumstance of the hiking. And you feel the sounds of the music that pour through your body and as you look around, behind, in front, and beside and you feel the warmth at the same time that it's cool. The warmth is satisfaction and the cool is comfort and it's really nice.

As you take those things that are so precious to you on that trip, you feel the flow and become part of that hike, that path. You find that it is exhilarating at the same time that it's restful. Because what relaxation really means is control .When you know that you have everything you need, you never really have to be worried about any of it because you're always going to be able to do what you need to do, at the right time, and in the right way. And the responses you have are those you can live with, because the competition that used to be of such concern, has been out-distanced and outclassed by your own classy attitude towards the kinds of things you want to do. That path is as long as you choose to make it at any one time. Because you pick your destination on that trip and you know how to get where you are going.

It doesn't matter if it rains or storms; it just shows the beauty of nature in there. It gives you the ability to understand that you can handle anything that you need to do. The music that you build inside you sometimes breaks forth spontaneously, because it feels so good. And the kind of power you tap into lets you really feel the potential that you deal with everyday. And sometimes you can coast and float because you are going downhill, and it takes half as long and you can look around a little more and you can really enjoy it. And it can be fun, and that's one of the things you need to know, because that satisfaction is almost a feeling of smug, because you've know *you've* got it made. And whatever it is, and wherever it is, it's really right for you.

It really doesn't matter that I know any of this. The only thing that matters is that you feel that challenge of change I talk about—the thrill, the anticipation and the excitement. Because the risk of that opportunity is so fulfilling, that you can feel so full of that kind of satisfaction of that potential. And you find that you do know all the things that you didn't know. You can get a handle on everything you need to and you can really get that in your hand and there are people who can reach out a hand anytime you need it. And you can do within yourself, without yourself, about yourself, all the things that matter. We don't really need to name them. They are nice, they're goals, they are objectives.

The real thing is having it all together because the music that you can hear out there, where you are so much your own person, is the greatest music you can ever want to play. I guess I think that's really what this message is all about. Because that's the kind of thing that each of us wants to do—to reach out and be better able to do whatever we need to do. And I wonder what it wants to do. And what it is it needs to do. And the rhythm and the power and the *real knowledge* lets you see that you can seize any opportunity to do it and that it's always the appropriate response.

And that kind of sensitivity is okay, because then you can handle not only everything that you know that you want to do, but also the unexpected kind of things that firm up and confirm that resolve. And this is a beginning of some things that are really good and it is okay because you let it be. It really is. And the amount of resolution can feel very much like when you have just gone through one of those famous Grand Canyon rapids. And the relief and the knowledge that you can do everything you need to do just really feels so good.

And you can hold onto those good feelings and bring them back to balance everything that you need to do in the way that you weigh all those things. Because the kind of work that is play is also progress and you are allowed to enjoy and that is really what life is all about. So as you become so much more sure, you find that you do what you knew you were ready to do, even though you weren't sure that you were ready to do it. And that's a kind of a reorientation and goal setting and resolution, even though it's not New Years. Although sometimes years can start at different times. Birthdays are always a new year for everybody, aren't they? At least I think so. I have a friend whose birthday is December 26, and I didn't know it until he was 30, because they always celebrated his birthday on July 26.

V: My birthday was Sunday.

T: Happy Birthday! And a whole new year.

V: That's a fact.

T: I'd rather be lucky, than good! I had no idea he had a birthday. It was very nice to have a birthday for me!

Question: In another setting, would you have asked him about his hands?

T: No, I made a lot of comments about doing whatever he needs to do, which could be communicating to me. Were you really listening to me? You can use me as a point to take off from and to come back to and that's fine.

Question: About when and why I used the term *appropriate response*.

T: I used it in response to his facial expression. The word appropriate was utilized deliberately as a grounding word. Remember where we are and the circumstances and appropriateness is appropriate.

Question: In this type of work, is there ever more interactional conversation?

T: My objective was to do conversational induction with spontaneous trance in a concise and obvious way as possible. In a therapeutic kind of session, we would have gotten into more conversation. I took over and started talking well before I would have in my office.

The advantage of a conversational induction is that the individual can go into trance and come out of trance and then you can teach him about hypnosis after that.

Second Demonstration: Sailing

T: He's from Hawaii. If I were from Hawaii and saw all of those lights on this stage, I would feel I was in the sun. What would it take to get you to be warm enough to be back there, rather than here?

V: To think about the beaches or hiking on a hot day.

T: You are not allowed to go hiking. We just went hiking. Sailing?

V: That's okay too.

T: I'm out of my element, I don't know much about cats. I have to stick to just ordinary boats. What is the difference between a cat and the other kind of boats?

V: Catamarans have two hulls.

T: Yes, that's as much as I know. You are in a trance. What is the difference between sailing in a cat and an ordinary one-hulled boat? What would I notice?

V: Speed. They're faster.

T: Do you jump between one hull to another?

V: Only if you are in big trouble.

T: I'm in big trouble. (*Laughter.*) Tell me about a catamaran and I would really love to go.

V: You have two hulls with a canvas or a plastic tarp and a metal frame around that. It's like sailing on a monohull boat. You have a lot more room to move around on and they go an awful lot faster.

T: What happens when there is too much wind?

V: There is never too much wind. You make adjustment in the sails. It's kind of fun to go up on one hull. You just climb up. If you are cruising, that's different than day sailing. I don't sail if there is too much wind. I think it's dangerous. I like the danger and excitement enough to be out in winds up to 25 to 30 miles an hour, but not above that. In that wind, a cat can go 17 to 20 miles an hour.

T: That's skimming. Wow! What you are talking about is an evaluation of the circumstances, so you are sure you can be in control. You end up with the recognition that if there is too much wind, the sails get too full, you get out of control.

V: Yeah. You can let the sheet out.

T: How long does that take, depending on your crew?

V: A second.

T: What goes into making the decision to use that second?

V: It feels like the boat is going to capsize.

T: So instead of going overboard, you do that.

V: You lean out.

T: How many people are enough to balance it?

V: You could take two but it was designed for one.

T: You are out there with the wind and the water and the control issue by yourself. How long could you stay out without being beyond nicely tired and staying out too long?

V: Two, three hours.

T: At the end of 2½ hours and the recognition that you have gone out pretty far and it was going to take a really long time to get back. What kinds of adjustments can you make both in your physical being so far as what you do, and with the catamaran itself to make it easier to come back in? Is there something you can do?

(*Pause.*)

And what happens when you think about all those things, you have to end up monitoring your entire system, not as though you are here, but as though you are there. It's all right to be there and still know you are here. You can do two things at once. And in doing two things at once, you can make the appropriate adjustment to respond to being here and understanding there is a message here, in terms of doing whatever it is you do there. So the kinds of control that are required when you sail the cat, generalize to the kinds of control when you are not in the water, when you haven't really pushed yourself beyond the limits.

When you can use all of your kinds of awarenesses and unconscious cues and bring all that kind of thing into play, and in that second that it takes you to spill, you can really understand exactly where to put your weight, exactly what you need to do, to get the results you need to get based on whatever it is you want to do. It doesn't make any difference whether you think about that.

Once you recognize that you access your unconscious that way, I wonder what kind of understanding of change is permitted to surface and work its way up to the conscious level. So you can acknowledge that you have these skills and it hasn't been necessary for you to use them very often, because as you say, you don't go out when it's too dangerous to go sailing.

You find that you started out not really knowing too much about her, and you had to work with her, with the catamaran to find out what you could do, and then you keep pushing the limits. And life is very much like that. And you take all of that and do the jigsaw puzzle of putting all the pieces in where they fit. And what I'm doing is saying, Hey, there are a lot of other places where you can use the kinds of knowledge and the monitoring to keep from going overboard, and to know when to let that wind out and to know when it's too windy, too rough to go sailing. You don't have to know why you know those kinds of things. That kind of control continues to get stronger and stronger without you really having to understand why.

I know you've heard me talk about knowing things that you don't know you know. But, I wonder whether you are going to spell the "know" one way or the other way, depending on what it is you need to know about it. And whether you really have to come out of trance to respond to that or whether you don't. Do you know?

V: I don't know.

T: Does it matter?

V: No.

T: Does it matter that it doesn't matter?

V: No, k-n-o-w.

One of the things that we were doing was responding to the question whether you could have a lot more interaction when somebody was learning about trance and hypnosis. He's in a very nice trance and so am I. Somehow, we are able to talk.

Question: Did he recognize when I started doing the talking?

V: It seems that it was when she started talking about coming back after 2½ hours. I was visualizing, seeing and feeling myself following the wind, because those were the circumstances she created.

Question: You didn't want to break into my conversation and start responding?

V: Didn't I respond?

Question: How did I know he was in trance when he came up on the stage?

T: The second question I asked him was acknowledging that fact that I recognized that he knew that I knew he was in trance. He looked different in the sense of expectancy. Besides, that's what he came up here for. There was a methodical element to the behavior that wasn't the free-flowing kind of thing that I would have expected under this circumstance. There was more of an attention kind of interaction, the same kind of alteration of perception when he went back into trance. There is a shift in focus that lets him respond, by being off somewhere else and to think differently. I picked up on the literalness of the responses. When I am in trance, I tend to respond very literally also.

This was fun. This was one of the things I wanted to get across. He was doing more work and was internalized a lot more. I thought it might be interesting to give an opportunity to see this could be a playful thing with humor and a lot more interaction. He picked up and went along very nicely. In return for him picking up, I really needed to offer him something for putting himself in this kind of position, so that's when I made some of the suggestions. I do appreciate him coming up here and being in this kind of situation. It's not the most comfortable place in the world to be.

Question: Did I know the different volunteers?

T: Yeah, I know the first person from the institute. I didn't know anything about him as a person. He said he had a special relationship, which was one of the things I was encouraging and supporting. With the second person, it was just, let's swing it and have fun.

Question: What kinds of strategies do you use for making it happen?

T: My expectation in terms of making the trance happen is to present a smorgasbord and see what the person is going to tune into. And then tap the potential that they have to go inside their heads and incorporate what I am saying, and the way they are responding to the need that they have expressed. Sometimes, the need is not expressed verbally. It is sometimes in a less threatening way, particularly the way I come on. They can leave whatever they want to leave. They are willing to share more than when I say, "Put your feet on the floor, we are going to get levitation." Then they dig their heels in.

This is more difficult to resist. They get the feeling that they are doing this and that's the way it has to be. That's what I'm after. I am the teacher, the catalyst. I'm here. I'll help. But, it's your job, you're the only one who can do it.

Chapter Twenty-two
Strategies of Hypnotic Utilization

Question: It's (hypnotic metaphor) like writing poetry?

T: I use a lot of poetry. I have some that are kind of neat. After a while you learn the subtle differences—the bottom line is that, you learn and learn. With every goodbye, you learn. Milton was involved with reading tremendously. When Milton died, I was in the Netherlands. After traveling for 24 hours, I hit Phoenix at 4 a.m. in the morning and I was asked to speak. I said I can't, but I did. People needed to cry. The other people had stonewalled it through their presentations. I said that this was what I thought Milton had meant to me. I had never met anyone who had ever heard of this piece of poetry. When I finished, the Erickson family came up and said, "How did you *know* our poem?" I think it is an excellent way of reaching people who are able to block a number of things. If you use this during trance, it is an extraordinary tool. One of the things that I am quite willing to have people see, that makes me able to reach them, is I let my vulnerability show and I don't have any problem with that. It makes it easier for them. Sometimes the poetry lets that vulnerability be seen a little more easily.

Question: What is the difference between hypnosis and transcendental meditation?

T: I think that hypnosis and meditation are the same to a point. When you meditate you have to be off by yourself and get yourself out of yourself. You need quiet and you need a little time. And it's a little hard to do in the middle of a party. Hypnosis can have exactly the same concomitants, but the difference is that I can go into trance in the middle of a cocktail party and nobody ain't going to know the difference. You can't meditate in the middle of a party. So the active alert variety is different from the meditative state. But deep meditation and the somnambulistic state can be very similar or identical. Margaretta Bowers (Bowers, 1959) did a tremendous amount of research on this. She found the states absolutely identical, except at one point she could activate the hypnotic state and be in the alert, kind of bright-eyed, bushy-tailed trance. She couldn't achieve that same thing with meditation because she would lose the meditative ramifications.

That's why I like hypnosis because it's so useful. I'm going to be in trance 90% of the time here. Because I can think about the points I want to make and remember what I have been saying, and can figure out where I want to go. I talk about it with a piano analogy.

This occurred when Bob Pearson, Ray Le Scola and I first worked with the dual induction. I am a mountain climber and had gone off to climb a mountain and came back in. Ray was practicing the piano. He is a concert pianist and he had one point in this piece that he was getting wrong all the time and he was going over it and over it and, *"Rrrrrr."* I stood beside him and said, "Just keep playing" and I started talking. I said it was absolutely amazing how very, very slowly and methodically he could play it in his head, and in the time it took his finger to reach for a key, he would be able to hear that note in his mind, decide whether it was in fact the correct note. If it was not the correct note, he could change it and modify his finger so it would go to the right note. All of this in a span of real time that it would take him to get his finger to start to move to the right key.

You would absolutely not believe, even I couldn't believe, the difference when he played it the next time. He went back home and his teacher said, "What did you do?" He said, "Nothing, just distorted time a little bit." And so this kind of thing is very useful, it's very productive. Nobody else needs to know that you are doing it. That's very useful.

Clinical Demonstration: Hiking

T: I want to know what you think we can talk about that might be useful for you. What should you share with all of us?

V: I've had trouble in my life when I'm told I made a mistake, it's like when I was a kid, it's panic. I'd like to be able to respond appropriately to making mistakes and not freak out.

T: Mistakes are learning opportunities.

V: Intellectually, I get it.

T: Still that little kid. Couldn't be rebellious? If I had a southern accent, it would give me the ability to sllloooww down like they do. That has its advantages. What do you like to do?

V: Biking, backpacking.

T: I once packed 100 pounds for five miles. We had a friend and the guy hurt his ankle. We took their packs while his wife stayed with him. I thought I'd die. I bitch when I have to do 50 pounds. I found out I could do a lot more than I really thought I could. *Uhh!* We went out and sent horses in for them.

V: Once, this guy asked me to hold his guitar and disappeared. I ended up taking his guitar up the mountain and so many times looked over and thought, goodbye, guitar. The guitar was lucky. (*Laughing.*) He showed up at the top of the mountain.

T: I have a friend who climbed Mt. Everest. One of the things I learned is that everybody who climbs at that level uses trance. When he came back he ended up losing 10 toes. He climbed again.

Ten toes is not really that bad a price to pay for having achieved a lifetime goal which few people could do. It's the way I looked at it, which was the reason he could listen to me talk to him about hypnosis for his toes. Everybody else said, "You idiot! Why did you do dadadada?" I said, "Nahh, it's only 10 toes, it could have been your life!" And we went on from there. The people who climb and recite poetry or count are all doing trance kinds of things.

V: I've done those things while biking.

T: You have to use trance to keep going, to get through the pain. There's a point where you're not sure it's worth it. What did you do with trance?

V: I've had those experiences you talk about with backpacking and riding my bike. I've used hypnotic tapes to go to sleep. I learned what it was to really be peaceful. I don't think I ever knew before what it was like to feel like somebody watching myself. I could make mistakes and say, "Oh, that's interesting and not be upset."

T: Where did it go? You used past tense.

V: It comes and goes. I haven't been able to sustain it. I can get in that space, lose it and go back.

T: So maybe a mechanism for deliberately accessing that space would be useful?

V: Yeah.

T: When you pack, you go up mountains?

V: Umhmm.

T: Let me talk about how I climb mountains. Some of it will be different from how you climb mountains. The goal is to get to the top of the mountain. But you find out when you start out, you complain a lot about the weight of the pack. You put it on and start out and know that you ought to go slowly. We tend to forget that when we start and walk faster than we should. You find out soon that you don't have enough air or wind. Your body says, this is not the way to walk. You are supposed to walk at a slow steady measured tread so you can keep walking forever. So you listen to yourself for a little while. What generally happens is the person in the lead has trouble staying as slow as they should. People who are following say, "Uh, uh, you are going too fast." You are setting too fast a pace. And then someone else takes his place and leads.

I don't know how long it takes, but you reach a point where you start to get your second wind. Until that time you have to watch the path you are walking. Sometimes, you take a longer step and sometimes a shorter step. When you get your second wind, you don't have to pay attention to the trail in front of you so much. You find that your feet can land on a little pebble or rock and you just roll off it and keep going without having to make the detours for it, which is an appropriate kind of learning. You begin to find that the little rocks that get in your way really don't get in your way, if your feet keep going in this very steady pace. You learn very quickly if you step on one, which slides with you, your body knows how to recover. You find that when you pound down a mountain more than when you go up.

You learn to make these little minor adjustments that make it easier for you to get in the pattern which says *I could keep this up forever*. Forever, with the people I climb with, means about an hour. Then it's time for me to eat my way up the mountain, because I walk for an hour and eat for five minutes and have a drink. That's where I evaluate whether the straps on my pack are too tight or need to be adjusted. I make a good follower as long as the leader knows what he is doing. When I am doing that following, I have the ability to put my mind in neutral. I can look down and look at the trees. I realize that maybe I've only been out for two hours and it seems that I just have been putting one foot in front of the other. If I turn around and look back and realize, not just see, I realize how far I've come. I look ahead and it looks like forever to get to the top. I know that based on my experience, I'm going to get to the top if I just keep up my very steady pace.

When you go out with some hotshots I usually find that they decide that they are going to break out and get ahead of the head of the pack. They do it for a little while. As you get to the altitude you get winded. They discover they haven't learned to pace themselves and end up having to sit down. If I keep going at my steady pace, occasionally, like the tortoise and the hare, I slowly manage to get past them. I sit down and look around and perhaps am above the tree line. I find out that the things that are growing up here grow in a little bit different way, because they don't have the protection and because they are exposed more to the elements. I keep going for a few more hours and it becomes lunchtime. We sit down and have a really nice view and a marvelous breeze.

I remember one particular time that I sat and looked and it must have been 10 minutes before I saw what I was looking at. There was this little flower that was growing there. I think I went into a trance because I thought about what it was doing there and how it got there. It was kind of like 10 years ago or 3 years ago depending on how long it took to grow. Someone dropped a seed there and there wasn't a whole lot of earth. There were a lot of rocks at that point. It got kind of beaten down into the earth. When that happened, it discovered that the rocks protected it and the snows came. And when the snows came, they kind of covered it and they protected it for a while. The next year, it managed to get a few tiny green shoots that came up out of the ground. And those shoots were very, very tender and very, very green.

And the wind and the rain came along and hammered away at those little tender shoots. But the nice thing is that the rocks that had made it so hard for it to find any earth to grow in, kind of protected it and moved around it and kept things away from it so it could grow a little bit taller and stronger. As it grew higher, the rain came along and gave it some of the nourishment that it needed. When the wind came along, it discovered that because it was so fragile and tender, it could let the wind blow it all the way down to the ground. As long as it bent with the wind and didn't try to fight the wind, it could, when the wind passed and the sun shone on it again, stand up straight and tall. Because it was young and flexible and it was able to learn and to grow.

It began to discover that that rock that had protected it for so long really was getting in the way. What it had to do was to detour as it stretched and it grew, to get out from under that rock so it could discover its own strength. The rock was very convenient while it was there but it was really holding it back. It made the detour it needed and got out from under. It also found that the rock had also been protecting it from those little green sprout eating animals. So in order to protect itself from those, it discovered it could grow some thorns. When it grew the thorns, all those little green sprout eating animals went away and let it alone, because they didn't like those thorns.

So it could grow even taller. The rains came along and the winds came along and blew it this way and that way and hammered it down to the ground but it maintained its curiosity and flexibility. Every time the sun would come out, it would reach for that sun and straighten up again, strong and gaining a little bit of independence each time, a little bit of reaching for the sun. As it did that, it was really kind of neat. It began to understand that that sun was there for a purpose and that purpose was to help it become what it was that it really wanted to do and needed to be. Every day people would walk past and never see it.

Finally, that little plant developed this tiny bud and the bud was there. Again we needed some rain, we needed some nurturing and nourishment, and finally the bud became a blossom. When that blossom opened up, it was a flower of such exquisite beauty and subtleness that all the people around there could look at it and exclaim with wonder, that anything that could have gone through what it had gone through, could grow in that particular climate. It was only the flower that sat there, saying to itself, "Of course, I knew I could do this all the time." You wonder, when you fold up the lunch stuff and move up the mountain, how many other little plants there are along the way that have done a similar kind of thing.

You walk for another hour and are really up where you can get into that rarified air. You can start filling your lungs with the purity of the knowledge that the oxygen up there is very special for you. You can work with the people who are climbing with you. You know that deep down inside that you really have the ability to keep putting one foot in front of the other. Looking at all the elements around you, you have to evaluate the best path to take when it is up around the rocks, and you have to look at the clouds and decide which direction the storm clouds are going to go.

And you have to decide how much of the weight you are carrying is a burden and how much is a protection. And the things that are a burden, you discover you can take out of the pack and stash them somewhere and pick them up on the way down. When you get to the top of the mountain, one of the rewards is to take that pack off for a while and get rid of that weight, that burden you have been carrying for so long. And reward yourself by finding the perfect place to sit and to relax.

And you look at the sun and the sun is under a cloud. And you know the sun is going to come out from under that cloud. And you find a place for your pack and put your head back against the pack and watch the sun. As the sun comes out from under the cloud, the shadow moves away and you feel the sun on your feet and feel the warmth and wiggle your toes and relax your ankles. And you get curious how long it is going to take for the sun to relax every muscle in your body that has worked up all that lactic acid from all that climbing today. And as you watch that cloud moving a little further, you explore those muscles.

Most of us don't realize that lactic acid is created from muscle tension and muscle strain. And you do have that lactic acid and what you do is you let the warmth of the sun moving out from under that cloud just work its way through every muscle in your body. And, finally, what I would like you to do is picture those muscles the way you would picture them in an anatomy book— each one of those muscles from your toes to your head, into your ears, and your jaws, and your neck and shoulders and your back.

Picture the lactic acid as a yellow oily liquid on the outside of those muscles. And you talked about learning to relax. This is one of those times you picture the lactic acid on the outside of those muscles, in front of your ears, and into your cheeks and jaws. Picture it here going through those jaws, into your neck, across your shoulder, down through your arms. Picture that oily light yellow liquid lactic acid running through the hands, down into your fingers and dripping out from the end of your fingers.

(Break in recording.)

It's kind of like a marshmallow. And a marshmallow sits out in the sun. And the skin sort of stays there in the powdered sugar. And you know how the marshmallow feels like inside, all kind of melty and soft. When that happens, the marshmallow really gets in this business of relaxation. And you can picture that softness, that mellowness, and that melty kind of feeling in those ears and the jaws and in the oxygen. Because every time that lactic acid moves down through those muscles and out your fingers, it has to be replaced by something. And that something that replaces it is oxygen, which comes in with that deep breath. It goes into your lungs, goes into your bloodstream, the hemoglobin, and is carried into those muscles through circulation.

Circulation is kind of like the streams you see and you hear as you decide to walk back down the mountain. And you can see the stream and realize that the spring runoff in that stream is kind of interesting. You look down in that stream. The current is kind of moving along and that is fine, but then you come to a place where it's flat and overflowed. Where it's overflowed, it's interesting because you discover that the oxygen and nutrients in the stream are pretty hard to get to. When you get to the pool which is overflowing, the banks are quiet and flat. And in the pool it is always safe to drink the water because all the nutrients have settled down to the bottom and the oxygen is there. And then you find that as you move on to the other end of the stream, back in the pool where it's quiet, the fish grow bigger, and the plant life is a lot bigger because the oxygen is available for that relaxation that you need. At the other end of the stream, the current picks up again.

And your body understands all about that stream and all about replacing that lactic acid with oxygen, whenever the relaxation says it's okay and appropriate. And as you continue the walk back down the mountain, one of the things you have to learn, is that a great number of burdens you picked up and thought you had to carry with you, you didn't really need in that backpack. And you can look back at that mountain and realize you don't have to go back there, you don't have to back down the mountain in order to back out of any of the things you don't want to look back on carrying with you.

391

And you can let yourself understand that the very smooth, stable, steady way that people learn to climb mountains is conducive to a great many other kinds of smooth, steady, stable ways they learn to do everything. It isn't always necessary to do ordinary kinds of things in the kind of perfection way that one would think was necessary. Because the idea is to get to the top of the mountain.

Sometimes you have to step on a few pebbles that are in the way, in order to find out that it's all right and you can keep going. That it doesn't matter if the pebbles interrupt or interfere for a little bit. Every pebble you step on, you learn something from and you find that it makes the next pebble a little easier. You never really sprain your ankle or end up having to stop the climb. Because each pebble is a learning experience in and of itself. Nobody else really ignores that particular pebble but they learn from your experience. You can be curious about just how much it is possible to learn and what direction you can go.

When you get back to the bottom of the mountain, you are aware that the lactic acid level has decreased but that there is a certain amount of tension. One of the ways you learn to deal with tension is to find out how to be really, really tense. When you walk around paying attention to the kind of tension, that doesn't tend to tone down the muscle tone you have; you can tune into that tendency to let yourself tend to get rid of the tension by paying attention to your body in a way you didn't tend to pay attention to it before.

One of the ways you do that is take a really deep breath and make your body as tense as you possible can. Now, count to five and let go of your breath and your tension. In a moment when you are ready, I'd like you to do that again. This time, hold your breath so hard you can feel it in your ears and count to five. When you let go, watch what happens in your hands and arms. When you are ready, take a deep breath, hold it to five. Feel the warmth in your hands. And feel the getting in touch with the opposite of that tension. Because your body doesn't know how to do that unless you help it.

I'd like you to practice every time you feel yourself getting uptight and wired. Every time you feel yourself biting back words or swallowing insults or berating yourself, you find that you can take that deep breath and make your body really truly tight. Then when you let go, you can *really* let go all over. You find that your jaws and your cheeks, your shoulders and neck and your back can look back on that ability to learn how to be comfortable and really in touch with relaxation. And you can access that capacity for enhancing the oxygen, eliminating that lactic acid, and letting your jaws relax and letting your body follow through.

You can practice that until you get so good at it that all you have to do to remind yourself is to pinch your thumb and index finger together. When you take that breath and sigh it out, and let go of those fingers, nobody around you will be any wiser about the magic you have inside you for being able to understand that you have the control that you really want. Because when you really have control, you don't need it; you can get it back anytime you want it. It's only when you don't feel you have control that you have to have control all the time because if you let it go, then you will lose it. Since you now have it, and you can practice it, then you can learn from the curiosity of wondering what kinds of new things you are going to experience, practice and learn.

Every time you get to the summit of every mountain, you will begin to understand that all of those little pebbles got you a little bit higher each time. The kind of high you have when you have done it and got to the top of the mountain is a feeling that is purely your own and is pure oxygen for your system. Just like that blossom was a flower of such exquisite beauty, that you really can't understand how it got there, except you know all the steps that went into getting high enough to be able to be comfortable with wherever it is that you are on that particular trip.

You can bring back with you all the understanding that you know a great many things you might not have known that you know. But now that you know them, it doesn't matter whether you know all the things that you don't know you know. As long as you know it's okay, because you do know that they are there when it's really appropriate for you to need them. You can take all that kind of understanding and put it back in that sponge that we call a brain that is absorbing and absorbing and absorbing.

Anytime you really want to, all you have to do is squeeze that sponge and you'll find that something is there that you might not have known was there. It doesn't matter whether you understand why it's there, as long as you know that somewhere inside you is the ability to know how to use that.

Just as surely as deep down inside you is the understanding that the pack you carry gets lighter, as you put down the burden you have been carrying, from the weight of waiting to find the way to carry the weight you really want to carry in the way you want to carry it. That's what this is all about. I think that that's the kind of thing that is a useful knowledge. I suspect a great deal more than you know that you know will be absorbed and filtered and gradually incorporated and utilized into all the different kinds of learning and climbing and remembering and forgetting, that you really know you want to do. When you are comfortable with the fact that your body understands and your mind remembers a great, many of the things you can know and use, I guess that's what this is really about and I would really like to thank you for cooperating. And you have all the time you need in the time you have...because the view is particularly *splendid*.

(*Pause.*)

T: Good afternoon. Do you have TMJ?

V: No, I got hit in a car accident and it screwed up my back and my neck and it's all tense and in my jaw too.

T: This is a particularly useful one for that, that's why I went into that. You were giving me some signals that there was something going on there in terms of tension. And this is absolutely great for that, it really is. And it's an exercise, like anything else, you practice it and you become more skilled with it.

V: I suddenly realized that you were starting it. You just started talking. I suddenly realized you were doing it.

T: No, you were doing it. You already knew everything you needed to know, so why waste time doing that? Makes sense.

V: It doesn't matter if you climb the mountain, how you get there.

T: You better believe it. And the view up there is worth the climb.

V: Thank you. I think the work you are doing is healing the planet. I appreciate it.

T: I practice everything I told you. I run a high stress life. Until I found out I could do this, I don't think I could have handled it. So practice. Talk to yourself, or go into your mountain climb or watch your flower grow.

When you get up into that rarified atmosphere, you really work for it. Scuba diving is interesting because all you have is the silence and the bubbles. I did that because I needed to find something to do in the sun and sand in order to stay away from the work of skiing. It's a matter of teaching yourself that it's okay. Once you learn that, you start to trust in your unconscious mind to do the things you need to do. As you get better, you are allowed to get more arrogant about it.

When you do technical rock climbing, you are awfully glad you have the rope around your waist. You hope you will never need it but you are awfully glad it's there. I like that because I'm not competing against anybody else, except myself. You keep increasing your skill and increasing your skill.

V: That would really be a form of meditation.

T: Absolutely. If you let it distract you too much, you end up hanging at the end of the rope. That's why you have the rope. It's a good feeling. It's constant upgrading of your skill and constant learning. There's always somebody who is a little better than you are and you can learn from them. But it's something you are doing yourself. And that's kind of neat.

Question: About your tears.

V: There was some sadness—the vulnerability of that flower. Not a painful sadness. You get to start over.

T: But when you blossom, it's *well* worth it.

Question: There are some kinds of fruits and flowers that don't bloom under ideal circumstances. Sometimes, it takes an occasional lack of water, people climbing on vines to be the stimulus for the beautiful blooms we see.

T: Yeah. How many of you thought of a rose? The original thing I wrote up was called the rose. That's my flower! I don't know what they [clients] are seeing. So it has been renamed, the flower.

(*Break.*)

That particular story I initially did for dental students who were taking boards (see Chapter Fourteen). You have to be flexible. You persevere and are stronger for all the trauma I used it for quite a while and it became appropriate for other problems.

If you take the mountain climbing analogy alone, you realize how many problems it would fit into in terms of development. And you take the rose, with this client who had gone through a divorce, I changed it from rocks to one rock which protected her and nurtured her and kept her from all the animals for a while. But then it got in the way of her developing her independence. So she had to get out from underneath it so she could discover she could grow and be strong.

So I was giving her some support for going through the divorce from being protected, having everything she needed and wanted, to find that she could work her way out from that. And there were all the people who were trying to devour her, so she could grow thorns and she could protect herself. The beating downs are the criticisms she was concerned about. She could listen to them and when the sun came out and they were over, she could straighten up again. All of those had multiple kinds of messages.

That was embedded in the other one of one step at a time. Any mistakes, any pebbles you step on, you learn how to roll with it, every pebble gets you a little bit higher. Every mistake you make, you are getting further up. You have to learn to deal with the elements, read whether it's going to storm, or whether the sun is going to come out, how far you are above the tree line. All of that was related to the work and the mistakes and the slow steady pace and stopping to take a rest and revaluate and going on again. As a climber, she understood that and that meant a lot and she could generalize to her other behaviors, by incorporating tension and relaxation.

She was giving me all kinds of cues about the muscle tension that goes with the climbing, the God awful aching in your feet. She had a ball with the marshmallow, as you all saw. You know, campfires and marshmallows, when you are out in the woods. I needed to give her some kind of way to deal with that muscle tension and stress, and the lactic acid is one I picture a lot and utilize and you replace it with the oxygen. All of her deep breathing was incorporating that. She gave it to me. I wasn't going to throw it away. I ended up putting bunches of them together. There were four different kinds of analogies that all tied in together; each had a separate focus.

Question: I noticed that the muscular exercise [tensing and counting to 5] seemed to be a deepening for her.

T: Yes, that meant something to her, right then and there! That meant something.

Question: Someone asked about the tear.

T: I chose to ignore it. Normally, I would have reached out and touched her arm or given her a Kleenex, saying, "I'm here and it's okay." I chose to let her deal with this because she has got to be able to deal with this. I was just vocally supportive. I think the sadness came from the divorce and the husband who had protected and the need to be independent. To be a little sad about that kind of thing, I think, is appropriate. I wanted her to do whatever it was she needed to do without putting so much emphasis on it, without her feeling obliged to have any stronger reaction to it.

Question: Do you usually refer to the tears?

T: Usually, I say, "And it's absolutely marvelous that you can let yourself do whatever it is you need to do."

Question: I was curious if the muscle relaxation was a metaphor and if the TMJ description was designed to stop her from thinking about what you were doing?

T: Moi?

Question: Do you often change the subject immediately when someone comes out of trance?

T: Sure.

I'm working with an oral surgeon who refers TMJ patients and I haven't found anyone with a straight TMJ problem. I have found everything from someone who needed to change jobs but couldn't because of his wife's needs to a blatant multiple [dissociative personality]. It's really interesting to think that all these people are showing up in oral surgeon's offices and periodontist's offices and the dentists don't know anything about the underlying causes. I have a way of talking about this. I say, "Before we had words, we evidenced displeasure by mashing our teeth, gritting our teeth, and showing our rage. We bite back words and swallow insults." I use a lot of body language kinds of things. Just as I talked to her about looking back on, using "you don't have to back down in order to back away to back out", in terms of muscle tension in her back. I think that with TMJ, there is a tremendous amount of rage and anger and hostility they aren't allowed to express. Most TMJ patients are women and they have been taught, you never do that!

People who grind get disc problems and people who clench get disc problems. In the joint, there is a cartilaginous disc. When you get too much pressure on the disc, you push it out of position and can't close the mouth or you will mutilate the disc. Cartilage disappears and it's bone rubbing against bone. You get earaches, eye aches, backaches, and toothaches. I had patients referred with low back pain from grinding their teeth. True bruxism only happens when you are asleep. Clenching happens when you are wide awake. I do direct symptom removal and if it doesn't go away, then I work with it on a more psychological basis. I give them three tries with direct symptom removal and then say, "Would you mind having a consultation with my friend down the street?" or I do it.

Question: How do you balance your therapeutic and dental work?

T: With great difficulty. I ended up being the only poker game in town for a long time. I got patients with whom I wasn't real comfortable. That's when I went back to graduate school and studied psychology. I could have refused to see the patients. That wouldn't have been fun. It is difficult. You simply have to know your own limitations. There are a lot of things I just won't touch and there are a lot I shouldn't, but feel comfortable with. And there are some I don't feel comfortable with, but feel I'm better than most of the people around working with them. Anyone with 35 years experience can do that, right? I'm flip with it, but that's by the virtue of a lot of experience and Milton Erickson saying Uuuuh! [Go!]

Question: When she was sitting next to you, you touched the client.

T: There was simply wanting to get with her to get that flow started in her hands, because she was having some trouble letting go of the lactic acid. It was a directional kind of thing.

Clinical Demonstration: Back Pain [21]

T: In your stomach and your hips, you can feel the support of the water. You can feel the buoyancy and lightness. It's kind of like when you first discovered that you didn't have pain back there after the surgery, that same kind of warm kind of light-hearted feeling with the warmth and glow that spread through your body with that kind of comfort. And as you feel the warmth moving up into your chest out into your shoulders, down through your arms, when you put your arms out in the water, it's fun to let the water hold them up. Then very, very gently with your fingers moving ever so lightly, letting that water slowly creep up over the tops of your arms and hands.

And the warmth penetrating through the water from the sunlight. And the sun finally moving completely out from behind

---

[21] Note: Tape begins after induction has already started—no prior discussion is available. Ed.

399

the clouds, and finding your chest, *and your shoulders, and your neck, your jaws, and your cheeks and your lips, and your tongue.* Muscles you never even knew you had. There's a muscle under your nose that makes your nose wiggle that people don't pay attention to and there are the muscles across your eyes and your eyelids and your forehead. And just picture yourself, not really having to swim yet, but letting yourself be supported and backed up by that relaxation and water. *That's good.*

As you feel yourself now, letting yourself move into the water further to the point where it's just the right depth. And you know it's not too deep. You can stand anytime you want to. It's deep enough that you can start to swim. You need at first to do some exercises, stretching, moving and testing the water and getting yourself comfortable and gradually moving out. So you can picture with the whole front of your mind that whole body and you can *feel.*

There was a study where one group visualized their exercise program and another group actually rode bikes as part of their exercise program. And what they found was that the people who really went into trance and visualized their muscles doing that exercise program, got the same kind of benefit as the people who actually did ride their bikes. That was hard for them to understand because they didn't understand what a marvelous thing your body is.

Because you are not your body. Your body is a precious physical plant through which you experience life. As you really want to enjoy a marvelous quality to your life, you can discover that you have the ability to respect and protect that body you inhabit. With that determination, it's going to be really supportive to know that it's perfectly all right for a little while to just relax and let go. To find out just how much that stress and that tension has been really, really wearing you down and wearing you out. That back support and backup that you have and need can be present in your own ability to know what's best for you, to know exactly how to take care of that body and that mind in a way you can be proud of yourself. And you can respect yourself for being able to do absolutely everything that you need to do for yourself.

That's such an important part of being able to look back at that back surgery and find out there are ways, away back there that you might have looked back and recognize that you can back out of so many things you really didn't back away from then. You don't have to back down from doing the things that are important to you. You can have strength in those muscles and guts in that kind of fortitude and perseverance.

And I really, really want you to feel that resolution inside yourself. You can learn to do absolutely every single thing that is going to be good for you. You have a right to make all those muscles and every disc in that spine so straight. It's your perfect right to get them to stand upright, to stand up for yourself in a way to give you the funniest kind of pictures. Every time you think about the back pain that sits there in the background, knowing that it's really good for you to learn that kind of control.

What I'd like you to imagine is that you have a hand that is transparent. And I'd like you to pretend in your mind, that you can see through the skin on the back of that hand. And I'd like you to imagine that you can see down in the tips of your fingers, under your fingernails, and see the little wires we call nerves and can picture those nerves, those little threads under the fingers. And you find that one or two fingers wiggle as they get more in touch with those threads. And picture them moving back from your fingers into your hand and kind of wind around one another and become almost like a telephone cord. They wind around so they can carry messages separately, but at the same time.

As you picture still more of the wires, coming together as main trunk wires, they move back up into your wrist. As the wires are so very, very fine at first, they are almost invisible like a hair. As more of them start twisting and getting together in the area of your wrist, you can see them more easily. When that happens, they move up into your arm. And they pick up even more as they move back through your arm. When they are at the elbow, it is about the thickness of half the lead in a pencil. It moves up still further and you can follow that kind of map, where it's the main road. And it leads up through your upper arm and into your shoulder. Then it goes across your shoulder and up into the back of your neck.

The fantastic part of that which most people don't know is that up there in your neck, is a telephone switchboard in your head. And you have all these wires that plug into the switchboard. You don't really have to know because any good telephone switch-board operator can look and they know exactly where the master control is for any switch. They can go in there and turn that switch off. If they are real good or real clever, it's like a rheostat and they can turn it down. What I'd like you to do is to get in touch with the switch that controls the feeling of pain, of hurt that goes into the back of that hand. And I'd like you to turn the switch off for a little while.

You need to get in touch with the fact that *you now* can learn to control the switches that carry the feeling of pain to that part of your body that you want to control. Of course, one of the things you learn from that is that there is such a big difference between feeling and pain. The ability to turn off the hurt doesn't mean you have to turn off the feeling. You can have a feeling of heat and cold and you can have the sensation of touch, the only thing you need to turn off is the hurt. The neat thing about being that telephone switchboard operator is that you have the ability with that rheostat to know whether it's safe to turn it all the way off, because it's not going to bother you to do that, or whether you need to turn it down a little bit, so you can tolerate the feeling of hurt you might have, that's necessary to protect it.

Because pain is a really important part of your life. It's a warning that something needs to be fixed. But our minds work in such funny ways. Once we get the warning we're afraid it hasn't heard it so the pain keeps going for a while, like a baby that starts crying and sometimes doesn't know it's okay to stop, even when the reason for the crying has left. What you need to learn to do is to trust in the back of your mind, rather than having that pain down in your back. Let the back of your mind understand how to back up all of this learning that you are doing. So you can stand up to anything that you really know is good and important for you to stand up to. That back can be such a marvelous back up.

And you can find that your exercises will strengthen you and will give you support. You know that just as you swim laps, that with each lap, you get stronger and stronger. And each time that you go into the water, you can get in a little deeper, because you can swim a little stronger and you can always keep your head out of the water. You never have to get under the water so far that you would be concerned or worried, because your strength increases, at knowing just how deep you want to get into that. You find that you know when it's time to get back out and to know that you can stand up to any of that kind of depth that you really, really want to. You know exactly how much risk it is appropriate for you to take in that back up system that you have, so you won't get in too deeply.

In addition to letting yourself turn off the hurt in that hand for a while, at some point down the road, you can check that out. You can keep it because your body didn't understand about the numbness in your back, when that kind of warning signal wasn't being listened to. And so it's time and your perfect right to be right about understanding that you can stand under so many misunderstandings in the past, that you can discriminate good feelings and you can have the strength you need and that you can develop.

In addition, I'd like you to think about some more of the parts of that brain, because you have a kind of master control switch for your blood supply. I like to think about it as more water, only this time, instead of a swimming pool, it's a river that moves through your body and grows and supports all the life systems that are necessary to respect and protect your body. As you picture that circulation system as a river. You walk along the river (see Chapter Twenty-one) and you notice that the waste products, all the leaves and stuff that have fallen in the stream get picked up by that current and carried off and discharged downstream somewhere—the same way that black-and-blue marks on our body disappear by the current going through them and carrying away all those waste products. The waste products get back to being tossed out in the air and disappearing, the same way we exhale them out of our lungs and let them disappear.

In order to prevent too many floods, we set up a series of locks and dams. Every lock and dam has this dam master that controls it and looks at the level of the water and decides when it is appropriate to let some water out from this dam here. And to let the boats through safely and let water out, as is appropriate, either to build up the level or let down the level.

And if you think back to when you were a little kid and were outside running. You remember on a really hot day … (This suggestion is repeated from Chapter Sixteen. To read the full text refer to page 294.).

So you already know everything you need to know about how to increase your circulation to carry the oxygen and nutrients to heal the parts of your body that need to heal. You know how to let that happen by thinking warm and feeling that warm flush go to that part of your body, not only to carry the oxygen and nutrients into that area, but to carry away the waste products so they won't get stuck there or stagnant.

Your brain is the most marvelous instrument because it's in touch with every cell in your body. It has all these clever little bits and pieces up there that have the master controls through the different glands in your body and the hormones you release. And you know that stress and tension mean that you squeeze out the ability of your circulation to carry your own natural pain reducing materials away. When you practice relaxation, practicing imagining, taking a walk to the swimming pool or taking a walk beside the river, you can tune in to the ability to relax and produce your own endorphins, your own interferon.

It doesn't matter if the front of your head knows what that means, because the back of your mind understands how to make those things that help your body. As you remember how first of all, it's okay to turn off hurt to the point where your mind understands that it is safe and still have all the other feelings that you need. And it's okay to increase the warmth and the circulation to the parts of your body that have been flooded and need that extra circulation to heal. And it's okay to have the backup system inside your head to be able to stand up for yourself straight and tall, and let yourself know that you have a perfect right to right everything that has been wrong and that has been left behind. You can correct these things in the sense that you move forward at your own rate of speed.

The real nice thing about learning this with all your body is that it ties in with that temporomandibular joint stress that I was talking to you about early on. This may be the last lesson that you need to put in that primer you have started today. That lesson is that most of us, particularly women, and I'm one of the people who learned to do this very early, tend to bite back words. Because we are taught as ladies that we are not allowed to say things, so we find that we bite our teeth, hold our tongue, and swallow insults, and do all these body language kinds of things that abuse our mouths and our jaws and teeth. That is very, very destructive.

What I'd like you to do is to turn destructive into constructive, because that is much, much better. Exercise is fine. I wouldn't care if you grit your teeth or clench them or grind them except that it hurts your jaws and hurts your teeth. You end up losing your teeth and have problems with your disc you already know about. Let's take that negative thing in your jaw and let you accept that every time your jaws come together to clench, that that's going to be an automatic signal. That's going to be a signal as if you have a magnet inside your teeth, to push them apart and send that electric current from here, this time through your arm into your hands and you can clench your fist.

When you clench that fist, that will take all the stress and all of tension from here, where it is destructive and move it down here where it can be constructive. Because it's going to build up all those muscles for your swimming. Clenching your teeth doesn't do a thing for increasing your muscle ability for swimming, but clenching your fist builds up every one of these muscles. You can take a habit, that has been really negative and build it into a very deliberate positive constructive kind of exercise. I know that this is a lot and know it is a heavy load and that there are people who would be perfectly willing to carry on with this teaching.

That's why I have chosen that you can handle this and all of this load of abilities I am tapping you into. And recognize that the same way you have used this clenched fist, when we started to get you in touch with relaxation, any time in the future, when that stress is coming back, you can use that same clenched fist and tightness, and then relaxing to get back in touch with all this stuff I have been saying today.

That you can use this to really, really move on with your life, to get on with it, in a way that can make you so pleased with yourself and so satisfied. Because the only way to get from today to tomorrow is by going beyond yesterday. You find to go from yesterday to tomorrow, you really start with today. You have listened to so much and so well that I'm real appreciative of that. I'd like for me to stop talking for a few minutes and let your mind kind of review and let your body remember all those things that it has heard and practiced and learned. So you can be comfortable that you know and trust in your unconscious to know the kinds of things it needs to know to help you in this future that you finally can begin to look forward to. When you know that, you can bring those confident kinds of feelings back with you knowing that you really do have the ability inside you to do and be and become exactly what it is you want to be for yourself. Because that's what this is really all about.

We probably could have taken a little less of a heavy dose all at once. She was ready for that, ready to hear it and has the skills and ability to do these things. Therefore, I just decided to go for it all. She can certainly sort out what she chooses to from the things she was offered, as needed.

Good morning! One of the neat things about waking up before you have to get up is precisely that. Not having to get up. It's almost worth waking up earlier!

I think you did a very fine job of listening and learning. I really appreciate it.

I would have a real hard time with that empty pool out there. I would want to spend most of my time in it.

V: (*Crying.*)

T: Part of that is coming from the fact that most people have not given you the option to be able to do a lot of things to help yourself. You have had to guess it out. The opportunity to help yourself can bring pretty strong feelings and it is perfectly appropriate. I think that what that tells me is just how good a job you did of listening.

V: Going from zero to 80. I've come home from the hospital and been there by myself. It seemed like you knew exactly how you feel. It was strange when you were doing it because, not because I was trying to think ahead of you. Right before you said you were at this place, I was there.

T: So you read my mind.

V: I thought I wasn't trying to be strong but I still was.

T: Sometimes that can get in the way. I meant what I said. I was hitting you with everything that you might want to take at a slower pace, because I know that there are people who can help you.

V: It would be nice to have a tape, I should use something every day. I want to separate things. When you go out into the body part, you don't really realize that you are your body.

T: You can't get away from it.

V: Once you've had surgery, you realize that you have a liver.

T: It's the way you put them together that matters.

Question: My sense is that you are more in your body, your presence seems to be more physical now?

V: Probably is.

T: Both curiosity and a safety there now, that might not have been there before. That it's okay.

V: What I discovered when you started the process was that every one thing relates to everything else. I realized how I really felt when I walked in here. I probably am kind of hostile and just sort of afraid.

T: That's reasonable.

V: That colors what I think of people and how I perceive them. After I started to relax, Jeez, she's so neat, she's so smart, gosh.

T: That works both ways.

V: I started to think these positive things. That always makes me cry, Wow! You have such a low opinion of everybody, or yourself, probably based on myself.

T: Maybe it's time for you to change that.

V: Where have I heard that before?

T: Inside your head?

V: Just when you thought it was safe to come out on the street, you know. (*Laughter.*) I was perfectly convinced when I came here that I really am in control. I'm always wanting to feel normal or something.

T: Where you are at any given time is normal, but that doesn't say you can't be more normal as you go along. I suspect that there are a lot of things that will keep popping up. You will think about what you heard and I'm quite sure you are going to use it well.

V: One thing you did say, I have always had a problem with. I can't, I never believed that about illness. I saw this book that says when your foot hurts, it means you want to kick your grandmother. People who have eye problems, you know what I am saying. For the first time, I had never heard that "backing away from". I heard lack of support. A book said if your back hurts, you are lacking support. "Backing away" in the situation, every thing seemed to fit. The way I felt when I came in here. When a negative thought comes, I'll say to myself, remember how you felt, and how it worked out. That's how I have to go, maybe everybody has to go that way.

T: If you go that way, then everything else can go that way.

V: Meditation and mental images are helpful with pain, having some kind of map to turn to is constructive.

T: Yeah.

(Break.)

T: In my office, I would have done this differently and wouldn't have given her such a load the first session. I would have talked with her. I feel uncomfortable that you hear me talking at, not with her, but that is a function of the limited time for this demonstration. I would have talked about the hand, particularly about the anesthesia and her switches. She gave me cues that she was doing these things. And I was paying attention to them, when she moved, saying that's right or that's better. I think it's appropriate to interrupt your sentence, right smack in the middle, and say, "That's better," and go right back to your sentence so she's very much aware of how in tune you are with her.

I would have done the needle in the back of the hand thing saying, "Do you want to do it or do you want me to do it to demonstrate to yourself," and learning control of bleeding. We would have talked a lot about that and talked about the TMJ thing. My effort here was to give you a broad variety of what maybe would have taken three or four sessions in this jammed together smorgasbord.

Comment: You were doing a good job of overlapping the multiple metaphors and integrating the metaphors. Even though each and every one could have been a separate branch by itself, they came together as if they were all one metaphor.

T: I think that's important. I have heard a couple of people tell story after story after story. Why bother? It's important you make that connection and transition. My mind is looking for ways to do that. All the while I'm in one, I'm thinking how am I going to work my way around to the next one.

Comment: I'm learning that I don't have to make a logical connection.

T: "It's kind of like" is a good way.

Question: I went to a workshop with this Vietnamese monk, Thich Naht Han. He talked about how everything is contained in everything. He talked about a piece of paper. He asked, "Do you

409

see a cloud in this piece of paper? Without the cloud, this piece of paper wouldn't be here. The rain comes down and the tree grows." In a natural metaphor, everything is transformed into everything else.

T: Russ has a really great generic metaphor about the universality of man and you end up out on some star somewhere, when you listen to that one. Russell Scott, a psychologist and friend of mine, is an absolute gem. He came to me referred for a dental phobia of 18 years standing. He could not park his car in front of a building he knew a dentist office was in. He got a job in a dental school thinking it might help. It didn't, hypnosis did. He's been involved in hypnosis ever since, that's like 25 years now. He and I are the ones who do so much work together and do a lot of dual inductions. He is extraordinarily creative. Just as I have the hemispheres metaphor I use as the initial one, he has the universality of man. It has a lot of the kind of things you are saying about the monk, which I think is really important.

About the client. When she was sitting on that sofa, I was really uptight because of her hostility. I was so pleased she acknowledged it. She had the appearance of a hostile, depressed, resistant person. I'm thinking, "Oh Lord! What am I going to do?" I was fishing. I couldn't get anything from her. She was just here. Go ahead, do what you can, despite me, not because of me. It was good I had talked about the first part.

I didn't have the feeling I could set her up with this group because I didn't have any sense of what she needed to have me saying. It was tough! I was concerned that nobody, including her, was going to get anything out of that. I gave into it. I thought, quit prejudging her. I was searching desperately, all the things I could do, looking for the something that would work. I couldn't do any of the physiological things I would lead into because of the back, like "this is going to be silly, but do it anyway" or "let me show you how easy it is for your mind to let something happen that isn't really under control of your mind", because people need *hope*.

Question: I used the sand bucket induction technique with two people who then complained about a lot of pain in their shoulders. What would you suggest?

T: I'd say, "Isn't that wonderful! I think it's absolutely marvelous that you have been able to so quickly create that pain and tension in your shoulders as your way of interpreting the message you were being given. I think that's wonderful." A lot of people do get tension in their shoulders while doing the sand bucket. I say, "That's wonderful. That's your way of your unconscious reminding you that you really did that."

Question: That they are in control?

T: Yeah, and that something really happened. I'm just so impressed when someone learns something that I didn't teach them. I say, "Oh! Aren't you wonderful! Jeez, that's great."

There were about four induction and utilization approaches that were intertwined, that I would consider using as separate kinds of techniques. The tension one was my way of doing a sand bucket. This is giving her hope. I pointed out the simple physiological changes that would take place. When they took place, I was right. I started something. She had done it. There's the foundation that I was beginning to establish. She said, "That hurts," and I agreed with her. I reinforced that and that was appropriate. I didn't say "the next time you don't have to hold yourself so tense." I left it up to her. When you can make it hurt worse, what is the opposite implication?

Question: About the metaphor of the network with switches.

T: That is my favorite one for anesthesia, with a child or adult. It's the easiest one to use, because in this semiregression that they do automatically, looking through your hand is sort of fun. It's transparent. We had this 9-year-old, who when we were talking about wires, said, "Do you mean nerves?" Yes!

Question: Why did you do it in her hands, instead of in her back?

T: Because her back is too emotionally charged. I wanted to put it somewhere where there was no risk in her learning and then she knows she can generalize it.

Question: You wouldn't do any other teaching? She could do it there and leave it to her to generalize it?

T: Yeah. And the emphasis of the teaching was not on the anesthesia. It was turning off one part of the feeling, turning off only the pain, which I think is important. She talked about feeling dead and feeling numb and that's a terrifying kind of feeling. Part of the reason for the anesthesia was not so much for pain control in her case, as it was for being able to discriminate the type of feeling. You can have hot and cold and sensation of touch and still turn off the appropriate amount of pain, which is where the rheostat came in.

You talk about pain and pressure or suffering and pain as being different, but people really don't know what you mean. I think it's very important because people give me the feedback, "Oh, I can *feel* without it hurting." That was a great deal of what went into teaching anesthesia to her in the way I was breaking it down into parts. I wanted to do the whole thing so you would hear the verbalization I use so much of the time. Did you see her big grin when I went to the switchboard in her head? She was having a great time with that. Part of the grin was, "Oh, my God, I really see it!"

The relaxation was important. I was combining the swimming pool and the cloud over the sun. I use the cloud moving away from the sun with people who don't get sunburn, and it gives a positive hallucination and you can watch the shadow disappear as the sun comes over your body and it warms you and melts you. I wanted her to be sure, moving into the water, that the water would be the right temperature and not too cold, because of the back. That's important. That was why I did it, so she couldn't tell when she was in the water, because it was just the right temperature. So she could choose the temperature and the whole progressive relaxation.

Then I went into therapy. I was talking about deciding how deep you want to be involved. The other thing she laughed about was when I was giving her spine this ability to stand straight and she was hearing those messages loud and clear and choosing to be amused by them. I was also doing a lot not only in terms of backing away and backing down, but to stand up for herself, to stand straight and to essentially confront in any relationship she had to. Getting her into the water, in terms of how deeply she wants to go was part of that message. That's why I was using the swimming pool, as well as her talking about the swimming pool. Every time she goes swimming, there will be that question sitting there, how deep do I want to go?

Comment: It was very powerful. She was crying.

T: She had tears running down here. I'd have gone for the Kleenex in my office. I did a lot of backing off. I didn't want the transference to be too strong, which is why I referred to other support systems. I didn't want her to rely on me. It was important she be able to trust and rely on herself. With the progressive relaxation, there was this approach to therapy, in terms of backing down, backing out, backing away, standing up, standing under so many understandings. Whenever I get too much of an acknowledgement, I would acknowledge her acknowledgement and move away. I didn't want to be hitting her over the head with it. I wanted it to be able to disappear as much as necessary. She was very complementary, considering where she started.

Comment: That was quite a transformation.

T: Yeah. She did some risking with the group and I was real pleased with that.

I used the circulation system with her because that's exactly what happens, especially with a surgical procedure. That works with childbirth in the same way. There's a breaking of the walls in order for the baby to get through this canal and there needs to be a reparative process. So you talk about the pooling and then you talk about the reparation and restoration and healing.

I had the feeling that there was a lot of little girl and used careful basic language. I kept wanting to mention the endorphins and interferon and kept thinking, *she doesn't want to understand that now.* I finally decided, okay, we'll talk about it and protect it and say it really doesn't matter, whether the front of your mind hears it. It's back there and she can do with that whatever she needed. I wanted to tie in for her the relationship of stress to their production. I did more direct relating of the river to her body. I did more of direct analogy, "it's like", but probably wouldn't have

413

done that in my office. I wouldn't make the direct connection. I was overloading her at this point.

Comment: With your word play, if it's relevant to her, she can take it in and use it. If she doesn't need that kind of intervention, it just goes right by. If it's too soon for her to hear, it sits there until she's ready.

T: Yeah, people hear what they need to. It's put in the background.

I didn't do the thing with the lactic acid today. I figured it was too much. The TMJ thing I did is the direct symptom removal I do, changing a destructive negative energy into a constructive positive energy. If it is a young person, who plays tennis, I justify it with saying, it's a neat way to improve your tennis. If it's an older person, I say it's a nice isometric exercise. I want them to have a *reason* on the surface for doing what I would like them to do.

The touching of her was grounding and appropriate under the circumstances. We needed to do that. She really needed some direct contact with me. I didn't want a full-blown tears and crying, because I didn't think it would be productive in terms of the rest of the work. I did the patting on her back, it's okay to do as much as you need, but let's not let it interfere with the other things you ought to be doing.

I think she did a marvelous job at the end, that she acknowledged that she was so surprised at the emotion that was there and what she thought she was doing and could admit that, demonstrated how far she had come. She had a lot of resistance to my suggestions about getting other support. She did say a tape would be nice.

And a lot had to do with the rheostat on this pain, in terms of having as much pain in any area, *any area* that she might need and being able to hear the warning system. There was so much tied in together. The themes I was using I would have broken down into a number of sessions and given her a tape and exercises in between times, for the tension and muscle release, the imagery of swimming and to practice the anesthesia. I thought she would challenge me about the study (imagining exercise was as effective as actually doing exercise) but she didn't. What I would want are deliberate periods of relaxation and I would try to make them as inconvenient for her family as I could.

Comment: Afterwards, when she got emotional and was overwhelmed and wasn't able to communicate, I noticed you didn't encourage her to express her feelings.

T: I spoke to her quietly and very deliberately about being in control and still say what she needed to say, as a way of reassuring her. I'm back into protecting the patient from the audience. I don't think she should have opened too much. She has to be protected.

Question: I was noticing you and what you were doing. Sometimes you would close your eyes and sometimes look down. I take it you were in trance?

T: Sure. I am aware of that even when people have their eyes closed. I am convinced just as when you answer the telephone, if you answer with a smile, people hear the smile. I go through this because it makes my sincerity easier than if I am just sitting there talking. If people have their eyes closed and can still be able to see, I am continuing the interaction that way. It eliminates any possibility for me that I am reading a script. It demands that I get involved and that's why I do it.

I did this whole thing one time about teaching versus training. If you look in the dictionary, to train is to demand obedience, as in teaching a seal to bark for a dead fish or to keep a lion at bay with a chair. To teach is to open up, and to expand and to educate. I have a real problem with training in hypnosis because I think the scales some of the experimentalists use are much more like the dead fish than they are the educational aspects of clinical hypnosis that we use.

The train comes back again into anybody's station. You can take any trip on any train in a couple of ways. You can get on the train and find your seat and be very impatient about getting on with your journey. You watch some people who sit there and tap their

415

foot and drum their fingers. If people beside them try to talk to them, they bury themselves in the newspaper. When the train finally starts and if it's on time, the person is convinced the train is really late and if they walk they can get the train to the station faster. They don't pay attention to the kids playing outside. They don't buy coffee because they are too intent on getting to the station. They don't pay attention to the trip along the way. When the train comes to their station, they are the first ones to gather their belongings and get off the train. I always feel there should be a brass band to greet and play for those particular people. When there isn't a brass band, they hurry off and get back on the train after they do their business to get to the next station. Because they are sure there will be a brass band that will appreciate the intensity they are using to get to their next destination.

I obviously think the other guy who gets on the train is a whole lot better off. He settles back in the chair and has a conversation with the good lookin' lady sitting next to him. He looks at the paper and yeah, he looks at his watch and thinks, oh isn't it nice that we are going to be on reasonably good time today. He has his cup of coffee and shares the journey with the other people in terms of looking out the windows, and talking about the flowers and the lay of the land and the kinds of things growing there and whether they are going to put houses in that particular area.

When he gets to the other station, that the first guy got to, it's with a sense that he has really already accomplished a great deal in terms of learning about the trip along the way-the people, the countryside, the different kinds of climate of the people them-selves, as well as the land. When he gets off the train, he doesn't need to worry about that particular destination. He doesn't need the brass band. He has the satisfaction of the trip itself. He knows that wherever he is, he's going to find people and places and friends he's going to be able to deal with.

I really think the training we talk about in terms of learning about hypnosis can be done either in the short, scheduled intense way or can be done with the satisfaction of enjoying the trip and the people you take it with. And the learning that goes on and the goal is important somewhere. If there is a nice place to stop, it's perfectly okay. When you drive along the freeway, you get so used to it, you drive 65 miles an hour.

All of a sudden you come to a detour and you swear because you don't want to get off the track and so you take the detour and end up on a little two-lane side road up a canyon and maybe there is a place where they sell strawberries or a little teahouse you have never paid attention to before. If traffic is pretty heavy, you decide, what the heck, to stop and have some tea.

When you do that, you find out that there really are trees and people and nice things to experience. Without the detour, you wouldn't have had the chance to experience that. When you go back to your car, the traffic has moved on, and rush hour is over. You know you can go back on the main road, anytime you choose. Sometimes, it's nice to stay on the two-lane road. The things you learn there are much more real and much more satisfying. You don't pass up the opportunities the way you do when you are up on the freeway. I think that in many respects, hypnosis is like that. We have that ability, that capacity.

You are not your body. Your body is the precious physical plant through which you experience life. I don't know how many of you have had a broken bone. If you have seen an X-ray of a bone that has been broken and healed, you recognize that it always overheals. The cells that create our bone structure, that create our tissue, when we cut ourselves and heal, for a little while there is an extra thickening of the tissue there, because we need to over-heal to be sure we heal properly. We sometimes forget we have overhealed and that gets callused and hard. We need to realize that in addition to those cells being there, that the macrophages are also present, the cells that eat up all the excess material that we have in the body.

You can picture, almost like a jellyfish in there. You know that a jellyfish kind of encompasses everything. It grows and moves by surrounding and eating up. After it eats, if you take your toe and dig a little ditch in the sand around the jellyfish, the sun comes out and the jellyfish can't go anywhere. The sun tends to dry up the jellyfish and it shrinks, and as it shrinks, it gets less able to hold onto the beach. Eventually, the wind picks up and the sun and wind gets the jellyfish kind of cell so thin and so light and it kind of floats away, leaving all that new sand and cleaned up area.

In the same way, every time the tide comes in, it washes away all those elements of the ravages, the things that have been thrown on the sand and get in the way. And the tide comes in and washes away, with every wave, all of the waste products, all of the rocks, all of the shells and all of the things that people have dropped there that have grown in their own way. So the tide washes these things clean and fresh and softens them up and lets all of that excessive material be washed out to sea, where it can be strained and drained and disposed of appropriately.

It's absolutely fascinating to watch that process of devouring all those foreign bodies, because that goes on in our body all the time and we just don't pay attention to it. It's kind of nice to sit back and to picture that in our heads and to feel that warmth of that sun drying up all of those excess kinds of foreign cells. And to picture that jellyfish phenomenon taking place, so it can become very light and very dry and very floaty and the ocean waves come in and wash away all those cells that are no longer necessary. And they can wipe everything new and fresh and smooth and soft and clean.

And it is absolutely amazing what happens when one begins to understand that in this matter of going into a hypnotic trance, it becomes simply a matter of focusing on one's ability to permit the conscious and unconscious mind to let something happen. As you review in your unconscious mind all of the things that are waiting there to be learned and understood, the conscious mind can let itself relax so the unconscious can do its own thinking and feeling and organizing. And you can begin to understand that you can become so entranced with learning how you can make the knowledge of this experience and the memory of this experience change into something that it wasn't when it began, only because you hadn't thought about it as being what you didn't think it was.

And when you think about it in that way, you can cope with it on any number of levels because you have the ability to take that ability and turn it into the most marvelous coordination of body and mind, of conscious and unconscious, of need and understanding. Letting yourself know and experience that it isn't always necessary to learn things directly. And you have the ability with your experience and your background to put to use all of the knowledge that you acquire in any way that you choose to acquire it.

The important thing is that you discover that it is okay to use it, even when you do not understand that you know how to use it. Because this trust and reliance on your own unconscious is one of the things that permits you to constantly move forward in this knowledge and this learning and this way that you have of finding what it is that you need and want, wherever you may be. Because this journey you take is such a delight when you choose to do it in that way.

References

Bowers, M. K. (1959). "Friend or traitor? Hypnosis in the service of religion", *International Journal of Clinical and Experimental Hypnosis*, 7 (4), 205–15.

Chapter Twenty-three
Pain Control and Healing Enhancement

T: This is a demonstration of the things I really do which is to teach people how to deal with pain.

V: I went to the dentist because I had lost a filling in my back tooth. He went to fill the tooth and hit a nerve. He was one of those, when you put up a finger to stop, he wouldn't stop. And he dug deeper and I had a full-blown anxiety attack, screamed, hollered and got up and left his office.

T: That was sensible. I might have done that too!

V: I found another dentist who packed it and filled it and said, "I don't know that it might not heal with antibiotics." I can't take any pain medication at all and have to suffer through anything that happens. I can't even take aspirin well, so no pain medication. It did heal. But now, periodically, once a month or every six weeks, when it flares up, it goes through the jaw and down the neck. There's enough inflammation inside that it goes up through the eye and out back up through the head.

T: You have just described the Gasserian ganglion.

V: Cool! Can you spell that?

T: There is a central nerve and it has five branches and you just described five branches. From the source of your problem, it's like hitting your crazy bone in your elbow and feeling it in your fingers. When you touch that tooth, it refers back to that central ganglion and goes to all those places. See, you just learned something. This is the source of a great many interesting learnings. You said, it's healed. How do you know it's healed?

V: It's taken a vacation for four to six weeks.

T: When you get on an airplane, it gets worse?

V: I've taken two trips in the past six months. As soon as I landed I've been in an enormous amount of pain.

T: Does the stress cause the pain or does the pain cause you to grit your teeth which causes the stress which exacerbates the pain?

V: I think it's stress. I'm going to take a wild guess. When the pain keeps me up all night, it's very possibly associated with stress because I'm gritting my teeth.

T: I understand why that happens. That doesn't necessarily come from gritting your teeth. That is a physiological response. You know about hypnosis. Do you know whether you have been using it to control the pain?

V: I wouldn't say for sure. I can dissociate the pain. When it gets to the point when it's so bad, I can do that.

T: That makes sense. Do you generally know when you are using trance? How do you know?

V: Yes, I hear better. I'm kinetic; when I switch, I go to audio.

T: One of the things that triggers for me was when Betty Erickson was doing a demonstration on autohypnosis. She was talking about a rather naïve person who did it and when asked how he knew he was in trance, he said, "My teeth fit different." We all have our own way of knowing. If you are so good with hypnosis, nasty question, why don't you turn your pain off?

V: (*Pause.*) If I am so smart, why didn't I get the tooth fixed before now?

T: I think I know why you didn't turn your pain off. I'm giving you all these motivations about why you should go into trance. She said she would like to experience my style. I'm not sure what my style is, but I'm working on it.

You see better. What do you see when you see better? Do you see the same things more clearly or from the same perspective?

V I don't think I understand your question.

T: Yeah, you do, because you just answered it. And the answer which your conscious mind gave me was not the one which I was looking for. I was looking for your unconscious nonverbal, when you went off to that side of the room and thought about it.

I threatened to do a formal structured induction technique so you could see my style.

That's what I'm going to do. Is that all right? I don't know what you are going to do.

Have you ever played the piano?

V: By ear.

T: So you know about running your fingers across the keys. Pretend your knees are a keyboard and put your fingers way out on the end of your knees. Take a deep breath and let it out. When you take your next deep breath, watch what happens with your hands and arms. See how they go up and down with the breathing. While you are breathing, I want you to do something you are not going to be able to do. Try to balance your hands, your fingers exactly evenly on your legs. What happens is that we're not made so we can balance them the same. So the weight of which hand is lighter and which is heavier, so the weight shifts back and forth from one hand to the other hand and fingers.

Gradually, I'd like you to discover which hand and fingers are lighter. Pay more attention. And discover with each breath you take, that hand and those fingers start to get a little lighter and lift away from the fabric of your pants. There it goes. That's good. And gradually with every breath you take, that hand getting lighter and those fingers getting lighter and the balance is the really interesting and fascinating thing about this. As the fingers get lighter, that hand gradually starts to lift into the air and the arm begins to follow. That's it. And the other hand can, almost as though the weight from this hand can go up through your arm and across your shoulders and down into that other hand and it can settle in your lap, so you can really focus on what's important.

And as the hand lifts higher and higher, you can be absolutely curious about where it is it's going, because obviously it knows something that you don't quite yet know. And somewhere there up in the air, there's a pillow of air. When that hand and those fingers and that arm get light enough, they will float and lift and float and the weight from that hand will go up across your shoulders down into that other hand. That's the way.

And it's almost as though the hand has a mind of its own. Because it does know a great deal about how to let that happen with the satisfaction and the learning and the experience that goes with it. And when it gets to that pillow of air, then we have the next step in that learning, which trance-lates early into the kind of knowledge and understanding, that lets you stand under so much additional learning, that your standards expand and increase.

And when that hand knows that it knows everything that it needs to know about how to make the memory of this experience come back for you whenever you need it, only because you had not yet thought about it as being what you didn't think it was, then to get on with the rest of your learning, the most amazing thing can happen.

That pillow of air can develop a tiny, tiny, tiny, tiny hole in it. And everybody knows what happens when a pillow of air gets a hole in it. And when your hand touches again your leg, that will be the signal to let all that knowledge just kind of reverberate through your body, so we can use it particularly around that silly Gasserian ganglion which I talked about earlier, because that's really what this is all about. When the hand touches, then you can let both hands relax and both ears really open up because after all they don't have any lids. And you can be curious about what it is that I know that you will be able to use. That's the way. Deeper and deeper.

And as I pointed out a little earlier, I know why going up in an airplane lets you have the experience of more pain from that plane, and its very plain for me to see that that pain is real and exacerbated by something called air pressure. Because when you have something that's going on in a tooth and you have some waste products there, waste products create a kind of putrefaction and with putrefaction you have gas pressure. When you heat a gas, it expands and when it doesn't have anywhere to go, it sits there and it throbs. And when you get off the plane, it's still plain to see that that pain from the plane is still there. And it will take a little while for you to be smart enough on the unconscious level, to take care of that pain by enhancing the healing, the circulation to that part.

Now when you had the original pain, my philosophy about it is demonstrated by your toothache. Because pain is a danger signal, it is a warning signal. Until you pay attention to the pain and do what it is that you need to do with that pain, then that pain cannot go away because your body needs to have that signal. And when you went to the first dentist, unfortunately, he didn't understand your pain. So it was plain to see, that you needed to do what you did, which was take care of yourself by leaving and finding someone else, who wasn't sure but at least made the appropriate effort to deal with your pain.

To deal with not just the physiological and physical pain, but also the psychological blow that first dentist inflicted upon you. Because that invasion of your tooth without taking appropriate care not to give you that hurt, was a very inappropriate behavior and you have every right to be angry with that dentist! But not with that tooth, because the tooth was not to blame. The dentist was to blame for that pain. It need not be a case of feeling that you need to suffer because of it, but a matter of knowing that you did what was appropriate.

But, sometimes, pain is like a hysterical child. And even when the reason for the crying of the hysterical child goes away, the child keeps right on crying, so you have to distract the child so it can stop crying and feel better. And maybe it's appropriate now that you have been able to distract yourself from that pain while that tooth made its effort to heal. The difficulty that I hear here is that back there, the dentist who did the second attempt to heal and help the tooth was not enough versed in your capabilities to be able to tell you what to do to heal that tooth.

And I think that it is my turn and job to tell you what you need to do to take the appropriate care of yourself. And to let you

425

understand that with this pain or any pain, when everything that can be done and should be done, has been done, then there isn't really any reason for the pain. Because when pain is a danger signal, if you use pain, when everything that can be done and should be done, has been done, then your body gets really confused, about whether that pain is just the hysterical child response of the pain or whether there's really something wrong. So its time for you to learn to discriminate and to be able to differentiate and help to heal that tooth, that ganglion, and that circulatory system.

Every tooth has one or two roots and yours has a couple of roots. At the bottom, at the very tip of the root, there is a little opening and that opening permits the nerve, the artery, and the vein to carry the nutrients and the sensation up into the tooth. And at the top of it, there is a little bit of a ballooning so you can get some extra circulation there, and that's the way it should be because it helps to keep the tooth healthy.

The interesting part of it is that as we age, by the time you get to be 85, that artery and nerve and vein have receded, they have pulled back, and you have put down an insulating layer of dentin between the enamel and that nerve. And sometimes, as with other physical things that happen with your body, you can do a similar kind of speeding up job of depositing that insulating layer between the outside of the tooth and inside of the tooth.

What I'd like you to do is picture that little strip of inner part of the tooth going from the root into the crown of the tooth, and picture that bubble inside the crown and picture the artery, the vein, and nerve that come up in there. What you have is the response to inflammation. Just the same way, when you have the inflammation anywhere else in your body, that circulation gets kind of engorged and slows down.

When that happens, there's more blood that piles up inside it and makes it more engorged and more inflamed. That's a warning signal. That is telling you that there's something wrong in there and what you need to do is tell yourself that you hear that warning signal and that the appropriate way to respond is to increase the circulation out of the tooth to carry away the waste products. That's the really important part of that.

When you do that, you let the tooth return to normal and you let it heal and you let all those little secondary dentin kinds of molecules settle down there right up against the nerve, the artery and vein. And the nerve, the artery and vein can recede, they can pull back and they can shrink back. And you are capable of depositing that secondary dentin layer of insulation right up against that nerve that the dentist so brutally violated. And you can insulate that and you can coat it.

And the other thing that you need to be aware of is that the second dentist, when he put the treatment in the tooth, put a sedative filling right over the top of that area to calm it down, to sedate it, and to encourage the deposit of the secondary dentin. It's just like any other part of your body if it's injured. If you ever had a broken bone or seen an X-ray of somebody else's broken bone, if you look at it, you can always tell because it overheals, it's not smooth, and it's not long, and it's kind of lumpy around there because you get extra bone just to make sure that it's extra strong.

Because what you are doing in the inside of that tooth is making extra dentin, which is composed of the same stuff as bone is, making it extra strong, and you are letting the artery, vein and nerve pull back so the tooth itself can have additional strength and additional healing. While that is happening, you can understand that your system knows how to carry away those waste products, it knows how you heal. You've done it all your life. In this case, no one explained to you what it is you needed to do.

It's kind of like in the spring when there have been those floods. You go out and walk along a stream and look down in a stream and see the current bopping along at a pretty little clip. You wonder how those little creatures that live in the stream and plants that grow there manage to get nourishment, manage to get any oxygen because everything is going along so very fast. They really have to reach out and grab that and get the oxygen and nutrients.

If you walk along a little bit further and you come across a place where there's been a flood and it's been a pretty bad flood, you can see rocks and all sorts of things that were moved by that flood. You know at one time it's been very damaging to the environment and the area around there. But when you look now, it's not a flood any more, it's a nice quiet pool. And you look at the pool and realize that the current has slowed down and the oxygen bubbles can come together and make bigger bubbles and that the nutrients that are carried in the stream, well, they're heavier here and settle down because the current isn't fast enough to keep them going. And they kind of settle down and go down to the bottom of the pool. And as a result of the availability of oxygen and nutrients, the things that grow there are healthier, and bigger and stronger and that's the way that it happens.

That's the way homeostasis that we see in nature all the time, takes place. And then if you walk on a little further you come to the place where the pool starts to narrow down and go back into the stream. You understand that's the way the waste products, the leaves that have fallen into the pool and all that stuff, get picked up by that current and get carried away to be disposed of someplace else. And this is the balance of nature and nature really understands this balance. And if we listen really, really well to that kind of balance, we find that most everything that we do has a similar sort of homeostasis. But sometimes we get so busy with the feelings we have and the emotions we have, and the lack of understanding of the physiology, that we really forget how well we are able to balance.

As you think about all the things that go into letting you know that you know a great deal within yourself about how to heal and how healing happens, and how you really really, really can understand that you can do the most marvelous things by taking the physical, physiological and psychological aspects of pain here. And the physical was the cavity you got the first time, and the physiological was the actual part of the tooth that had the difficulty, and the pain and the psychological was dealing with the concern and the guilt and the anger that came with the dentist. And you're thinking, well, maybe I should have done it sooner, and maybe I deserve for him to be so mean to me, and did I do the right thing by getting up and walking away?

I think that it is important that you know that I *know* that I believe that you did everything properly. That it was appropriate for you to get up and leave because he did not understand and he really did you a disservice. And it's important to me that you do not take it out on your tooth because that would not be fair. Because it's appropriate for you to be fair to yourself and to know, whether or not you had a reason for the pain back then as a warning or the danger signal, now you can really let that pain settle down.

And as that happens, the circulation that soothes that nerve has the branches that go from just in front of your ear, to down into your lower neck, to your lower jaw, your eye and behind your ear and up our head. You can *feel* them being washed and soothed with the circulation that carries the oxygen to help them to be really, really comfortably balanced, really, really comfortable and at rest, because it's been such a long time.

And we know that when a nerve has been irritated, that there has been muscle tension with it. You know that I asked you if the pain came from the stress of the grinding or the grinding came from the stress of the pain. It really doesn't matter which it was as long as you will permit it to be over, to be done. And to recognize that any time you have muscle stress, anytime that you grit your teeth or grind your teeth, clench your fist or curl your toes, you are putting strain on those muscles. If you do that, and you do that for a long time, those muscles get tired.

When those muscles are stressed, the muscles create a lactic acid as a byproduct, because the lactic acid makes it hurt, makes it ache. I always picture that lactic acid as being kind of a smooth oily yellow liquid that I can bounce out of those muscles by pushing oxygen into them. When the oxygen displaces the lactic acid, those muscles can be refreshed and invigorated and relaxed. You can see the lactic acid drip and roll down the outside of the muscles, and in this case down across your shoulder, down through your arm and drip out the ends of your fingers.

I really, really think that it's time that you decide that you don't need to have that toothache any more. The only reason that you had it was that it was a danger signal. As long as normal healing is progressing, you can be absolutely amazed at how very comfortable you can be. As you let yourself realize how much your mind missed when it managed to make that motivation for letting your toothache go away, turn into all these things that you hadn't thought about it being. As you let yourself go into that space where this is all so much more clear, even though it may be confusing to the conscious mind. But the things that are important, the things that matter are the things that you may not have known, but your body has known. Your body has so much experience at healing. It has had so much experience at knowing and it knows how to heal.

By putting in perspective all these other kinds of interferences, you can let yourself get that balance back that is so important for you. And I wonder and you probably know, just how long it will take for those things to get reoriented and settled into the place where you can deal with them. And I will give you all the time you need, in the time you have to do whatever you need to do with what you have learned, and then we can talk about it.

T: I'm a very patient person. I've given her permission because I gave her a lot of information to take the time she needs to reorient. And also I know that she knows we are here for a purpose and she's not going to push that time. So the trust comes in.

V: The little Pac-Men were in there. I'm totally pain free. You know what?

I didn't know I was so mad at my tooth. And you didn't even do anything.

T: I knew. That's right. But once you figured that out, that was all you really needed to do, wasn't it?

V: It was a perfect clear picture. The Pac-Men came in with little buckets of calcium and went to work and they cleared a canal and watched it flow.

T: Your dentist may have trouble with that. But you can tell him on good authority that it works.

V: But I am totally pain free. Totally. Very comfortable.

T: That's great.

V: You guys know how good this feels?

T: How good it feels to not feel? Because when it doesn't hurt, you're not aware that it doesn't feel. It's only when something hurts that you're aware that it feels.

V: Are you intuitive to little things that I said? You used certain words that fit me, little things that you used that fit me perfectly, in just three minutes.

T: I get inside your head.

V: She got inside my tooth, trust me!

T: I spend all my time inside people's heads, remember? Gasserian ganglion. Questions?

Question: What kind of words helped you (the client) stay with her?

V: Medical terminology, and I understood what they meant. It was almost like she knew me personally so I was really just tuning in to her.

Question: I'm not going to be able to give medical terminology for all the pain problems. How will I address the pain without knowing the terminology?

T: If you cannot use the medical terms? I know her background and I hooked her with Ganglion. I have in my bag, a tablet and pencil and would have drawn what we were talking about. The metaphor I used of the stream and the pool and narrowing and carrying away the waste products is the one that I almost always use for healing with my patients. And that doesn't require any medical knowledge at all. I wasn't sure that she needed it. It's a good example and good imagery to utilize.

Question: How will you know that the pain is gone?

V: I'll know in six weeks or will know when I land in Florida. She tapped into my belief system. When I go in the airplane, it will increase pressure. If I land in Florida with pain, I will have to go to a dentist and get this fixed.

T: Two sentences that I used that you heard but you didn't hear. When everything that can be done and should be done, has been done, there's no longer any reason for the pain. That does not imply that the patient is going to get well. It can be a terminal pain that they are dealing with. And if everything that can be done and should be done, has been done and they want to enjoy a good quality of life, at that point they can turn off the pain. But the other thing that I put in there is: You can be pleasantly surprised at how comfortable you will be as long as normal healing is progressing. What's the opposite of that? If normal healing isn't progressing, lady, it's gonna hurt. I don't have to say that. I'm building in the protection for her. As long as this is healing normally she can remain comfortable, but if it is no longer healing normally, she will have difficulty. She will have pain. But it's giving that protection in a positive way.

Dentists are very careful. We tend to tell the patient, you only have a 50–50 chance because we don't want to take the responsibility. We do informed consent by telling them all the terrible things that can happen. You can get a broken jaw when we take this tooth out, you can get a dry socket, you can bleed or any of this sort of stuff.

You have to recognize that some of your most vulnerable patients are those patients who will do all these things because you told them to. So that you give them the informed consent and then you say, but here are the things that you can do to help yourself to be certain as possible that you will heal normally and naturally. You protect them. You build this protection in. It's hard to get that way of speaking when you have been taught the other way for so many years. But it's really important because those patients who hear the words you say for healing are going to go out and do it. She doesn't need to know the mechanism, but she understands the principle.

Question: Do you use the same language with migraines?

T: Yeah, I use a variation on the circulatory system. How often I explain depends entirely on the feeling I get from the patient. I don't have a real sense of that. Every patient is different and the way I work is different. I use the same stories. I can't make up a different story for every patient and I don't need to, but the story will vary according to the patient. And I made an effort to get into her head.

Question: About your playing with words.

T: When I play with words, I'm appealing to her earlier learning set and getting her to play with the words. That means that her whole body is going to be involved in them and see them and hear them and feel them at an earlier response level, when Mommy could kiss the booboo and make it better. And so I'm going to have more credibility with what I say at that point.

V: You have my full attention. The rhymes draw me into it comfortably. Right now I'm going to be nurtured, I'm going to be rhymed.

Question: Do you find confusion technique especially useful in pain issues or specifically working with her?

T: I'm being accused of using a lot of confusion techniques and here I thought I wasn't using very much at all. Do I find it especially useful in working with pain? Yes. You need to know that she was never confused. So much of what is called the confusion technique is confusing to the people outside listening. Because she and I are in the same place, she can follow me on an unconscious level. I have no question about that. [Speaking directly to V] I don't think that you felt confused?

That's an important part of the misconception about confusion technique. It's not just playing with a lot of words to get her to have trouble following me. It's to get that message and to get the attention, so she will really focus in on that, and recognize that I believe that she's going to do what I am saying that she can do.

V: This was the first time that I felt as nurtured and taken care of. She was very kind and gentle and loving and it was almost like a parent and it was authoritative. She knew that I was going to comply. It was a very nurturing experience, one of the most loving experiences I have ever had even though it was highly directive.

T: I believe that there is a time when I need to take charge. When somebody has been having pain and has not been able to do anything about it and they are looking to me to do something about it, I'm not going to sit here and say, "Well, if you really want to …" No! I know what you need to do and I want you to do it!

Question: If you were working with some other kind of pain, like a facial pain, would there be another way to describe the Gasserian ganglion?

T: I would make it relevant to the particular pain. I might be more metaphorical than I was here. Recognizing that we have a sophisticated person sitting across from me, I offer more sophisticated options. I'm a good one for drawing and getting the person to focus in and just almost translate that into the idea of the hypnotic induction, using that as dissociative imagery.

Question: How much information do you need for this physiological work?

V: I let her know that I was a visual person. I closed my eyes and did my own surgery. I specifically chose to close my eyes. As she talked about the swelling I could visualize and this is what she is telling me to do. For me, the exact physiology was very effective.

T: For very young patients, I'm not going to do that. For patients who want to be out on a raft on Lake Erie during surgery, I wouldn't do that. For someone who didn't trust me and wanted to be right there during the surgery, then I would do that. It's a judgment based on the information I get from the patient. It varies. There is no one way that any of this can work.

Question: Could you speak to your use of "I" and the personal?

T: I get involved with my patients. One of the things I said early on about Dr. Erickson was that I know that people are supposed to remain objective when working with patients, but that doesn't mean you cannot be compassionate. There are some people who can do both and I think he exemplified that extraordinarily well. I'm quite capable to convince them with my own commitment. When I say to someone, "I know you can do this!" the conviction I have from my own personal experience, transmits itself to that individual. I've heard this as a response from people. That's the way it works for me. I'm willing to let people know that I use this and I believe in this and they too can do this. They are at least as smart as I am.

Question: What were you paying attention to?

T: We didn't have an audience after the first few minutes. You don't matter. I was focusing on her and on my words and watching very carefully her nonverbal communication, thinking about what I was saying to make her imagery clear. The best way to do that was to do this in trance. Do I need to cut this short? Then I would lighten the trance state and would use it to see where we need to go. I am functioning in trance, almost as though you are driving a car and looking four cars in front. I am making an effort to do that here. Where am I going to go next is based on how she responds to it. It is constantly changing, based on her response—wiggling an eyebrow or clenching a jaw or relaxing the muscles on that side. All of these things I am paying attention to.

Question: When you are in trance, are you refreshed after the session?

T: I am exhausted. I am working hard. My brain is thinking. I don't know how anyone can do this for 8 or 10 hours a day. You need to put all your commitment to it. If you aren't making that commitment, the client will know that I am just saying words and they don't mean what they feel. I felt what I meant and believed everything that I said. That's the important part of it.

Question: About rapport through e-mail.

T: I think a lot of people who use e-mail and the computer are eating time. The way they eat time is that you go into a trance when you go in there. You determine the purpose for which you sit down at the computer. There's no reason you couldn't sit down at the computer for the therapeutic reason. I suspect that in the next few years, there will be an explosion of information on this particular version of focused attention or altered states, whatever you want to call it.

I didn't have any idea how this was going to work out. I just had faith that it would. You gave me an opportunity for us to teach a lot of people how to generalize things about pain. The most important part is that you learned to turn off that pain in your tooth.

V: You brought up yesterday in your workshop that there is a trust issue. I sat in your workshop in advance and saw your technique and I believe the healing had begun yesterday and today it was completed. I admired your philosophies and techniques yesterday. It was almost pre-set-up.

T: If you don't have that relationship, then you better learn how to establish it really well and soundly with the person that you are going to work with.

Chapter Twenty-four
Clinical Posthypnotic Suggestion

First Demonstration: Time

We have enough time in our lifetime to deal with the kinds of things that we have to deal with. The problem is we tend to get impatient much of the time. We talk about peripheral vision. I don't know whether he knew that I was watching him as he was sitting in his trance, but we talked earlier about the fact that he had been given a suggestion about having enough time. In order to ask him to come out of the trance he was in, in order to have the opportunity to go into another trance, all I had to do was say the word time. And I got his immediate attention.

T: Did you know I did that?

V: No!

T: Did you know you did that?

V: No.

T: Do you now?

V: I believe you.

T: Why are you here?

V: Even though when I am working and thinking I can go into a trance, I have never had a good responsive experience in trance. When I go into a trance with someone else my experience is I get real scared and don't respond well to the other person. On my own, I move in and out quite freely. The last time I worked with Dr. Erickson, he said, "You need more time." I told Kay, it's been a number of years. More time is relatively open ended. I'm curious, have I learned what I need to learn?

T: More time is really open ended. If what you need is openness in that time, then how much time does it take to learn to be as open as you need?

V: Well, the thought that comes to mind is that I heard Erickson say, "We think things have to be learned slowly. But they can be learned very very quickly, in an instant almost." That somehow doesn't make sense. No.

T: That's right, it really doesn't. In an instant, you can do so many things. I'm sure you have heard him talk about, when you are waiting for a bus on a cold and windy and rainy day and the bus is on time. And you have been there 10 minutes and it seems like an hour, and the bus is really really late, but it isn't, it's on time. It's only that your perception of the waiting has been very long. With a nice pleasant day with the sun and breeze and with the right kind of people, waiting for the same bus you may have been waiting a half-hour. When the bus comes, it seems like you have been there only an instant.

The *real* time has nothing to do with the time that is reeling by in your head. That kind of instant in universal time takes a universe to move. But you can move worlds in the time that it takes you to talk about that kind of item. You find that it's really kind of timely when you are ready to realize not that you have to respond to the other person, because the only person you have to respond to is you. You do it in your own way, but you do it with an openness that lets you understand that it may be the time you have been looking for, rather than the time you have been waiting for. The time you look for is the appropriate time to do what you need to do. You have all the time you need in the time you have.

It doesn't really matter whether it is cold and windy and rainy. You can do the same amount of work in that instant that seems like an hour that you might do in that hour that seems like an instant, when the circumstances are better. Does it *really* make any difference whether that time takes a long time or a short time, from where you are right now to where you were, or does it really only matter, that the way that you get from yesterday to tomorrow is by going through today? It doesn't make any difference where yesterday was. It only matters where today is. In this kind of universe that we have, it is almost as if there is a universality of man that we have always been and will always be.

The message for the individual is to be able to take the time to go inside and to look around and to understand that when you *really* have control, then you don't need it. It's only the people who don't have control who have to have it all the time to be sure they don't lose it. When you are sure you really have it, you don't need it because you can get it anytime you want it.

That time is the right time to recognize that the readiness you have has been involved in the work you have been doing. And the acceptance of the understanding that the time is now and the time is then, and it is time to take the time to look back in absolute surprise and amazement at all the things that have gone on and all of the things you have absorbed. And to recognize that as you let yourself become more absorbed in that kind of absorption, it's all right there where it's been all along. It's just that you haven't looked in the right time frame. Because you do each reel of this movie of your life, frame by frame by frame. The time framework that you are working in at any one time lets you flow forward or back with the ability to stop the frame to examine it to see the things you might have missed the initial time you went through it. And to realize that you can take all the past experiences and run them by in the mirror of your mind very very quickly in terms of using them in that future time that you will need them for.

It doesn't matter what kind of responsiveness you have to anyone else because you are the center of this wheel that revolves around you. You can permit all those people their impact on your center, knowing as they change and move in that wheel, you have the stability of being the core of yourself. You can permit them to change without changing you except in the way you let them look at you. No matter what happens outside, you have the ability to decide whether that time is appropriate for you to move forward with that wheel or simply to let it move around you and let you remain in the place you need to be at that particular moment. The ability to accept whether the wheel is marking time or whether it is moving forward really doesn't make any difference.

The only thing that matters is that you understand that in your own good time you find that you have known all along the things that you really didn't know you knew. You can accept this universal reference to time as being any moment now. It doesn't make any real sense to not accept, and so you find that you can be really comfortable as you anticipate the things that you didn't know that you knew. And it's all right for you to know now that you don't no any longer because you have suddenly found out you can say, "Yes," and that's nice, isn't it?

Question: About ending up at the same place.

T: It's interesting that we ended up at the same place. Because I was headed for "yes" at the same exact time that he started to nod yes. And I thought that was absolutely so nice of him. I really did. I don't know and I don't need to know all of the things that went into that situation being presented, because it really isn't any of my business. He was giving the assignment to work on this and what I was doing was being very open about his needing to let himself be more open. When he is open in this way, he is still safe and private and protected and it's okay for him to decide that it's time to accept that kind of thing. And that can be very nonspecific and very, very general and still let him do the things he needs to do, which I think is more appropriate in a situation like this. But there were an astonishing number of posthypnotic suggestions given in that which I assume you were hearing.

One of the things I teach is that when someone terminates trance I do not immediately turn to them and say, "How was that?" Because they need time to get it settled within their own head. For anything they choose to let fade away to fade away like a dream and for anything they choose to bring forward to bring forward. So I come up with some innocuous chatter here to give him time do that. And has anyone counted the number of times I have said "time" since I quit talking about time?

Question: About what I was saying about the posthypnotic suggestions that were given after the trance was ended.

T: The trance hadn't been ended. Although I appear to not be paying any attention, I watch when he changes his glance from his hands to looking at me or looking out at you people or being reflective again. And I gauge that kind of internal responsiveness and I reinforce everything that I have said. That serves two purposes. It bridges the gap between the trance work and the usual distracted state and lets people understand there is a bridge there that they can utilize, and it reinforces the things that were said while he was doing this work.

Question: How did that compare with his expectation or his sense of where he wanted to go, which was verbalized as learning to be able to be more comfortable with someone else working with trance rather than simply relying on himself?

V: The nice thing about this trance experience is that after watching Kay this morning, I knew if I had the opportunity to go into trance with her, I was going to see what happens and follow her. That was the big difference between this one and the other ones. In the other ones I had reams of anticipations and paid a great deal of attention to subtle suggestions. With this one I was just looking at Kay and listening to her.

T: One of the things that I was not about to do was make any effort to get him to close his eyes. I used a lot of facial expression. I was giving all sorts of nonverbal reinforcement to the things I was saying. When I wanted him to be more introspective I would think with my face. When I wanted him to be more reflective I would put that kind of an expression on, just mirroring really what my words were saying in terms of getting him to recognize that he does have all these skills. Hear them and let's use them!

This is why it's so hard for me to talk about posthypnotic suggestion. You see it in action and realize that all of that was taking the past and orienting it toward the future, so it was all posthypnotic suggestion work from my frame of reference.

Question: Would I ever explore emotional things that came from the past?

T: It just occurred to me that one of the things I should share with you is that when he asked me about this, I asked him if he was willing to do this as a demonstration. I said this is a fairly straightforward kind of thing. We can maintain your integrity. Did you get that sense that you would be safe doing this? [Volunteer said, "Yes."] That was part of the contract. I would not violate my portion of the contract and would permit both of us to work in a safe situation. What I said at the end of this was "it really isn't any of my business and I don't care," because the work he has to do is work he has indicated he can do on his own.

One of the things I am doing while talking is monitoring him (the volunteer she worked with) and making sure everything is going well with him. That's the kind of responsibility you have when you offer someone these kinds of opportunities. Erickson said that when you teach someone this kind of skill, you have the obligation to teach them how to handle it. That's not hypnosis. It really isn't.

Second Demonstration: Getting Rest

T: I was going to say, why are you here? When I listen to the possible answers, I will have to assume that she understands the one meaning I am asking her to respond to before I say, why are you here?

V: I'm here because I want to learn either to go to sleep when I want to or not to need sleep I've missed when I haven't. My preference is to go to sleep when I want to. I have had problems with sleeping off and on for 20 years. I was thinking that part of the reason is probably that I don't have enough time right now by myself. I have a reasonably full practice and a 3-year-old child and after she's gone to bed, there's my husband to talk to and there isn't any time.

T: And there isn't time for you? And that's important. And you said something about energy. Do you teach your patients trance? Do they like it? Do you like it? She likes it a lot. I'm asking yes and no answers so you can see the answers. What do you do with trance, yourself?

V: Sometimes, I use it to go to sleep. In the area I live, I don't know anyone who uses hypnosis, who I trust as a clinician. As soon as I came to the conference and someone did a trance with me, I remembered how much easier it is to go into trance with someone else and experience it. I've used it myself to plan what I was going to do for the day and to get rid of a psychosomatic stomachache, things like that.

T: One of the things that we are doing, here and now, is taking turns. I talk for a minute and I give you the microphone and you talk and give it back, and I think that life is kind of a series of instances of taking turns. And sometimes it seems as though you really think your turn will never come, and that's really pretty tough and it's not fair. One of the things that I think that it's fair to say is that everybody needs to know that they do have time to take their turn and it's time for everyone to recognize that it's only fair for you to have the time to take your turn.

You are saying that trance can be useful for so many things. And yet I hear a void in there for using it for the one thing that you really need it for, almost as though there was some question about whether you deserved to use it for your own time. Because the void I hear is being able to use it when it means doing things for other people, when it means accomplishing things you need to accomplish, but not for you, pure and simple. You find that it's easier to let someone else do it in terms of teaching you to go into trance. But I wonder whether it's really true, because all you do is bounce off the words someone else says to accomplish your own objective.

You talk to yourself all the time so you've learned how not to listen, which makes it harder to do for yourself. But I wonder what your mind would listen to, in terms of having it be your turn to sit down with a tape recorder on that other chair? And to put yourself on that tape recorder in your mind and to fill that avoidance you have been utilizing, by talking to yourself and saying the things that you need to hear, because you know better than anyone else *what it is that you really need to hear*. And when you are finished telling that tape what it is—*that's better*—that you need to hear, then when you rewind the tape, that will be the signal for you to go into an even more profound trance.

So as you listen to that tape of your own words coming at you from outside your head, you will find that it will be even more effective than just having someone like me talking with you in this circumstance. You might be really curious as to how very, very quickly you can learn to turn off that tape, when there's something that you want to think about, so you can turn on that ability to turn off and to let yourself go wherever it is you want to go with such skill. It will be kind of funny to wonder why you waited so long before you found out that you know everything about turning off and putting to rest all of the things that need to be given the opportunity to recharge and regenerate during that rest period.

And it can be arresting for you to think without having to think about that void that you have avoided filling in terms of knowing that quiet time spent in a car, driving, thinking can be your own precious private time or that quiet time spent is not so much quantity necessary as quality necessary. You know how to teach time distortion. So the quality of time that you experience in time distortion can be so great, that your mind can accomplish all the things it needs to accomplish without avoiding the necessity for the rest that your body needs, in order to fulfill the rest of the things you need to do with that body.

And that the energy that you store up when you are resting in that sleep that is so very comfortable will be of a higher quality, because you know it will give you the time you want and need in the quality of private quiet time distortion that can be so long in such a short time. Because it's been such a long time that you've had anything but a short time to turn into the quality of time you really want. And as you let yourself listen to the things that you know that you are going to say that you need to be able to see, that you can hear, in order to understand that you have all the skills and abilities that you really want and need, and that you trust yourself on that unconscious level to be able to put the things on tape.

And to find that the most amazing thing will happen, that when you turn on that tape and listen, it can be so productive that you might not need to remember what is on it. And it can be fun to realize that the tape is there whenever you want it and you can deliberately choose not to remember, or to not remember the things that are on the tape because they are your own private secrets. Because that private time in that secret place can be of such quality that it will suffice to let you get the rest the rest of the time that you have arrested yourself from getting.

And as you need it, you know that the amount of time that you rest will be the amount of time that you need to sleep. And you can be comfortable with that in a way that you have never come forth with before. And as you become more comfortable with that becoming, you can feel how very becoming it is to become what you wanted to be all along. Because that's really what it's all about. And take all the time you need in the time you have.

And nobody really heard me say anything about insomnia, because I don't think that's important. She said a lot of other things in a very short time. I was giving a lot of those other things the space that I think she doesn't have time to give them in other circumstances and situations, and a method for reaching the space she needs to do those things that are in that place, because there's nobody else.

But in the long run, is there really ever anybody else? They can help and support and say, "Go, girl!" but you are the one who has to do it. And making the doing of it more practical, more realistic and more reachable is all we can do—the catalyst in the structure of the learning situation. Now again, I am monitoring both my time and her time. And she knows that. And when it gets to be time, she also is aware of that.

Question: Was I being literal about the tape?

T: When I speak to her about making the tape, I intend that literally, and I would recommend it to anyone here who is out in the woods as a missionary all by themselves, because you do know better than anyone else what you need to hear. And you talk to yourselves all the time but you have learned how not to listen.

Right? And it's very difficult to not listen when that tape with your own voice is coming in from outside. It's very, very potentially productive.

Question: Did I take that statement as a multilevel communication?

T: There were a number of messages in that statement and the way I said it was, "Very, well, of course, that's a fact." Isn't it? She decreed that it is. Therefore, it is. At least think about the fact that when patients come in, they bring in all sorts of posthypnotic suggestions. Everything that you hope they will accomplish in the future is a function of the posthypnotic suggestions that you have given, rather than making it a narrow segment of the hypnotic trance experience, because it certainly is not that.

Part VIII
Ethics in Caring

Kay Thompson was renowned for many things, including her integrity, the integration of her ethics in all aspects of her life. She didn't take time to teach about ethics; she lived them, modeling and inspiring ethics in caring, in the same way she modeled so many of her teachings.

Thompson saw people when they were in need and did whatever was necessary to help them. When she made a commitment to help someone, serve on a committee or work for an organization, she was fully and completely there. When clients needed four hours for an abreaction, she stayed with them. She often worked well into the night, seeing patients, students, and colleagues, even while attending congresses and workshops. Her respect for the privacy of her clients was so important to her that she said that she refused to do therapy during clinical demonstrations, when almost all of her colleagues were doing so, because Erickson also had refused. She truly "walked the talk" and deeply respected the same in others.

She gave her time, energy and skills generously to her patients, students, colleagues and friends. Her commitment to community was equally significant; she worked tirelessly for professional organizations and was an active politician and leader in many, besides being a board member for numerous professional and service organizations. She only charged $50 per hour throughout her career, when she could have charged multiples more, even as her fame increased.

Thompson was perfectly aware of most people's shortcomings, but saw through to the core potential within. Her dedication to awakening the potential of others guided her throughout her life. This simple commitment was fundamental to all her teachings and yet she recognized that it was hard for many therapists to grasp and embody.

Kay Thompson's integrity was the very foundation of her being.

Chapter Twenty-five
Ethics
Selections from Panel Discussions

> Today responsibility is often meant to denote duty, something
> imposed on one another from the outside. But responsibility, in its
> truest sense, is an entirely voluntary act; it is my response to the
> needs, expressed or unexpressed, of another human being.
>
> *Erich Fromm*

*In this simple but profound introduction, Thompson defines the ethical
premises for her work.*

Ethics is not a genetic trait. Ethics has to be learned. Working with
hypnosis has the potential to demand more of an awareness of an
ethical sense, because you need to recognize the vulnerability of the
people you are working with, and it becomes your responsibility to
behave in an appropriate way. Utilization of hypnosis opens the
gates for abuses in ethics in unique ways.

The words that always impacted me with what Erickson did were
"respect for the patient". He was going to where that patient was.
When he picked me out and started working on me, he was encou
aging women. He encouraged women and minorities. His sense of
what was right was so strong. I wished we could build it into all of
our therapists and health professionals. So many of the people who
are writing stories, and books and are teaching about him only
knew him in the last years as a teacher. We knew him when he was
strong, dynamic, authoritative, Machiavellian, whatever he needed
to be for the welfare of the individual.

If you have this respect, concern, this absolute conviction that this
person can improve and get better, then the ethics are obvious; you
don't have to think about them, you have them. If you can handle
yourself in an ethical fashion, then you can handle clients.
(Thompson 1994a.)

In the following panel discussions and workshops, we have a unique opportunity to hear Kay Thompson discuss a wide range of ethical issues. Remarks include her introduction, clinical vignettes and selections from some of the question-and-answer segments.

I tend to be very simplistic. I am out there doing. I don't have a lot of time to get inside their heads before I go inside their heads to do my work. I don't have a lot of time to build transference, to worry about transference; to build trust, to worry about trust. When I started, I was getting all the disturbed patients from most of the psychiatrists in the city, because I was the only one willing to work with them as patients—not the psychiatrists, their patients.

I didn't know very much about psychiatric situations and circumstances. But I realized that even disturbed patients get toothaches and that somebody had to deal with them. And I recognized the psychological significance of the oral cavity with these people I was working on. It was easy for these people to say to me while they were in my chair utilizing hypnosis, "Why don't you make me some suggestions for x, y and z?" Recognize that it is very tempting when you first learn hypnosis and you start doing hypnotic phenomena, to think that you are making them do these things, because enough patients have not spit in your eye to tell you that you are not making them to do it.

Consider the patient who has been coming to me for dentistry and is a really good patient. And she says, "I'm doing pretty well with Weight Watchers and I can't lose that last 15 pounds. While I'm in trance, if you just make some suggestions about my eating, I would really appreciate it." She's a good patient and I can justify my suggestions. She'll be eating things that are good for her mouth, and she won't be snacking between meals because that's not good for the teeth, and I can justify it from a dental viewpoint. Right? Okay, I might make a couple of suggestions.

What I don't know is that she and her husband are having marital problems and that extra 15 pounds is what keeps him turned off to her. And so she doesn't have to say, "Sorry not tonight, I have a headache." It's the extra 15 pounds that accomplishes the same thing. What happens is that the hypnosis suggestions for the weight loss don't work, because they shouldn't; because I'm not dealing with the real reason why she isn't losing her weight. And when she comes back to me the next time, I become a lousy hypnotherapist, our relationship is destroyed and I can't even use the hypnosis for the dentistry. (Thompson, 1994b.)

You need to make sure your clients understand the suggestions you give them. Errors of omission, rather than commission, occur when people stray outside their field of competence. It gets really tempting when you first learn hypnosis, and go to a party and someone says, "I hear you've taken a course on hypnosis, I want to stop smoking." Instantly, you have this crowd around you, saying, "Oh yeah! Yeah! Hypnotize him, make him stop smoking!" If you have listened to anything I've said, you can't make stop them smoking. In the second place, the party ain't the place to show off. And in the third place, you are outside your field of competence when you are playing that kind of game in that kind of situation. (Thompson, 1995a.)

A lot of people really tried to get me to do these things. I had a really good teacher. I didn't stray outside my field. I went back and studied psychology. The ethics of the circumstance becomes a lot wavier. Back when I learned hypnosis, it was only taught to physicians and dentists and PhD psychologists. That was a strong rule. That would have eliminated most of the people at this conference. The ethical responsibility the doctors have to their patients, is to make sure that the ancillary people who are going to be working with clients have an understanding of the power that the other speaker was talking about, when they are using hypnosis.

I am really distressed by the fact that ethics are not being stressed enough. Our technological capacity has far outstripped our social conscience, and we are not paying enough attention to this. We need to have more emphasis placed on discerning the appropriate ethical circumstances in the utilization of hypnosis. Because it's really easy to justify what it is we are doing, by virtue of the tool we are using. It ain't the tool, it's what we do with it. Give me a pair of forceps and I can do the right thing with a tooth. Give you a pair of forceps and you are going to destroy that mouth. Hypnosis works very much the same way. It is a very powerful tool. It is the precision with which it is utilized that we need to be concerned with.

I say a lot of outrageous comments to my patients. I am willing to push a lot of boundaries. I am willing to make a fool of myself. I am willing to have them in my home for the therapy they need. The bottom line is that we should do what is fair and right for the patient's best interests. That ain't easy to determine.

The ethics involved in this whole issue, concerns how we are able to determine within ourselves what we are doing for the patient and client, versus what it is we think we ought to be doing, to get them to do what it is we think they ought to be doing. That is a sticky issue because who knows best? The motivation and insight we can provide will become more and more relevant as the ethical issue becomes more apparent. Other countries have different standards about who can learn what kind of hypnosis. Many of them are much narrower than the generic kind of teaching we are doing in the United States.

Question: About ethical issues with a psychiatrist using hypnosis to retrieve memories about alien abductions.

T: Stage hypnosis is a clear violation and everyone knows that. I hope we are going to get some laws about it and draw up an educational level and at least say where we are going to use hypnosis. Memory retrieval is much trickier. We don't really understand what the boundaries are in terms of hypnosis.

A physician called me and he wanted me to see his wife who had been seen by the local psychologist. The psychologist thought it was in her best interests for him to have sex with her and he would put her into a trance (I don't believe she went into a trance), and then he would have sex with her. She became addicted to the man and couldn't break away from him.

The ethics are real clear. Somehow, because he did this with hypnosis, it had a different aura. The disciplinary boards get very, very mixed up when they make statements about theses cases. The other place we are having trouble with hypnosis is with the legal profession.

In some states, if I use hypnosis for hypnoanesthesia and my patients have to testify in court, I will have contaminated their testimony. That is as ridiculous as anything I have heard. But this is the misconception people have. Has anyone here been in the witness stand and testified? Do you realize you were in trance? If we can't identify when people are in trance, how can we restrict it? This is the educational responsibility we have to take on. As upstanding citizens who are using hypnosis, it is our responsibility to educate everyone we come in contact with.

Comment: Erickson mentioned that a person can't be hypnotized to do something that is against their moral or ethical code.

T: I don't believe that at all. I used to. When it is used appropriately in a clinical or a therapeutic situation by an ethical practitioner, it is true. I was involved in giving expert testimony for a case against a lay hypnotist, who used hypnosis to teach people to stop smoking and lose weight, and in the process had sex with them. He had a person come in who was a dependent personality and who was out of her element. The first time he saw her, he "hypnotized her" and proceeded to have sex with her, and gave her amnesia for the experience. She broke the amnesia with the usual traumatic episode you would expect.

The district attorney pursued a criminal conviction. We fortunately had a judge who asked the right questions and we got a decision against the lay hypnotist. He is going to jail. But she did something against her will. The question is, what was her will? What was he able to do in her vulnerable state to make her do that? He was a large man and she was a small woman.

No ethical person would ever do what he did. Nevertheless, she, through the hypnosis, did something against her will. She dissociated during trance. It was clear that she was screaming up in the ceiling and said, "No!" And the other aspect of hypnosis is brain washing and involuntary use of hypnosis with drugs. We need someone to make some rules and when they are violated, discipline people with them. You pushed my hot button.

Question: What about using hypnosis without a formal release?

T: I had a child, screaming, biting, kicking, having a tantrum with an abscessed tooth. It was a Saturday afternoon and I used hypnosis with her and it worked. The next week, her mother said, "Don't you have to ask me if you are going to use hypnosis with my daughter?" I told her, "I have treated your other children. I do what is appropriate. I don't ask if I should give a local anesthetic or use a cement base in the restoration. This is part of my treatment." Her mother said, "I'm awful glad you didn't ask me, because if you had, I would have said 'No'." In this case, I had a generic informed consent in my practice. And this was for a clinical purpose. What kind of informed consent you need depends on what you are going to be doing. (Thompson, 1994b.)

Question: How do we handle the sticky problem of informed consent?

T: In this country now, the absolute law is that you must tell your patient all of the possible negative side effects of any intervention that you make. And they must sign a statement that they fully understand the potential side effects of this treatment. I have a friend who is a neuroradiologist who talks about informed consent. He has to say, "The side effects of this procedure are blindness, stroke, and death. Do you still want this done?" What do you say? How do you convince them to do this anyway?

With molars, you have to go in with a hammer and chisel and a drill and there's all this noise and they see all this stuff coming at them and it's terrifying. And you have to tell them the potential side effects are permanent nerve damage, a broken jaw, dry sockets, infections, all of which are not nice.

I say, "Jeannie, I'm sure you have heard a lot of stories about having molars out. And with a horizontal impacted tooth, there is always the possibility when removing that tooth, of fracturing your jaw because there isn't very much jawbone there. And you have heard about how people have bled and had their socket packed. And if you don't have the right kind of socket, you get an infection. And if the nerve is wrapped around the canal, you can have some nerve damage that can affect your lip and the side of your face. Those are all things that have the potential for happening. And you know we are going to make every effort to keep those things from happening. And here are the things you can do to make sure that this procedure will proceed uneventfully and you will heal as rapidly as possible."

You are taking advantage of this last in, first out process. The things in the informed consent come first. And then you say *but*. They hear the "but" because they don't want these things to happen. Here are the things which are your responsibility, which you can do to help to be certain that these things will not take place.

I'll give some other examples in terms of terminology.

Dentist A: "Gee, I just did this really big deep cavity preparation. It was so deep when I finally got all that decay out, that I could see the red of the pulp chamber through the dentine and I'm not sure if the tooth is going to be all right. I don't want to put a permanent silver filling in because if the tooth blows up, we'll have to take it out. So I'm going to put a temporary filling in there until we see whether the tooth is going to be all right. If it is, we can put the permanent filling in sometime in the future. In the meantime if this tooth should start to hurt, call me right away, because it will only get worse."

I have given all the appropriate informed information about that restoration. For the patient, the question is, "Is it hurting yet?" Not whether or not it is going to hurt, just is it hurting yet?

I go to a different dentist because I didn't like that. I have exactly the same cavity on the other side of the mouth.

Dentist B: "Gee, that was a pretty big job we did today. I'm pleased we got all that decay out of there. That made me feel very good. You know when you put a silver spoon in coffee and in ice cream, how fast it transmits heat and cold? If I put a metal filling in your tooth, every time you eat something hot or cold, it will hammer that tooth and you'll feel the jolt from the temperature. So I'm going to put a sedative filling in there in order to give the nerve and the pulp chamber a chance to pull back and deposit an insulating layer of dentine. After a month or six weeks we'll put the permanent filling in. In the meantime, if you have any questions, give me a call."

Which dentist would you rather go to? You have exactly the same information in both situations. I have been harping, listen to what you say. Trance-late the negatives to positives and start practicing them. I wasn't born speaking positively. (Thompson, 1983.)

Question: About teaching people hypnosis who are not professionally trained in hypnosis.

T: Karen Olness, who is a pediatric physician, has addressed this in all her teaching. One of my things is teaching language for patient management and pain control. It is not my decision as to whether or not the patient goes into a trance. I don't think that teaching people in the health professions about the power of their words, about verbal and nonverbal communication, and about responsive behavior, has to come under the category of hypnosis. A colleague said that when she is going to use formal induction, she uses a formal consent. When she uses indirect induction, she does not feel she needs to get an informed consent. It is an interpersonal working relationship.

When you are using indirect induction techniques, you don't get any feedback from the person and you don't really know if they went in trance or not. I would use that as my answer. I am telling the story. If they choose to go into trance, I just presented them with the opportunity. That's kind of the way I would go about this. I'm sure this is not an easy problem to address.

Question: When can I start utilizing hypnosis in my practice and what do I have to tell my patients?

T: When I took my first course, I came home to my first client who had a dying nerve. I said everything wrong, but it worked because she was motivated. It's better to start with easy circumstances, like utilizing hypnosis to relax.

When you are using it to get a specific result, you need to get an informed consent. At this point you are simply teaching them to be more comfortable. When I teach them how to relax and they say, "You were trying to hypnotize me, weren't you?" I put on my wide-eyed, bushy-tailed expression. I reply: "No, Mrs. Jones,

I was only teaching you how to relax. Of course, the ultimate is hypnosis, but I didn't know that you were so good!" It's all in the way you present it. This is my personal belief system. This is what I am teaching to my patients. Always have the best interest of the client as primary.

For that reason, I believe that it is worth trying to help patients. The worse thing that happens is that nothing happens. We've gotten into some fairly interesting kinds of things. Why not? Because frequently, the mental distress that the patient is under increases the tension, thereby increasing the neurological response and making the deficit worse. If all you do, for instance with a cerebral palsy patient, is teach them how to relax and be more comfortable, they will have better control.

If all you ever do is teach your patients how to relax, which I think is only the beginning of the hypnosis and not always necessarily the beginning, but rather the ending, they are going to benefit from that and so are you! Let's face it, working on a nice, easy comfortable patient who is not having spasms and sitting all tensed up and making it difficult to get into his mouth, makes your work a lot easier. And that's part of the reason for using hypnosis, isn't it? (Thompson, 1994b.)

In this workshop, Thompson suggests that we have an ethical responsibility to suggest positive outcomes. Her ideas have been substantiated by recently published research about "nocebos", or the effect of negative suggestions.

T: Our whole orientation is negative toward bleeding, toward hurting. Tell the person the worst thing that can happen, because if it doesn't happen, you look so good. The really good suggestive patients go out and fulfill your highest expectations. They have all the worst things happen because you told them they would. Do you have the right to do that to your patients? I don't think you do. I know I don't. I have the right to give them the opportunity to have the best things happen. I have never, in 30 years, had a patient come back and say, "You didn't tell me how bad this was going to be!" That's what we are all afraid of. I'm not so afraid to be unwilling to take the risk.

T: It's okay to have this conscious level of wondering concern, it's your unconscious that we need to be dealing with. Every time it works, I say, "Thank you!" Culturally, I still have this fear. On an unconscious level, I don't let it stop me. It's okay to be afraid as long as you can go ahead anyway. It requires some trust in the patient or client. (Thompson, 1983.)

In this workshop, Thompson emphasizes the obligation of the therapist to do whatever the client needs.

This was what Erickson was willing to do. Be uncomfortable yourself if that's what the patient needs. I used to take myself by the scruff of my neck and go into a private room and talk myself into doing something I'd have to do, like what Erickson did with the German man in a wheelchair. It's tough to be that confrontational and have a Machiavellian relationship with someone who has come to you for help. They need the help. It doesn't matter if you are uncomfortable with it. If being tough is what they need, that's what you have an obligation to do. (Thompson, 1995b.)

Thompson received the Pennsylvania Dental Association Annual Award weeks before her death. The following brief remarks about orga- nizational ethics are from her acceptance speech.

Our high priests are being defrocked—old laws are changing. We must adapt or perish. We must establish a caring form of power, not a power of manipulation and exploitation. Compassion, coopera- tion and patience must come from within and bring us together. Strategic planning involves not only the direction, but the energy with which an organization must move, and the responsibility those managing the association must accept. You need to do what is right and decent and honorable. Be a volunteer and take it seriously.

At the ADA (Kay was the second woman to serve on the Board of Trustees of the American Dental Association in 134 years), Dave Whiston called me the "Conscience of the ADA Board". I owed no one any favors, political or otherwise. I was outside the usual polit- ical process of deal making. I had no hidden agenda or further aspi- rations—although many people did not believe that—so I could maintain my integrity. I was free to make the best appointments, not the most politically expedient, for people to serve at the ADA, especially since I got very few suggestions from the districts when I requested them.

And I could fight for what we on the Board believed was best for the profession. The chance to make a difference, that's what this is about! I did my best and that's all anyone can do and what everyone should do. (Thompson, 1998.)

References

Thompson, K. (1983). "Pain control in traumatic situations", workshop at the Second Erickson Congress, Phoenix, AZ.

Thompson, K. (1994a). Case presentations/discussion/ethics, Supervision Panel, Sixth Erickson Congress, Tracking Ericksonian Methods, Phoenix, AZ.

Thompson, K. (1994b). "Ethical issues in Ericksonian therapy", Panel discussion at the Sixth Erickson Congress, Tracking Ericksonian Methods, Phoenix, AZ.

Thompson, K. (1995a). "Introduction to hypnosis", workshop at the 24th Annual Advanced Workshops on Clinical Hypnosis, cosponsored by the Minnesota Society of Clinical Hypnosis, the Behavioral Pediatrics Program, Department of Pediatrics, Medical School, and Department of Continuing Medical Education, University of Minnesota, St. Paul, Minnesota.

Thompson, K. (1995b). "Patient management and pain control", workshop at the 24th Annual Advanced Workshops in Clinical Hypnosis, cosponsored by the Minnesota Society of Clinical Hypnosis, the Behavioral Pediatrics Program, Department of Pediatrics, Medical School, and Department of Continuing Medical Education, University of Minnesota, St. Paul, Minnesota.

Thompson, K. (1998, May). From Dr. Thompson's private papers for an address she gave to the Pennsylvania Dental Association 130th Annual Session, Pittsburgh, PA.

Part IX

The Personal Impact of Hypnosis

"How I Got to Be What I Am Becoming" is from Thompson's private papers. In this article, she summarizes her personal relationship with hypnosis and illustrates, in several inspiring metaphors, how hypnosis is an art form.

In the brief question-and-answer segment that opens this chapter, Kay Thompson passionately conveys the personal impact of hypnosis on her life. "Why Do We Learn about Hypnosis" is a delightful passage in which Thompson explores several critical reasons for learning about hypnosis.

Chapter Twenty-six
How I Got to Be What I Am Becoming

So far as my history is concerned, I always knew I would be a dentist. From before the time I was 10, I began assisting my father in an office he had in our small town, where he worked evenings for the convenience of the townspeople. For difficult extractions I got to hold the light and the suction and the sponges etc. I was fascinated, and impressed by the good he did for these very poor people.

Despite my very introverted nature, and the discouragement of everyone I talked with, I was determined to go to dental school—something women did not do in the dark ages. But I made it.

Well, back then, everyone knew that a woman dentist would be kinder, gentler, more understanding … so I got all the phobic patients in the city of Pittsburgh! And, because I didn't have a lot of patients, I had a lot of patience with the patients I did have.

Because I listened and spent time, the patients were better. But I didn't know what was happening. About that time a brochure came across my desk on "Seminars on Hypnosis". This seminar was being given in Philadelphia, so I thought I would go take the course, zap all my patients, and end all my (and their) problems! Wrong! That one beginning began what long ago lengthened into a lifelong learning lesson.

What instances reinforced my continued study and use?

One primary reinforcement was my first patient after I took that seminar. She was 9 months pregnant with a "hot" bicuspid, and an obstetrician who refused to let me use a local anesthetic. I said everything wrong, "I just took a course in hypnosis, let's try it and see if it will work," but she was motivated! As I devitalized the tooth, she was fine, but I was a nervous wreck, so I had to go back to another seminar to try to learn what happened. If that procedure had not worked, I assure you I would not be here today.

Back then, when I began my own experience with hypnosis, and Erickson, through these seminars, I could not have realized where I might be today. Ted Aston, that gentle, caring dentist, was the reason this particular mouse came back, again and again. Meanwhile, my patients kept doing these wonderful things I asked of them—like not bleed! And heal in half the usual (no, I did not say "normal") time. And stop grinding their teeth!

And all I knew then of Erickson was the fear, the sheer terror, and the curiosity of him. But Milton Erickson saw through the people I kept hiding behind, and singled me out, and the changing process began. He taught me things I do not yet know I know. But I do know I'm still learning.

The introvert I was then is one you would find difficult to recognize, or even imagine today, and that, too, was part of the change. He taught me that it was right to be myself, to dare to do whatever it was that I had inside me to do, to be the person I wanted to be. This challenge is the one I choose to pass on to my patients. I give patients confidence through my belief in their ability. They learn to dare to risk the chance for change.

How did where I am today happen? I read, but mostly I practiced. Those of you who know me know I practice and I preach, "Practice, practice, practice!" All my teaching includes heavy emphasis on practice in induction techniques and motivation of the patient, two things I consider most important. And I practiced, with literally thousands of patient visits and teaching workshops.

One of the most important things I personally learned from Erickson was to trust in and rely on my own unconscious. As I improved in what he taught me about learning to observe, formal structured induction techniques often evolved into informal trance where the emphasis was on the language of communication.

I learned that anything communicated in a therapeutic situation contains many multilevel messages. When a word or behavior charges out at me from my current unconscious listening, I take the energy it has and utilize that spark from the person's polarity, offering positive potential, even if sometimes in a negative way. I can use opposites to neutralize: just as I can generate a case for "pain interferes with healing", so too can I amplify one for "pain stimulates healing", depending on the circuitry needed at that moment.

One of the principles of hypnosis is that at the start of hypnotic work, most of the time you don't know what it is that will be most helpful and contribute constructively to the healing process. As I learned to be more comfortable with the patients, I could allow them freedom to know that it is their trance, because I no longer needed to know what to expect—I couldn't. But I could handle the unexpected, and would have an appropriate response. Now as I approach a fuller understanding of the power inherent in trance, I can have confidence that the power will add to healing, to comfort and to physiologic changes.

My investment in my patients is to help them realize their own potential. It involves making them want to hear the things that need to be said. If I read the situation correctly, I am able to get inside the patient's head, and go to where they are—at least this is what they tell me. I know that it is their interpretation of what I say that is helpful.

This is the difference in motivational factors. I believe that it is not the instruction in trance that brings about change, it is the difference in the state of altered awareness resulting from the motivation. We must look at the purpose of the trance and the motivation of the practitioner and patient to understand the differences. My belief that motivation makes the difference comes from clinical responses of patients who have experienced different types of trance, on subjective responses from patients and experimental subjects, and on my own clinical, experimental, forensic and demonstration experiences.

I read much of the early literature religiously. Now I consider what may be possible. I appreciate the work of the people I have learned to respect because of their work. Fred Evans was the first researcher I heard admit that just the presence of the safe experimenter might bias an experiment, and he said he would like to be able to have the researcher go up in a puff of smoke during the experiment.

465

Spiegel's work in the clinical situation expands the potential of utilization of trance. The current emphasis on investigation into memory is interesting to me. Helen Crawford's work with PET scans I find fascinating, and the findings of people such as Candace Pert help me understand what my patients have been doing for all these years. But I continue to learn from my patients.

In much of the experimental research on trance, the experimenter induces trance in a standardized way, and then observes the behavior. This helped to establish standards for research which includes scales of hypnotizability. When the method of induction is held constant, any variation in the subject's response is assumed to be a result of the actions of the experimenter. Motivation of the subject and the level of his involvement are discounted. My clinical experience convinces me that if the motivation can be developed, and if the individuals involved are willing to spend the time necessary for the learning experience, everyone of normal intelligence can go into trance. The question then is how much is the involvement worth?

With my clinical orientation and emphasis on language and motivation to determine the achievement of trance, part of my own interest in research and literature involves a curiosity about the ways to determine and enhance motivation. These techniques can then be integrated into the utilization of the trance experience.

This, then, is part of what encourages me to continue to study and use hypnosis. But there are a combination of other reasons. Mostly, it is fun, a challenge, and an incredible benefit to my patients and myself, both from a physiological and psychological perspective.

I have learned so much from the things my patients taught me. I recognized that hypnosis enabled my patients to do things they did not understand that they had the potential to do. And I learned to clinically use hypnosis for myself. I'm at least as smart as most of my patients, and if they can do it, baby, so can I. When that happened, my understanding of trance deepened, and the realization that it gave me personal control over my physiological response was significant.

I learn by teaching—the 30-year course at the University of Pittsburgh, the 14-year course at West Virginia University, and the years of teaching and then chairing the Education and Research Foundation (ERF) workshops for ASCH gave me ongoing experience. The best way to learn is to teach. I am committed to my conviction that hypnosis should be a part of every health care professional's armamentarium, and that teaching it to as many people as possible would help that become fact.

I am intrigued by the challenge of moving beyond "ordinary" trance work, of always looking for a better way, a novel way or a different way to teach. That curiosity resulted in the development of the dual induction, first done in the early 1970s with Robert Pearson and Ray LaScola, then refined with practice.

I respond to the challenge of others regarding my work with language, integrating induction into everyday conversations through appropriate use of words, and my subsequent and ongoing efforts at the refining of this use of words as a motivational tool. After all, the ears have no lids!

I am intrigued by the unfolding scientific knowledge regarding energy fields and even synchronicity, as described by Jung and David Bohm, relative to their future in the art of healing is concerned. The merging of such influences with the understanding of the continuum of trance or altered states of consciousness predicts some exciting advances in knowledge.

As far as words and motivation, meaning this matter and manner of mutual motivational manipulation is manageable but mandates mastery of many methods—which may be considered an art.

The use of hypnosis is in itself an art form. I get my inspiration from my patients. I consider it akin to surfing. The board is the vehicle, but the rider must do a multitude of things to stay in balance on the board. He or she must consider the currents and the tide, and must choose carefully which wave to ride. Every wave is different. It takes skill and speed to adjust and not get knocked off the board. It requires many different kinds of balancing on the board, depending on the vagaries of the wave, as well as the winds, which can influence the direction and intensity of the wave. And the wave may not last long, but there is another one coming, which requires more adjustment of balance depending on the size, the length, the intensity of the new wave.

The surfer cannot know what each wave will turn out to be, but that is part of the challenge and excitement—developing enough skill, after some falls and false starts and modifications in technique, to know she or he will be able to finally adapt to the oncoming wave and modify his behavior to stay with it and ride the wave to its destination, for a safe and exhilarating landing. And the elegant surfer makes it look easy!

The fun, the creativity comes with the conscious or unconscious resistance by the patient. It is a game, a challenge, presented to me by the patient who hopes that I will help them to fail in their resistance, so they can learn to succeed in their desire to change. My skill is to use words and actions that can open the patients' options and opportunities for change.

The sculptor takes a chunk of material and begins working, curious about what the final product will be, marveling as it takes form, often outside his or her direction and control, and changing the sculpture to fit the progress. The painter has a canvas, and an idea, begins, and is often surprised at the forms that develop and demand expression. The results are left to be interpreted by the observer, since each of us sees the artist's creation, the sculpture or painting, from our own perspective.

My words are the chisels, the brushes used to attempt to reach the inner block of material, the canvas of the individual, modifying the story as the cues demand, and waiting for the message that change is ready, leaving the creation to be interpreted by the patient, the one who commissioned the vision in the beginning.

Art is best when shared to be appreciated, offered for evaluation and understanding. As Erickson taught, utilization of hypnosis, not induction of trance, is the art form of hypnosis. I offer it for the potential understanding of the individual who comes to me for help. I work to create an atmosphere where there is the possibility for growth and change. Then I expect and watch for the miracle, or the magic within the patient.

I am not what I was, nor am I what I will be, but I am becoming, satisfied with the moment and the movement.

Chapter Twenty-seven
Why Do We Learn About Hypnosis?

Comment: As I listen and watch your communication, I feel you are giving the gift of expanding horizons and consciousness.

T: That's the absolutely nicest thing that anybody could say. I think people find out they can expand their own awareness and their own sensitivity and just reach that kind of potential. What is this all about? We talked about this during lunch. Someone said they wished people would say more openly, that it's how to live hypnotically. I really think it has become a way of life. I can't not do it because it's so great. It lets you look through the rose colored glasses even when the world isn't so rosy. Someday, that fog is going to burn off and the roses are going to be out there again.

So thank you.

Why do we learn about hypnosis? What does it do for us? It's important to meet with other people and brainstorm with them. We are doing pioneering work in the truest sense. Science is going to catch up to us someday. I'm convinced of that and I hope I'm going to live long enough to see that. We are on the edge and you need the support and encouragement of people who think like you do.

I think that that knowledge is what we are doing and sharing. We can't stay up on this peak forever. We don't need to. Once people have learned hypnosis, it's real hard not to do it. When you don't do it, you know you are not doing it. There is an awareness that changes the effect and the impact of what you do, what you are and what you've been. That's a really important part of it.

How is it going to change your life? It's going to make you a little more aware. You are going to be a little more tuned in. Maybe you are going to enjoy yourself more. It makes for more fun and more ideas. We use more of the brainpower we normally use. We can go out and expand our own minds by reading.

How do you get new ideas? That's an interesting idea. My immediate reaction was to be on a path. It wasn't a green kind of spring path. It was a rocky path that opened up into a fairly wide open area. As I saw myself moving out into it, part of it was scary because I didn't really like the area. But part of it was the recognition that it's okay to be scared as long as you confront that fear and don't let it hold you back. Go ahead anyway. Moving out into that area and just looking.

One of the things I find most interesting and intriguing is Marilyn Ferguson's *Brain/Mind Bulletin*, because that's kind of a summary of the fringe research that is going on. I get a lot of ideas by reading that and reading about alternative therapies, and then letting myself just percolate. I don't do formal kinds of trance. Sometimes, I only realize I've been in trance after I've been in it. I am so convinced that my unconscious will do what it needs to do, that I don't any longer use the formal stuff, unless it's a matter of three hours of sleep that night and I really need six.

In terms of mind expansion, I think that you get in these conversations and then little bloomers of things get bigger. And you think, what if, what if?

Free association with "What if?" is one of the fun ways to get your brain to move forward.

I'm thinking of the time when Erickson worked with a woman who wanted to have a trance experience, but not know she had it. She woke up one morning and she came home and she didn't remember anything that happened in between. She knew she must have done something, because she had gone shopping and there were bags and packages. It was scary for her because it had been a couple of weeks before, that that suggestion had been given to her, that at some point she could enjoy knowing that she didn't know she was in trance. It took two weeks for her unconscious to choose the time to let her go for a whole day in trance, and not know that she had done it until that evening, when she couldn't remember doing it.

But she had all these products that demonstrated that she had spent the day shopping.

I'm able to say to people that I don't know, and that's okay. With my patients, I know that I won't have the absolutely most perfect answer in the world, but I know that I will have an answer we can live with. That's, I think, all we can ask. If we get that, then progress is being made.

Hypnosis helps people understand that no matter what anyone takes from them, they can't take away their dignity. I think that's the key that hypnosis gives to people who may have been looking for that dignity for a very, very long time. What we are doing is enabling and empowering them in the very best way that we know how.

Appendix I
Kay Thompson Remembered

A Memoir
Ralph Krichbaum

Kay was the only child of older parents who were very active. Kay's maternal grandfather came from Scotland as a young man. He worked hard, prospered, and owned a coal mine in the Pittsburgh area. The family was affluent and had nine children, including Bertha Porter, Kay's mother. Only three survived into adulthood. Kay's father, Lony C. Thompson was raised on a farm on the Ohio–Pennsylvania border.

Lony was in the Air Force in World War I, and after the war he worked his way through dental school. Bertha was prim and proper, but she was also a fun-loving person. Bertha and her mother traveled extensively, and once they went around the world. Bertha drove a car, which was unusual for a woman in the early part of the 20th century, and enjoyed driving around the state. Lony was independent and assertive. Shortly after their marriage, Bertha's mother became ill, and to care for her they moved into the family home, where Lony opened a dental office. Most of those patients were from poor coal mining families. He also had a dental practice in downtown Pittsburgh, where his patients were more affluent.

Kay's parents traveled extensively and collected antiques. They took Kay with them everywhere. She started helping her father in his dental office when she was 9 years old. She excelled by working hard and long, showing her father that even though she was not the şon that he never had, he could still be proud of her. She skipped one grade in elementary school and her father, who was superintendent of the local schools sent her to a high school, which could better prepare her for college, than the one in their community. She didn't know anyone in this new school and was very tall and younger than most of the other students. She didn't make friends easily and was somewhat introverted. I think she took all of her energy and put it in her studies.

College and Dental School

After completing grade school and high school in 10 years, Kay went to the University of Pittsburgh intending to get into dental school in two years. She was an overachiever. She got into dental school with only two years of undergraduate work and was the youngest person and the only female in her freshman class. At one time she was the only female student in the dental school. Most of her classmates were World War II veterans. Seating in the class-rooms was alphabetical, but they made an exception and put her in the front row. There was only one locker room at that time. To avoid embarrassment the men bought a cowbell and asked her to wear it. She wore it one day, and then hung it on her locker door so that when she opened it, the men could know she was in the room.

Kay's mother had been a teetotaler throughout her life, but started to drink alcohol when Kay was in college to encourage Kay to loosen up. Kay became interested in caving and then backpacking, rock climbing, and skiing. Kay rock climbed the toughest routes with two of the best male climbers in the East. Most of her social life at that time was with this climbing group.

Dental Practice

After dental school, she went into practice with her father in his two offices. Before the invention of the high-speed drill, a lot of people had been hurt by dentists and wouldn't come back. They thought maybe a woman would be kinder and gentler and she started to get many dental phobics. She pursued ways of helping her patients, including psychology and became infatuated with hypnosis. She started studying with Erickson in 1953 and soon became one of his favorite hypnotic subjects in his teaching courses.

Marriage

I met Kay at Seneca Rocks in 1958. She was a climber and I was a caver. I wanted to learn to climb in the sun, and even though I showed up several times in the morning at the climbers' camp with all my equipment, her group ignored me and left me at the camp. They finally decided I might be interested in joining them and appointed Kay to cultivate me. She invited me to climb with her and I invited her out. After I returned from two weeks on a canoe trip, we were almost inseparable. She did such a good job cultivating me that we got married five months later, January 10, 1959.

When we got married I was a union sheet metal worker. I had become bored with college and was tired of being broke, so I dropped out after two years. I made good money and was able to take vacations when I wanted. I would take two or three weeks skiing, a week deer hunting, a week duck hunting, a couple of weeks on a wilderness canoe trip, a week trout fishing etc. After we were married, I completed college and became interested in computers. I went to work for Westinghouse as a programmer and helped install a pioneering telecommunications system and later was promoted to manage it. There were periods when I was working very long hours. At Westinghouse, I had over 35 people reporting to me. I was very busy and so was Kay.

Interests and Adventures

Kay and I were both skiers and we continued this along with rock climbing and caving during the 1950s and 1960s. Rock climbing has become immensely popular now. We were the first ones to white water raft on some rivers, including the Gauley, one of the most challenging rivers in the East. One of her climbing buddies moved to Boulder, Colorado, and we frequently went backpacking in the summer with him and his wife, and went skiing with them every winter. We went scuba diving in the Caribbean in the early 1960s when it was an infant sport. We worked hard but we played hard. We enjoyed these activities during the first half of our marriage.

I remember in particular one mountain climbing trip that we took in the West. We were going to climb Mt. Moran, the second highest mountain in the Tetons. We approached by the back and attempted to climb by two glaciers. We were tentatively cutting our steps with the ice axes. When we got in the middle of the first glacier, a rock avalanche caught us in the middle of the glacier. There were rocks falling all around us, some as large as three feet in diameter. Rocks were falling from 3,000 feet above which had been bound up about 100 years. We were totally powerless and couldn't run. By the grace of God we survived.

As soon as it stopped we got off the glacier. We retreated and moved our camp to another site. We chose another climbing route. We camped and it rained and the rocks came down again. That glacier was so covered with rocks, no one in their right mind would cross it. We tried to reach the summit by another route but it rained so hard that we stopped short of the top. We didn't make it down before dark and spent the night on the mountain tied to some trees. Dawn the next morning was one of the most spectacular I have ever seen. The clouds were all below us and you could only see the tops of the highest peaks.

Seneca, West Virginia, where Kay and I met, also attracted people from Washington, DC who enjoyed caving, climbing and other sports. With them we also enjoyed white water boating on streams in the area. Our most exciting trip was when we were the first group to go down the Gauley River in West Virginia, a classic rafting river now. We did it in the spring in high water when the snow was melting off. Each of us had a six-man raft with large oars so we were very maneuverable. We got to one place where there would have been two 10 foot waterfalls in dry weather. In high water, they were steep rapids. We wanted to avoid the left hand shore where there was a narrow passage that was too narrow for our boats. However, there was a huge rock on the right. I went over first and stayed toward the rock on the right. I actually hit the rock and with one strong stroke of the oar and went over the rapids backwards.

Kay was the fourth one to go through. Kay also hit the rock but she got stuck against it. We found later that half of the stream was going under this rock. She realized that the water was pulling one side of the boat down and could see that the boat was going to go under the rock. She took a deep breath and jumped overboard. She got swept through and twisted her leg; somewhere she got the opportunity to get a mouth of air and washed out at the bottom. Her boat was stuck under that rock for a long time. She later told me she thought, "I hope whoever finds me knows artificial respiration." It's crazy what you think at times like that. Standing above and watching her go through, I was thinking, "What am I going to tell her mother?" All I knew was that she disappeared under water in a very turbulent stream. She came up below the two rapids. When we came back, she was hospitalized. She was in a wheelchair for about a week due to an embolism in her leg.

Another memorable adventure was rafting with the Kennedy family. Robert Kennedy and Stuart Udall considered making the upper Hudson a wilderness river and wanted to come down it and see what it looked like. They contacted some white water canoers in Washington, DC to help make arrangements. They wanted to take their families. They had done this out West when it was warm, but when we did it in New York there was still snow on the ground up at 1,000 feet. It was cold.

This was an expedition with the Secret Service overhead and *Life* photographers in a helicopter. There must have been 12 or 15 rubber rafts and canoes. Kay and I had a surplus 15-man assault craft that was the biggest and became the party boat. We had a bunch of the Kennedy kids, Udall's family and one of the first climbers of Everest on our boat. Robert Kennedy was in a wetsuit and started out in a kayak. He was "game" and spent a lot of time in the water. The first part had a lot of rapids and as we continued, it was much calmer. Kay and I had put some clothes in a waterproof container. At the lunch stop the Kennedys were soaking wet and Ethel put on a pair of my dry pants. Kay used to joke, "I remember when I had to ask Ethel Kennedy for my husband's pants."

Bobby came in the boat with us after lunch. Kay was rowing the boat. It was big and you had to start rowing early to get out of the way of the rocks. I think he thought it wouldn't look good to the *Life* photographers with a woman rowing so he offered to row. We hadn't gone far before Bobby got the raft hung up on a rock. Kay and I had to get out of the boat and help him work the boat off the rock. When we finally got it off, his kids started to tease Bobby, "Dad,

Kay didn't get us hung up on any rocks." As big as that family was, it was obvious it was a tight-knit group.

Dental Students

Not having children of our own, we kind of adopted some of her dental students, mostly girls, and often had them coming over for dinner. She was their mentor and role model. One female student knocked on our door asking to be adopted by Kay. She was an undergraduate and belonged to the dental club. She asked the faculty advisor how to learn the politics of the dental school. The advisor told her to get adopted by Kay Thompson. Kay also worked in the psychology department at the dental school where she did a lot of therapy with students who had problems, including dental and test phobias. One student who was in dental school had a test phobia and was about to flunk out of school. His advisor sent him to Kay and she talked with him for one hour before a test. He did so well he was accused of cheating. They made him take another test and he got a similar score.

Love for Dogs

Kay loved dogs. She was very concerned about dogs on freeways, because they got on, but couldn't get off because of the fences and would get killed. She would always carry milk bones in her car. When she saw a dog on the freeway, she would get them in the car and take them to a place that would keep them and try to find a home for them. One day she picked up a German Shepard and left him in the car while she went to class. When she returned the dog had become possessive and didn't want to let her in the car.

Barry Bishop, a close friend, returned from climbing Everest with frost-bitten feet. The historic treatment for frostbite was to amputate everything that had frostbite, because it could become gangrenous. You don't know what has been frost bitten so you have to cut back a lot. *National Geographic* went to the government and found a naval surgeon who was doing research on frostbite. He prescribed a different treatment. In order to save as much of the feet as possible,

Barry had to keep the area surgically clean. Twice a day, they would unbandage his feet, and put them in a bathtub with a whirlpool and special soap in order to kill any bacteria. The problem was taking the bandages off his feet. It was very painful. He was on morphine for the pain and didn't want to get hooked.

We would go to visit them in Washington, DC every other week and Kay would hypnotize him and make a tape which he would use until she returned. She got him off the morphine and we did this for two months. They had a Lhasa Apso dog named Ama, which came from Nepal and didn't like strangers. After our many visits he began to tolerate us.

When the Bishops were about to leave the country for an extended period, they asked Kay if she would take Ama because no one else would. Of course Kay said yes and within six weeks the dog had us trained and ran the house. There was a period when Ama was in pain and I noticed one pupil was very large. Kay took Ama to Ohio State where there was a specialty clinic at the veterinary school to evaluate animals' eyes. He had glaucoma. They would do surgery, and so Kay reluctantly left Ama there over the weekend. When she returned to the clinic to pick him up, Ama went to her and started to bark as if he was telling her every indignity he had gone through in the two days. When he was done, Ama turned around and walked to the door. The vet said he had never seen anything like that in all his days.

When that dog died, Kay was severely depressed. Ama would always greet us happily when we would get home and now it was like a tomb. When we got another dog, I got a second one so that when one died, we would still have one. I swear that one of our other dogs could read her mind. Kay would be sitting working at the desk and would decide it was time for a break. She wouldn't say anything and the dog would get up and jump. I swear it could read her mind.

Hypnosis

Kay told me that when people came to hypnosis courses, some were skeptics. She finally decided that she had to do something dramatic to get their attention. Kay carried surgical needles. She would hyp-notize a student and run a needle through the back of his hand. She would tell the student, "When I remove this needle, I want you to bleed out of the right side, and not out of the left side." More than once, someone would run up from the back of the room to the front to see. She would then say, "I want you to stop bleeding out of the right side and start bleeding from the left." When they saw that, she had their rapt attention.

At one time, her mother had taken glass shelves out of a cupboard and they were leaning up against the wall. Kay bumped into them and they fell down and hit her on the arch of her foot. It was a very sharp edge. Normally, you would have had instant swelling. She sat down and went into trance and there was no swelling, no bleeding. I remember the exchange she had with an orthopedic surgeon one day after she was in a serious auto accident. When she told a nurse that she thought that she had broken legs, the surgeon examined her and said that they couldn't be broken because they weren't swollen. Kay looked him in the eye and said, "I don't swell. It retards healing." They X-rayed the legs and they were both broken. The things she could do with her body were amazing.

She used hypnosis on me, quite effectively, twice. The first time when I had my gall bladder removed. Before the surgery, she talked to me and told me that I would have little bleeding or pain. I had no problems. I didn't need any morphine. I healed relatively quickly. When I had my hip replacement she talked to me in the preparation room. The next morning the surgeon came in to see me and asked me what I was doing for pain. Kay was sitting in the corner and I pointed to her. I didn't take any painkiller at all for that. She asked me to hypnotize her on a couple of occasions. I knew a little about the technique. She was so conditioned that it didn't take much for her to go into trance.

Organizational Politics

She was competing in a man's world and in many cases she was the only woman or one of the few women in an organization. She was trying to command respect. Kay was very conscious of how she dressed.

Kay was never casual about anything she did. She was active in several hypnosis organizations when I married her. Shortly after our marriage, she and others did not support the person nominated for president in one of the organizations (ASCH). They ran Kay against him in a write-in campaign, and even though she was "only" a woman and a dentist, she won.

She held numerous offices in various organizations and won many awards for her contributions. One of her many achievements was her selection as the first woman to become a member of the American Board of Dentistry.

She loved to play the dumb blond. She would ask questions to lead you down the garden path and first thing you knew you hung yourself. This was a common tactic of hers. She loved it. It was a match of intellect and she had a great one. She was very ethical and preached ethics. She had little tolerance for people who would accept offices for prestige and then let the staff do all the work, write the speeches, and make the decisions. No one could accuse Kay of not doing her share. When she accepted a job or an office for an organization, she was committed to the time and effort required.

Kay was infamous for her dinners. When some people were invited, they knew they were in trouble, because they knew that Kay had ulterior motives. If the dental society had been unable to get someone to run for office, Kay would invite them, their close friends, and colleagues for dinner. She would rig the guest list so they could hardly refuse. No one ever did. They were pushed into the office. Kay was a fantastic cook. We enjoyed entertaining and had a lot of dinners and wine tasting parties.

Kay made every effort to introduce new blood into organizations. She disliked the old boy system. She thought that it discouraged and turned off the people that organizations needed most, the bright young members with lots of energy and ideas. Kay used to agonize over the appointments she made to committees. When she became the first female president of the Pennsylvania Dental Association in 1989, she broke a barrier that had stood for more than 100 years. Instead of automatically reappointing the existing committees, she started with a clean sheet of paper and created what she felt was a proper balance between experience and young enthusiasm.

Kay had a network that reached around the world. People would call and discuss issues with her because she was a valuable source of information. She had a memory like a computer and the political savvy not to share information that would cause dissension. She had a love–hate relationship with the telephone. She was able to use it to communicate with her friends and colleagues but it was time consuming.

When she became involved in organized dentistry, as well as hypnosis, we had time for little else. Our vacations became one or two days after a dental meeting or perhaps a week, if it was an overseas hypnosis course. Often she would conduct these courses by herself, and would be totally exhausted at the end. While she was working and her adrenaline was pumping, she was the bubbling, vivacious person you saw most of the time, but we had to start scheduling a day of recovery as we got older. Kay wanted to slow down and would not have run for the ADA trustee, had the Pennsylvania Dental Association not nominated someone who she felt in no way adequately represented the state. She ran for office and became the second woman, in 134 years, to sit on the Board of Trustees of the American Dental Association.

When Kay was a trustee, she was concerned that there weren't any women who would follow her in office. Kay decided that a woman could be elected to a vice presidential office because they are elected at large. She identified six women dentists who she felt were qualified for the office and got one to run and she was elected. Kay was a leader and proud of it.

Few if any realized how sick and weak she was during those last months. A few weeks before her death, she attended the Pennsylvania Dental Association meeting, which conveniently was held in Pittsburgh, and actively participated in discussions for all of the four days. She carefully selected which meetings she would attend, rationing what little strength and energy she had. I would drop her at the hotel before a meeting and pick her up as soon as it finished. She accepted an award at the banquet and gave a fire and brimstone speech on professionalism.

Permission to Change Their Lives

After her death, I received letters from many people about what she had done for them and meant to them. These were unsolicited testimonials. Some people described being able to do things they wanted to do all their lives, but weren't able to do. They wrote that Kay somehow gave them permission to change their lives. I wasn't aware of how much she had affected people's lives.

Wheels on the Concept of Love: "Well, If You Can Do Something Good for Them, Do It!"

Russell Scott with Saralee Kane

Saralee Kane

Russell Scott knew Kay both personally and professionally for almost 35 years. They were very close friends and taught hypnosis together for many years. However, the unique aspect of their professional relationship is that they frequently worked together on difficult clinical cases, often utilizing the dual induction. This brief chapter is the first discussion of their work together by Russ Scott.

Kay Thompson refused to do therapy during clinical demonstrations, because she believed that would compromise the confidentiality of clients and "because Erickson didn't". As a result we only have these demonstrations to review for understanding the depth and sophistication of her work. Dr. Scott's comments, therefore, are an especially important perspective on the "weave" of her work, besides including a wide range of wonderful stories and delightful personal recollections.

Russ was 70 when he was interviewed for this article; he had been diagnosed with MS five years earlier. Although his health was deteriorating, he was committed to completing a discussion of their relationship and work together. Learita Scott, his wife generously supported and encouraged him during this process. He had a wonderful sense of humor and his "heh, heh, heh" laugh is clearly one of genuine pleasure. As the reader will notice, his language is unique and folksy, almost poetic in the tradition of Mark Twain and Milton Erickson. He clearly loved Kay very deeply and was pleased to finally talk about her. We hope that his generosity, creativity, humor, playfulness, intelligence and genuine warmth are evident in his story.

Russell Scott [22]

Well if you can do something good for them, do it!

Kay did for me what had to be done. She not only did it for me, she taught me how to do it for other people. Even today, I have that knowledge. It truly is a knowledge. This is what Kay Thompson taught me to do.

This is the first time since she died that I'm going to talk about Kay. I met Kay in the early 1960s and knew her for almost 35 years. I am astounded how influential Kay was in my life and how profoundly she has affected me. Every goddamned thing I touch is somehow related to her. Most everybody I know and like I met through Kay. It has been a startling trip. She was bright as hell. Her intellect and intelligence were astounding and she could talk about anything. She talked in a way that drew you in. She was always, always very conscious and cautious about hurting your feelings. She could be very, very careful about hurting your feelings too. She was very passionate. She didn't do things by half measures. If she liked you, she could go all the way. If she didn't, you were in trouble.

We had a very special relationship. She would never say, "No." That was one of the marvelous things about her. There was no question about the way things went. She had a big heart and she would never say, "I quit." I don't give a dang what it was, who we were chasing down, or what the consequences were, she would never say, "I quit." She always stuck to things to the end. There would be

---

[22] Saralee Kane interviewed Russ Scott over a period of a year, and this memoir derives from those interviews.

times when she would get mad. She would give me hell frequently. I learned to keep my mouth shut. Sooner or later I got a chance to say something and she would always appreciate it.

She was a marvelous, wonderful woman. People were jealous because she had a gift. When they would accept it was in the genes, they would get jealous of me because I knew her. I probably knew her better than most anyone. She was a delight.

She could move back and forth between the theoretical framework and the practical. "Let's get this done." She had a goal orientation and she knew how to do it. You worked hard (when you worked with her).

How would I describe Kay Thompson in terms, as a person? She was inspiring. She inspired a fabulous amount of trust. When Kay said something, you didn't wonder, "Is that true?" You said to yourself, "Oh, my God, that is true." You sort of decided, I'm going to go along for the ride. You settled in and had a tight grip on your hat and you never knew where you were going to go. It was the same thing, whether she was talking to you about some absolutely unbelievable event.

She was spectacular in what she did but she wasn't spectacular in doing it. It was done so unobtrusively. Sometimes, you'd have to wonder. I don't know what she did, but it worked.

Kay was an exceptionally honest woman. All the time I knew her, I never knew her to consider anything that was dishonest or crooked. She would get furious, like, "Hell hath no fury like a woman scorned," which is what Kay was like when people messed around with ethics.

I happen to be very fortunate. I never asked a question she didn't answer. When Milton Erickson died, it was am amazing experience to go through that with her. She talked about him. She idolized him. She never did a thing in any way that would reflect negatively on him. She was amazingly close to his family.

To know Kay Thompson, was to give her your life. With Kay, it probably was the most important relationship in my life. It, she sort of takes over your life. You become so dependent on her, so trusting. Everybody you talk to, it's the same way. When you were as close to someone as I was to Kay, just because they died, doesn't mean they are gone. I find I talk to her on occasion.

She was widely known for her hypnotic abilities. She said that people thought of her as a witch, probably because they thought that hypnosis makes you do things you don't want to do. She thought that was funny and would play with that. She would frequently wear a black cape. She was a very impressive woman and made use of it.

She ate like crazy. She could eat like a pig and not gain weight. She told me that when she would eat, she would go into trance so the food wouldn't turn into fat and so she wouldn't gain weight. When you knew Kay, you threw out all the rules. She was a different world.

Dental Phobia

I had been hired by the University of Pittsburgh dental school as a psychologist. A colleague who learned of my dental phobia referred me to Kay. When I was about 10 years old, I had a bad tooth, a molar in the upper left quadrant. I went to the dentist. My family was cardboard shoe soles poor—we defined the lower limit for income. I went to see this dentist and he put me in the chair and his anesthesiologist, a pharmacist, gave me laughing gas.

He's fiddling with my tooth and all of a sudden, it hurt like an atomic bomb. I screamed and I kicked and kicked the dentist in the stomach. I started to swing and hit the anesthesiologist. Both attacked me. They did the towel technique, where they take a folded towel and put it over your nose and mouth as if to asphyxiate you, and don't let you breathe. That's what they did. As I was struggling, I thought I was dying. I finally lost consciousness. On the way out of the office, the dentist told me not to come back. That was the beginning of my dental phobia.

After that, I couldn't open my mouth. I never brushed my teeth after that. When I would go to get a haircut and sit in the barber chair, I would get anxious. I wouldn't get my hair cut. I was a classic.

When I was in graduate school, a friend told me about Kay. I made an appointment with her and went down to the building for my appointment. I walked into the revolving door and walked right out the building. I gathered up my courage in the street and walked back in the lobby. She was on the second floor and I had to take the elevator up. That required all my courage. Finally, I got up to the second floor. I found her suite of offices and had a seat in her waiting room and was the only one there. In a few minutes, she popped into the waiting room, dressed in her blue uniform. She said, "Good morning" and I said, "Good morning," and she said, "Come on in." I went in but not to her dental operatory. I went into her office and sat down.

I told her the story and she listened. There was a strong building of trust. She did a trance induction with a left hand levitation. I thought, "This is as silly as hell. There is no balloon attached to my hand." I watched my hand going up higher and higher. I thought, "I'll be damned, the damn thing is floating." I realized my hand was up for 15 minutes and it should be tired, but it wasn't. I was hooked into hypnosis. Each time we would do some hypnotic work and she did her magic.

She said, "Let's take a look." I walked in behind her into the dental operatory. I opened my mouth and she picked up an instrument and touched my tooth. That was a big deal. Nobody had put anything in my mouth since I was 10 years old. I was in my late 20s then. She prescribed a mouth wash. I realized she would be spraying water into my mouth when I came the next time. That week I desensitized myself by spraying water into my mouth while showering. I came the second time and she found a huge cavity. She was able to work on me.

She did glove anesthesia. I thought, "This doesn't follow what I know about physiology," but it worked. I was surprised and delighted. I turned off the feeling in my hand and touched my cheek and transferred the anesthesia to my face and gums. She used to tell me, I had a tooth in my head and it was a nasty tooth and needed some work. Every time she would touch that tooth, it would hurt. She said to me, "I'm going to take that phone call and while I'm gone, you get that thing turned off." I said, "Okay," and when she came back in, that tooth had been turned off. She did a root canal. She opened it up and worked on it and I didn't have any pain.

Learning Hypnosis from Kay

Shortly after meeting her, I asked her about whether I should take my young daughter to see the movie, *Mary Poppins*. Kay said, "Superkalifragilisticexpialadoshes. I can even say it backwards, sehsodalaipxecitsiligarfilakrepus."

She knew I was a smart-ass. She got my attention. She was smart and she also had fun and it established a connection between Kay and Mary Poppins in my head.

I am a curious man and expressed an interest in hypnosis and she suggested I take her hypnosis course. There were dentists and physicians in the course and I was the first psychologist in Pittsburgh to take her course. Later, other psychologists took her course.

Each week, one student would have to do a demonstration and perform an induction on another student. I waited and didn't volunteer. I managed to duck out until the last class. I approached that class thinking, I would have to do it today. Sure enough I did. I had this other student as my subject.

I went through one of the inductions I had learned and looked over and Kay was in trance. She decided to take a free ride. I was astounded and couldn't believe it! My subject was in a nice trance and so was Kay Thompson. That was another increment.

S: She was fully aware that you were very anxious about performing, and that you had waited to do this until the very last class. There was no greater gift that she could have given to you, than to have gone into trance while you were performing the induction so that you could see her. Kay did that purposely for you.

R: Yeah, absolutely! I thought, "Me? I did that the first time I was practicing in public?" The fact that Kay was a subject taught me several things. It did a tremendous job on my confidence. What the hell, if it lives and breathes, I could probably hypnotize it. Equally important was what it did in terms of our relationship. It touched a level of our relationship that is typically unavailable to people. I was her equal (at that moment). It made me realize that from her perspective, too. It was one of the most important moments of my life.

S: When you were doing the induction in her class, no one knew and no one had to know that she was in trance. It was just for you, just between the two of you?

R: Yeah, you could say, "Thank you. I appreciate that." She would know. That's one of the things that makes her so hard to talk about. There's a sense of awe that comes over me when I talk about her.

Pain

The things I learned from her were rather astounding. I'm 70 years old. When Kay taught me to turn off pain, it was another gift. I used to have headaches. I haven't had a headache in 30 years. The pain itself has become a stimulus for turning it off. I couldn't figure that out and one day, it hit me. Kay taught me how to control pain. She taught me to turn off my teeth and proceeded to do nasty things like root canals. I didn't feel them. If I didn't feel that why should I feel anything? I got to the point where I could turn off any pain. Having learned it from her, I could teach it to other people and I did. It was a gift from Kay once removed.

Managing Blood Pressure: Letting it Happen

Later I went into the hospital. My blood pressure was high, up to 180 to 200 or something and they couldn't get it down. They were plying me with medication and nothing happened. One morning, a nurse took my blood pressure and it was close to 200. Kay came to see me at the hospital and said, "We are going to work." I went into trance and we worked for the better part of an hour. She had an immense confidence in the body's own devices. She got me in a very deep trance and I was very relaxed. I tend to be amnesic for the work in trance. When I came out I was able to control my blood pressure. She said, "Don't go in there and mess it up. You know how to do it. You don't know that you know. It's just a matter of letting it happen."

The nurse came back within minutes of when Kay left. She took my blood pressure and I was down 30 points or more. It's been down within reasonable limits ever since. I have no idea what I'm doing, responding to a posthypnotic suggestion? I'm enjoying and I'm having fun. By the same token, I would help her anytime I could. It's nice to have somebody in the world like that.

MS: Another Challenge

I passed out in my office about five years ago and luckily had a surgeon in my office at the time, who did cardiac respiration. She helped me get to a hospital. MS affects my balance and I get tired very quickly. My reading is very poor because I have lost my visual acuity. And I have to use a magnifying glass. MS patients maintain their sense of humor very well. I had a lot of MS patients when I was a therapist. I'm pleased with that. I get a little bit discouraged and use trance a lot and I don't have any pain. I lead a relatively normal life. I can try out all kinds of hypotheses. I understand very well about the myelin sheath and what it does.

I was at a hypnosis meeting and one of my friends who was sitting at a table in the front of the room had a stack of books, but I couldn't read the titles. I decided I was going to invent an electrician who has rolls of myelin and wraps neural sheaths and insulates my nerves. I did that and when I looked again, I could read their titles. I was astounded.

S: What part did Kay play in your creative adjustment to MS?

R: Kay did that. She taught me hypnosis. Give it a shot! If you don't try, you don't know.

I made up my mind, I wasn't an MS person. I was simply a man who happened to have MS. Please don't think of me as a poor MS victim. Who knows? I may win.

Responsibility to Learn Hypnosis

She taught a lot. We would teach together sometimes. I've seen Kay refuse to teach certain people. After the first session, we would go over the list of students. She would say, "I don't trust him," and give me reasons as to why. I'd be alert and watch.

We were teaching a course and Kay wasn't comfortable with one of the students. When Kay decided that you shouldn't know, forget it, Charley. You weren't going to know. She alerted me to this person who turned out to be a sleazy kind of character. It sounds like playing God. What the hell, somebody has to do it! Of all the people I know, she was the best person to do this. She would minimize contact with somebody if she decided they weren't the right stuff.

Helping Colleagues and Students Informally

We were going to teach a hypnosis course together. She was worried about one of the students who was having trouble finishing her dissertation. She said, "We're going to have to do something about that!" One night during the course, we were at a party. Kay started to talk with the woman and I realized what Kay was doing. I slipped in, we did a dual induction, and the girl got a trance. Kay talked to her about obstacles, how they come and go. How nice it is when they went away, they weren't an obstacle anymore. It was sort of nice to know what was an obstacle now, wouldn't even be an obstacle later. Maybe she wouldn't even know it was an obstacle anymore.

That kind of thing happened frequently. People wouldn't even know it. I was involved in that quite a bit in social situations. It was startling how frequently it happened. She was a master about picking up on what someone wanted and needed. You didn't have to spell it out for her. You dropped a cue here and there. Suddenly, she had the whole story. And she had a key to unlock it. Sometimes, they would realize what happened and thank her.

Where I ran into it most was when she was teaching hypnosis. She got pretty tight with some of the students. When she got close and knew they had something on their minds, she would do that same kind of thing.

I was involved as a coconspirator and as a target, a subject. I would suddenly realize, "Oh my God, this happened because of what Kay said to me in trance." I eventually got to the point where I didn't trust Kay much. I'd realize and say, "You son of a gun, you are trying to hypnotize me. I'm glad you are trying to hypnotize me." She would laugh and say, "You're getting too smart." I would say, "That's because I had such a good teacher."

She was so kind and such an inspiration.

Pregnancy and Delivery

One of her students was pregnant and was planning on having natural childbirth. Kay would talk to her about all sorts of things and there were always some suggestions in there about natural childbirth. Kay called me up one day and told me that this student was in labor at the birthing center and asked me to go along. We went to see her. She was having a particularly long and difficult labor. We did a dual induction. She knew when talking with Kay and me, she was safe. We talked about shoes, ships and sealing wax (reference to Jabberwocky), meaning we talked about everything. We talked around issues in her family and a relative who had died. Later on that day, she gave birth and moved back to the hospital. Later she understood we had helped her.

Clinical Partnership: Therapy Training

Kay was a two-way street. She got interested in teaching at the dental school and in the university. She talked to me about her activities in the American Society for Clinical Hypnosis (ASCH) and how some people discounted her because she was a dentist. Dentists, at that time were not looked on as very intellectual people. I was a grad student in psychology at the time. I suggested, "Why don't you consider taking some courses in the ed psych department?" She wanted to go back to school and work on a master's degree in psychology. She had an amazing lack of awareness of her own importance. She was very quiet, never pushed herself on you. She questioned whether she could do the course work. She needed someone to remind her that she was able to do that.

I knew the chairman of the department and knew that he would like her and do what he could to help her. She took many graduate courses in psychology. The chairman allowed his graduate students to get credit for taking her course on hypnosis and some even did their dissertations on hypnosis and used her as their faculty advisor.

Kay had been studying with Erickson for about 15 years when we first started working with clients together.

Kay was my teacher! When I got my PhD and was no longer a student, I realized I had no backup any more and Kay filled that role. She and I used to work together quite frequently, sometimes with one of her patients, sometimes with one of mine. It got to the point where we could schedule appointments for each other without having to say anything to each other. After we made the appointment, you'd call the other up and let them know. She always was there. Although I didn't answer the phone when it rang all the time, I never missed a call from Kay Thompson. It was validation of my sense of knowing what was important.

Our work together gave her the opportunity to do kinds of therapy that weren't part of her "normal" dental practice, and she did this beautifully.

You never knew when Kay was doing something. She would run it into a story, anecdote, a theoretical discussion you had. She made me intensely aware of how very, very important every word is—don't ever figure that any word has the same meaning for most people. You have to be aware of that. She used to say, "It always starts before it begins and it never finishes when it ends." You have your first contact and say, "Hello," and you have to remember that it (the relationship) started before you said, "Hello."

You had to stand in awe. She always gave me the responsibility for myself. I never had the feeling Kay was in control. She would make a suggestion and I felt I had the freedom to decide whether to do it or not. There were few times I would decide not to.

You got to be careful not to jump in and do something. I got that from Kay Thompson. If you jump in and do it, it doesn't give the person a lot of confidence. Sometimes, you have to go through a lot of tears. It's always nice to say, "See what you did! I didn't do that for you, boy. You did that." Kay could leave you hanging. She'd say, "What are you going to do?" She had a great deal of faith in the person. And if Kay Thompson knows you can do it, you can do it! I'm doing that for my kid.

Client with Qualities Suggesting Multiplicity (Dissociative Disorder)

I had a client with qualities suggesting multiplicity and asked Kay to work with her. The client got to my office first and I told her about Kay. She was nervous. Then Kay came and I introduced her to the client. My client began to express ambivalence about working with Kay and finally picked up her coat and started to leave my office.

Kay got out of her chair and said, very loudly, "What do you think you are doing? I'm a very busy woman and I've taken my time out for today to talk to you and work with you and now you are going to walk out on me! What do *you* think you are doing?"

At that point, the client turned around, sat down in the chair, and we proceeded to work for the next four hours. We did a dual induction. The client got a very deep trance. I positioned several adhesive thermometers on her forehead and she abreacted an event from her childhood. It was a complete abreaction and then it came back down to normal.

I used thermometers with clients sometimes to make sure their temperature was going up and to see how hot they got. I had some physical proof that something was happening, some measure, independent of the subjective. It told me two things. I could keep an eye on it and not let it get too high and it assured me that something was happening. We worked for four hours with her.

After I went home, I got a phone call from the client, who sounded skittish. I invited her to my home. She was still in trance and spent the next three or four hours with my family. She wanted to plant flowers and then she settled down. She took some leave from her work and was fine.

S: Can you talk more about what Kay did in this case?

R: Kay was marvelously supportive of the client. She moved into the mother role and the client fell in love with her and remained friends with Kay for a long time.

Kay could manage the depth of trance, deepening it and making it lighter; she was a marvel of manipulation of trance. She was marvelously talented at being indirect and yet could be direct; it would startle you because she could shift gears so easily. She could take a simple phrase, or a word, *back*, and use it as time dimension, physical dimension, relationship or to give back something. You could never be sure what she was saying to you.

During therapy, she would intersperse suggestions in the induction. There was a lot of ego strengthening, a lot of encouragement, and a lot of support. "Go ahead and do it!" Both me and the client always knew you had a backer.

S: What else did Kay do that was significant in this case?

R: What matters (in that work) was what Kay meant to me. It was a very safe place to be. I thought whatever I did was okay. She seemed to be able to instill a sense of confidence in me. There was another "me", Russ Scott in the sessions. It was having absolute faith and confidence in Kay. I felt invincible by the union with Kay. It's an amazing sense of power. The power was to help the client.

S: Could you talk more about there being another "me", another Russ Scott?

R: I had a sense, a feeling, I have it now, when I talked with and interacted with Kay, a sense that there was more there than I thought. She inspired me. There was a sense of energy. I believed her when she used to say she was a witch. I had an expectation, if not perfection, damn near perfection when I was interacting with her. She wouldn't let you make a mistake. That was the way it was. It was a pleasure to interact with her. You always found there was more there than you knew. She was an awe inspiring woman.

S: Awe for her, but more importantly, awe in yourself? A part of you not accessible before you met her?

R: It seemed she knew me better than I knew myself, and was more than willing to let me see that part of myself. It was an astounding thing. You got to, I'm going to see Kay; it's going to happen again.

S: How did her belief in you affect yours in yourself?

R: I assumed that if Kay Thompson said it would happen, it would. I accepted.

S: You accepted her authority?

R: You're not supposed to hurt if Kay said so. I stand in awe of myself and that is primarily because of her. You have to be a cat to appreciate it. They have nine lives. It takes that many almost to understand Kay. Being a data-oriented man, I kept looking at the data and it happened. We have faith and confidence in things and wonder, where does that come from? That shouldn't work, but it did. You move from, "Oh, my God, I can't try this," to, "Oh, what the hell, I might as well try this." And then you move to, "I'm going to do this." It builds on itself.

If she was working on someone and they would start to cry, that didn't mean stop or go away. She would keep right on going and they would keep right on working too, until they finally got the thing finished. It was almost as if she was inside you, knowing what you were thinking and feeling.

She never said, "Now, you listen up, boy, I'm going to teach something about you!" I just accepted it. Sometimes, it would sound too much like fiction. There was a hell of a lot in Kay Thompson that flew in the face of reality. Sooner or later you learned to accept it.

Dual Induction/Regression—Posthypnotic Effect of Dual Induction

Kay had a friend who said there was something about him that made him uncomfortable. He asked Kay to hypnotize him. We put him between us and did a dual induction. We were talking about shoes and ships and sealing wax, or everything. When you worked with Kay Thompson, you quickly learned not to have any expectations. She could talk about anything. He went off into trance. He was astounded and went back in time. He regressed and experienced some things that happened when he was a child. All I did was to follow Kay. Then I saw him in therapy.

The effect was astounding. In our therapy, when he heard my voice, he also heard Kay's.

S: Kay's voice in the dual induction almost operated like a posthypnotic suggestion?

R: Yes, like a posthypnotic suggestion for him to go into a deep trance, a very deep trance. We were able to talk about the thing in his childhood, which had been originally elicited during the dual induction with Kay.

A Marvelous Hypnotic Subject: Automobile Accident and Body Scan

Kay was in an automobile accident and called me about 7:30 in the morning. I came to the hospital and she asked me to take a trip through her body. Kay was a marvelous hypnotic subject and could do all kinds of things and got a very good trance. In the trance, she said, "I got a broken bone and they missed it."

We took a trip through her body to see what was broken. I asked her to go inside and look. "Tell me what you see. Does that hurt? Is everything okay there?" She got a good trance. I started with the head. "Check out that head. Is everything okay? Does anything hurt? Are you sure it's okay? Let's move to your neck, and chest."

I think she could see inside and look around. "You know what it's supposed to be like. You've been there lots of times." I feel that people can visualize inside their bodies. "You know what it's like when it's normal. You know what it's like when it hurts."

Most people don't know when they have a broken sternum. They missed hers when they took the X-ray. She found the broken bones in trance, even though she had been through all the X-rays and everything. She insisted that they look again and they found the breaks.

Wild West Riddle: What is She Going to Come Up with This Time?

She called me up one day with a question, "Russ, what do you know about the Wild West?" I answered, "I don't know anything about the Wild West." She said, "Well, I have a mystery about the Wild West." She proceeded to tell me about something that had happened around the 1850s, which involved two men and a robbery and a shoot-out. She got the story from a friend. The story was that both men had died in the shoot out, but had left a message that somehow pointed the way to a map.

498

I said, "A map? Two gunmen dead and it happened 150 years ago. Sure, I'm interested." We started to poke away at it and that was as much as we had. We ended up finding the location where they had died and their bodies supposedly pointed to a map. So we reconstructed and deconstructed. By taking the positions of their bodies when they died, we drew lines and the lines intersected and pointed to a map. Somebody actually dug the map up.

She figured it out. The person who was interested was a friend of Kay's and he got us involved in a few things. I used to wonder, what is she going to come up with this time? I always knew that when Kay called me up, it was to help somebody. How can you say no?

ASCH: Politics and a Controversial Issue

On controversial issues we found ourselves on the same side. I got the ASCH Board of Directors upset one time. We had a meeting in New Orleans and Kay had one position and everyone else had another position. Of course, Kay was right. Of course, I took her side. I finally decided not to go to the meeting one day and wrote a paper. The paper dealt with various events and demonstrated rather conclusively that Kay was right. We presented that to the Board and I got accused of being Kay Thompson's lackey. But we won.

It was about who was going to be taught hypnosis and who wasn't. We were teaching hypnosis to policemen. We were being accused of being unprofessional. That was when they wanted to make it an exclusive club of physicians and people with doctorates and they didn't want to teach social workers. Social workers couldn't be trusted. They didn't want to let in riffraff.

Some people get very protective about hypnosis. You've got to be careful. People can do a lot of damage with it. They question teaching hypnosis to the police. You couldn't trust them. They would be using it to tell some people what to say. That is true. We did have cases where we ran into that. You can't teach women to drive because they'll have accidents. It happens every day but the payoff is much better than the cost.

Kay was very much in support of other professions, like social workers. She knew what I knew, that the police were already using hypnoticlike techniques. It was a matter of teaching them so they would know what the hell they were doing. Some of the brightest people you ever will meet are police. You have to face that fact. You can't deny it. You have to accept the fact that their hearts are in the right place. The things that they face and do are so uncommon to the rest of the world, that nobody has an idea what it's like. She was very supportive and nonjudgmental. If you are going to give the crook a benefit of a doubt, then you have to give the cop one too.

Police Connection

I was Director of Planning and Development for the City of Pittsburgh, taught part-time in both the undergraduate and graduate departments of psychology at the University of Pittsburgh, and maintained a private practice. You need to know about my police connection. I had a contract with the city police to develop and implement psychological selection procedures for policemen. While working with the city police, I met members of the FBI, CIA, ATF (Alcohol, Tobacco and Firearms), US postal service and IRS. I even taught at the police academy. All of these organizations contacted me for forensic work.

Torture Victim: Strength and Mothering

Kay and I worked with several clients who had been tortured. I had a client, B, who accidentally uncovered some very dangerous criminal activities by a cult. When the people in the cult discovered this, they tortured B and used hypnosis to install "fail safes" (conditions, behaviors or words that would automatically cause him to do something). In his case, when certain subjects were brought up, he would stop talking. They also gave him amnesia for the torture and for what he had uncovered. A concerned colleague was suspicious and referred him to me. I realized I was in over my head and called in Kay.

Kay supported and strengthened B, when he was reexperiencing the torture, and helped him get past certain memories. There were extreme political and criminal activities related to the case. I even became very frightened for my own safety. Kay never got scared. It didn't stop her. She was there with me and the client through it all. I always had the feeling that she was invulnerable. She became B's "mother", something she did frequently with clients who had been traumatized. B would call her up and talk to her sometimes. She was so adapt.

S: How did she develop such deep rapport with B?

R: She would tell you (the client) all about herself. I am somebody just like you. How could you not like somebody who was like yourself? With B, they had put in a variety of fail safes. Whenever you would talk about something you shouldn't, that would elicit a fail safe. Kay taught me how to work with fail safes. She would support the client while I did that.

Kay was the epitome of strength. Nothing frightened her. She always encouraged. She would say, "You can do this. You can do it well. You can do a good job. And you better do it (for me)."

After Kay and I worked together, I would often see these clients alone. I was seeing another client who had been tortured, and one day he attacked me during the session. I calmed him down, left the office, and called Kay on the telephone. Miraculously, she was home and answered the phone. I said, "G tried to kill me!" She said, "Well, Russ Scott, [*pause*] … what else is new?" I laughed. My knees got their rigidity back. I talked to her and then finished my work. I thought, she meant, "Well if you are playing with such big dogs, you have to come off the porch."

501

Forensic Hypnosis: Murder One

We had one case where a man was going on trial for murder. He had confessed to the murder but his attorney didn't believe the confession. I told the defendant that he had only three friends—me, Kay Thompson and his attorney. Everybody else wanted to see the man hang. It was Friday. That's a rather chilling thing to be hearing when you are sitting in jail waiting to go on trial on Monday. We did a dual induction in which Kay said, "The judge and the jury have already decided you are guilty because you confessed. There are only three people in the world who want you to live to be older."

He popped off into trance. And he started to describe the murder scene and he got to a point where the murdered man was lying on the floor. He stood up and got scared. Here's a man whose life was literally in our hands. All his previous confusion was terminated. He was able to make sense out of nonsense and reconstruct what had happened. Everything fit together very nicely. He had a rope tied on the wrist of his right hand. When he came to the trial, he was describing the rope. The prosecutor asked, "And where was your left hand." He said, "At the end of my left arm, sir," because he was in trance.

S: Kay has briefly discussed this case in some of her lectures. It's amazing to me how easily we could overlook how important it was that you and Kay were at that trial. And the defendant was in trance when he was testifying. It must have been very important for both of you to be there. And I'm understanding the deep commitment and dedication that both of you had to your clients.

R: Kay was the one who suggested we go to the trial. The detective who took the confession was at the trial. While testifying, the defendant would look at the detective, then he'd look at us and give his correct testimony. The detective was also there, perhaps trying to get him to corroborate the confession. Kay knew very well that a person can be in trance and it's not obvious. There's more than one way of skinning a cat. She knew them all.

Kay and I were there in order to keep the boy straight. When a man is up for murder one, and you are on his side, you do what you got to do, baby. We were there to support him. As long as we were in court there to give him support, it was an amazing thing. It's similar to group psychology. When one person is supportive of you, it's more likely that you will stick to your story. It's hard to be the only person to take a position. It gets real lonely. If there is just one other person who supports you, it's a tremendous advantage. He was looking at us and touching base, "Are you still there?" That's what he was asking, when he looked at us. "Where are you? Now, when I need you, where are you?" He was obviously in trance during the testimony. He was found not guilty of murder.

Courtroom

R: She used hypnosis in the courtroom on several occasions.

S: Her presence was enough to facilitate trance?

R: Enough to have an impact. They would go into trance and give more detailed testimony. We had a case where an attorney was on trial. Kay and I had worked with him. (*Laughing.*) I had video-taped our dual induction and presented it in court. The court reporter screamed, "Oh, my God, they are talking at the same time!"

S: Did you purposely show it for that reason? Were you always together in court?

R: Most of the time, yeah. We had fun with that. I was focusing primarily with the judge. It went our way. People went along on free rides all the time. You have to play the game by the rules as you understand them.

S: You were doing dual inductions outside of court. The clients had that cue with both of you in court. Did you ever talk about that? You and Kay in court was a dual induction in and of itself?

R: We never took on something we intended to lose. If we got involved, we got involved to win. Once we taught a course on hypnosis to the judges and told them what we knew. They are the ones that have to make the decisions, not me.

The Greatest Miscarriage of Justice

The only thing that made me more angry that seeing someone get away with something was seeing the wrong man convicted. We both were very conscious of the danger. There was a case where a man was convicted of murder and had already served 10 years. We were contacted by the DA. Kay and I worked with the guy. I learned a lot. I couldn't get a description of the other person present during the murder.

We got him back to when it had happened, to the physical setting. Looking at the scene from where he was positioned, sitting on the steps, helped him remember. She was supportive and making suggestions. He kept going deeper into trance. She was very pleased because we got him off. We hypnotized the guy and he was eventually found innocent. The governor said it was the biggest miscarriage of justice in the state's history. I was more proud of that than all the people I sent to jail.

Voices: With Kay Beside Me, I Could Take On the Whole Damned Army

Once I worked with a witness to a crime and after recording the session, the chief of police and I listened to the tape. We could hear a little child's voice on the tape saying "over here, over here". It was on the tape in three places. If you want to see two surprised people, you could have seen it. I called Kay and we went over the tape together.

She was amazed and fascinated. She confirmed that I did everything correctly and did not lead the witness. You have to be very careful when doing hypnosis with a witness. She admitted she didn't know what the voices were. That made her invaluable. She would never make fun of you. She was an utterly accepting lady.

When you get something like that, it's hard not to get scared. She didn't get scared. There was no question in my mind that with Kay beside me, I could take on the whole goddamned army. I took the tape to an engineer and he enhanced it. The voices were still there. The chief of police hand carried the tape to the FBI. And they got the voices too. Kay was interested in the FBI's estimate of it. We didn't know what we had. We never did figure it out. We had experts look at it from every reasonable point of view and even matched all radio stations programming at that time. I always want data.

Working with Children

She knew about working with kids. She would touch the middle of their forehead (both an induction and utilization) and say, "You are going to see something there. And you can watch it. This is your special TV screen. Now do you see it?" She would keep her finger on the child's forehead. And then, "Now you are going to watch your favorite TV show. You can laugh, do what you want to do, and tell me what is happening." She used the television screen and had them watch a children's movie. And then she would flash back and forth from the movie to what we were working on. "Let's switch channels," she would say. "You can go back and watch the other movie." Kids are great in hypnosis. They laugh as if they are watching TV. That was something she was so good at.

She could use something as an induction and as a utilization. She was very alert to when the child was anxious or restless, "Let's go back and watch the other show." She would say, "Isn't that funny? What do you think of that?" Always a lot of support for the child. The kids responded very well.

Doing What Needs to Be Done: What Should Be Done and Can Be Done

I had a client who was a teenager. The mother had come across drug paraphernalia. He had gotten kicked out of several different schools and had failed many classes. He was experimenting with drugs and we got him off the drugs. I developed a relationship with him that was very intense. I helped him through high school and college and girlfriends and then marriage. He decided not to have children because he didn't think he could be a good father. A few years ago, my wife and I gave him and his wife a pair of dogs. He grew up and they had a little boy. Recently he and his wife had a second child. He's a good father, a good dad.

S: Kay rescued dogs throughout her life. Giving him the dogs was a lovely gift, perhaps influenced by Kay?

R: It was like when Erickson kept a dog for one of his patients. Kay was quite impressed with that. I don't know how much it was Kay emulating Milton Erickson or Kay just being Kay. It's a strength. You do for me and I do for somebody else. Giving him a dog was a Kay Thompson kind of intervention. Kay did for me what had to be done. She not only did it for me, she taught me how to do it for other people. Even today, I have that knowledge. It truly is a knowledge. This is what Kay Thompson taught me to do.

S: She was manifesting love and encouraging you in so many ways.

R: She gave me the opportunity to experience it myself. I can say, "I love you and I am aware that you love me." The love was already so huge, I felt she felt about me. There were no limits. She had a way of overwhelming you with kindness. That's what made her moments of anger so impressive. She was so kind, it was always a surprise to see her angry.

There's a sense of awe that comes over me when I talk about her.

Kay put wheels on the concept of love. It becomes a tangible thing. It's more than a feeling.

Personal Vignettes

Kay Thompson, the Consummate Educator

Karen Olness

Kay Thompson was an outstanding educator. The term to *educate* derivés from the Latin word *educere* which means "to bring forth". The consummate educator brings forth the desire to learn in students and motivates their interest in and commitment to continue learning for a lifetime. An outstanding educator is generous with her time and knowledge, patient with the novice, and mindful of the shoulders on which she stands. Kay was all of these. Her goal was to facilitate learning for individuals whether they were clients, clinicians, academicians, or researchers. Her students knew that she cared deeply about them.

Where did she teach? Everywhere. She taught patients and students, but she also taught at local workshops, international meetings and during fabulous dinners in her home. She even taught while riding in the car with colleagues to attend a meeting. Her extraordinary skills, warmth, and generosity kindled love and respect wherever she taught. She taught for many years at the University of Pittsburgh and the University of West Virginia, gave lectures at other universities and was in great demand to teach at workshops and conferences throughout the United States and Europe.

How did Kay teach? She seemed to be intuitive about the learning styles and preferences of her students. Sometimes, she was direct and authoritative; more often she was indirect, choosing educational metaphors that suited her audiences. Kay didn't hesitate to use her own experiences to demonstrate teaching points, most notably when she allowed filming of her own facial surgery for which she used self-hypnosis as her sole anesthesia. This extraordinary film, which was shown for many years at workshops, was unforgettable. It was the impetus for my decision 15 years later to have my own surgery with self-hypnosis, also allowing it to be filmed.

Kay used demonstrations of hypnosis as a major teaching tool. When she encountered the occasional abreaction, she handled it with sensitivity and skill. Many of us who were subjects in her demonstrations considered these opportunities to have provided our most meaningful learning experiences about hypnosis.

As I read the transcripts in this book, I recalled Kay's voice speaking conversationally during inductions. Her voice was never monotonous and deep like many hypnotherapists, but full of life, humor and careful inflections. She avoided drama and sudden voice changes. She spoke naturally, quickly eliciting the interest of her audiences. She could speak to anybody about anything. This was especially evident in her work with children. Her childlike curiosity and playfulness spoke directly to their hearts. She spoke to children as if she took them seriously, which she did. Kay was never phony.

Students eventually understood that Kay "walked the talk". She believed in the efficiency of hypnotherapy and she used it for herself. She had no time for professionals who taught hypnosis, yet did not learn to apply it in their own lives.

In her superb article, "The Curiosity of Milton Erickson", she wrote that, "Erickson had the skill of the master teacher, who lets us think we have discovered things for ourselves." It is not surprising that Kay was also a master teacher, who selflessly encouraged, challenged, and guided her students to become everything they could be.

Kay's teaching and therapy impacted untold numbers of people, many of whom have shared fascinating vignettes about their interactions with her. One former patient who had suffered severe oral trauma was having some dental work done. At the end of the dental appointment during which Kay had talked to her throughout the procedure, she turned to Kay and said, "Kay, do you ever work with normal patients?" Kay looked at her, turned a 360-degree pirouette on one foot and answered, "Now! That wouldn't be any fun, would it?"

Kay lectured throughout Europe for several decades. A Dutch colleague shared that Kay had the amusing habit of screaming loudly when people in her presence talked in another language. Years later, he and his wife still laugh about Kay's emphatic message.

It would be impossible to share all the wonderful stories and vignettes we have heard about Kay. These brief personal vignettes illustrate aspects of the complexity of her therapeutic communications and share some of the profound effects she had on so many of her students and colleagues.

True Friendship

Roxanna Erickson Klein

A true friend is one whom you can depend upon to guide you into being a better person. Kay took on the role of friendship seriously, giving selflessly. I would like to think that ours was a two-way street, that I was as true a friend to her as she to me.

We first came to know each other well, after my husband Alan, my dog Earnest and I moved in for a prolonged visit, the result of a job relocation. What struck me initially, and what has remained with me, was the genteel largesse and the gracious hospitality that permeated the home. In the weeks that we were there, and in the two years that followed, my husband and I were "adopted" by Ralph and Kay.

We felt fully accepted despite the failing and foibles of our own youthful behaviors that I can clearly see now. During our month-long stay in their home, Earnest misbehaved constantly, yet there was not a single word or indication of fatigue from either Kay or Ralph. It was as though they loved being gracious hosts long after the usual time for hospitality had passed. Many times I heard Kay take advantage of the opportunity to introduce us, and by carefully explaining that my husband is a physician, I am a nurse and Earnest a blue heeler, she transformed a simple introduction into an artful commentary conveying the thoughts that good friends and good medicine are sometimes troublesome, but healing is always worth the effort.

A long line of wayward comrades were welcomed into that gentle environment. In fact, one of Kay's "projects" was nurturing a series of needy dogs, most of them short and furry "mops". Rescued from a variety of circumstances, then nursed or fostered into well-being, Kay managed to modify behavioral problems and to pair many homeless mutts with masters, some of whom did not even know they wanted a dog.

In a visit to the remarkable home where Kay spent her childhood, I learned about her father's powerful presence and sudden death. Kay's father, Dr. Lony Thompson, also a dentist, had died unexpectedly of an abdominal aneurysm some years before I had come to know her. Although her father had clearly been supportive, influential, and loved, she rarely mentioned him. My own carefully tutored upbringing guided me to not question her reticence. One day, in the home she had grown up in, she surprised me by sharing what she had previously been unable to. We sat on a bed together as she vividly described what a strong presence her father was, personally, professionally and physically. She emphasized how important he was in the community, in the family, and to her. I realized then why she was so quiet about the father whom she so clearly loved. She said that one day he hadn't felt well, and lay down to rest, "Right here, where we are sitting." She pointed to the spot where he had fallen after he got out of bed, his life gone in an instant, a precipitous and totally unanticipated moment.

The deep pain of that event sat heavy in the air, punctuated by the unchanged décor of the room. Antique furniture, dated wallpaper, meticulous positioning of art objects gave the room, gave the whole house the feel of a museum. We held hands, and, at once, I understood her previous silence about a wonderful man.

After our talk we sat in the kitchen, drinking tea from delicate bone china, and reminiscing about the joys of her growing up in that fine, stately old two-story home south of Pittsburgh, where her mother still lived. The original wallpaper was a print of English ivy climbing around the kitchen. I marveled at the 1920s décor, at how unchanged a home could be over a span of more than 50 years. What a unique experience, for me, to be able to drop into the past so fully. Kay's mother, Bertha, was proud of her own good taste and her ability to select enduring furnishings that genuinely still looked good! We laughed together at my surprise that the home seemed to be suspended in 1920s, and at the contrasting perceptions held by both Kay and her mother, of the normalcy of it. Bertha had left the home almost entirely as she had originally decorated it, only adding regularly to her marvelous paperweight and fan collections. These items, all of superb quality, were displayed on every flat and vertical surface, each one treasured for its uniqueness.

A wooded area buffered the home from a roadway, across from which arose an enormous landscape feature that Kay unceremoniously referred to as the "slag pile". With exquisite clarity, she described the spectacular night views of glowing red-hot embers being poured atop the mountainous heap of tailings from the local mines. Her verbal images of these events were so powerful that all of us present laughed heartily at the paradox of the splendid disposal of waste.

Collections

Kay's mother's magnificent collection gave unique character and definition to the home and the circumstance that Kay was raised in. Learning the value of collecting, Kay was able to apply that to other aspects of her life. Starting in childhood, Kay amassed a collection of elephants of every imaginable art form. Most had been gifts from friends, relatives and colleagues who knew of her passion for the strength and beauty of those intriguing animals.

Though she never even encouraged it, I thank Kay with influencing me to start a collection of my own (eggs). The pleasure she emanated over her role as custodian of the elephants, and the wonderful images associated with each treasure, made a lasting impression. Similarly, though he never acknowledged Kay's influence, my father developed a passion for collecting Seri Ironwood carvings. The very first gifts from his collection were made to Kay Thompson and Bob Pearson. For Kay he selected an elegant carving of a conch shell.

Presentation

Kay presented herself with a thoughtful elegance that spoke of a cultivated ability to enjoy the moment. Her home, her wardrobe and her quiet demeanor were all examples of the understatement with which she usually appeared. However, when she wanted to make a statement, she was equally comfortable dressing with a striking and dramatic flair. Physically, she was a rare blend of bold elegance and delicacy. Her statuesque features, combined with lithe and graceful movements, created an intriguing sense of juxtaposition. Her meticulous grooming, exquisite selection of clothes, unfailing attention to details of hair and makeup, brought forth delicacy, which seemed almost out of place when she displayed her unfaltering ability to stare down an opponent or to pursue a professional objective.

In contrast with the stately home of her youth, Kay and Ralph built what looked from the outside to be a modest home. Located on a residential street, with a gravel circle drive in front, the seemingly small home greeted visitors with a flair—next to the bright red entry doors was a prickly pear garden. The cacti unexpectedly thrived in Pennsylvania, finding just the right light and shelter for regrowth after burial in deep winter snows every year, and displaying stunning yellow flowers in the summer.

Inside the house, the large living area was the color of sunshine. The main floor was open and bright, with a long line of windows that revealed a beautiful view across a green valley. It turned out to be a three-story home that was welcoming and comfortable, as well as spacious enough to accommodate vast numbers of people for both business and entertainment. Perhaps in an unwitting metaphor for herself, Kay explained that the key was to find property on a hill, where only the modest entry shows: if one accepts an invitation to come inside unexpected resources and treasures reveal themselves.

During our prolonged stay with Kay and Ralph, Kay and I were able to work at play, and play at work, because of our well-matched energy levels and interests. We shared in-depth conversations about word use, health care trends, and organizational structure while we peeled potatoes and put together an "elegant but easy" meal for dinner (she planned—I helped). Those multitasking undertakings gave us a platform for companionship that was already well positioned on the firm foundation of family friendship. Amid the hustle and bustle of my finding a job, Kay doing hers, and Ralph and Alan attending to their own professions, we managed to come together for daily life activities that we shared with relish and embellishment. All of Kay's endeavors were undertaken with an air of relaxed dedication, as if the time involved in a task was irrelevant and only the outcome important.

A Most Valuable Gift

Perhaps the most valuable lesson I learned from Kay was the result of her quiet and careful planning at a party. She orchestrated the circumstance so that I was able to experience myself in a way I had long hoped for, but felt was outside the realm of possibilities On several occasions, we had discussed the value of being "noticed" as opposed to being unnoticed. Kay could present herself in a variety of ways to meet the circumstances: strong, forceful, quiet, demure or shy, but she spoke of an inside desire to just fade into the background, and not to be so central in activities. She acknowledged that her distinctive looks precluded her from being a wallflower—she was going to be noticed and that's all there was to it. Although she had learned to use that inescapable quality of her life in a positive way, she revealed to me that she had longed to be less conspicuous at times.

We compared these feelings with my own: my growing up always being recognized as Erickson's daughter and never being able to experience anything vaguely related to hypnotic work in a "normal forum". I had long wondered about the mundane and typical questions that students ask each other about hypnosis. I complained to Kay that each time I entered a room where individuals studied hypnosis, I was accompanied by an introduction of being Erickson's daughter. I told Kay about my perception that immediately the atmosphere of the room would shift and I would find myself with a private audience of interested professionals who had "prepared" questions. I never minded the interrogations, and had long ago learned to answer the inquiries, no matter how invasive, in a manner with which I was comfortable. What I lacked was the basic and ordinary experience that other people have—what it was to be in a "regular crowd" where people are sharing energy in an equal way and where people work together for a sense of discovery.

I told her that I too, longed to be a wallflower, but couldn't even hope to accomplish that since my educational qualifications (at the time) wouldn't even permit me entrance to professional hypnosis meetings. The conversation was in passing, nothing I took seriously or expected to be remembered or acted upon. But months later, when Kay hosted a party for the local chapter of ASCH, the extent of her sensitivity and responsiveness revealed itself.

Having arranged for Joe Barber, PhD, to speak at the dental school about pain control, Kay helped me slip unobtrusively into the back of the audience. The lecture was followed by a reception for both dental students and for the local hypnosis society. As it was just before the holiday, Kay and Ralph prepared for the event with a spectacular Christmas tree and an elaborate selection of hors-d'oeuvres.

A tremendous cold front blew in that afternoon and penetrated the air with unusual intensity including a chill factor of minus 10°F. Activities proceeded punctually despite the chill, but gas service to Carnegie [where they lived] was interrupted, leaving the entire community without heat.

Never considering the possibility of cancellation or postponement, Kay, Ralph and the guests followed through with the day's plans as scheduled. Blankets and quilts were brought out and candles lined up in case of an electrical outage. The idea of holding the meeting "under blankets" was approached with great enthusiasm and adventure, and the only concern expressed was that "if the electricity goes out, we won't be able to heat the food or enjoy the decorative Christmas lights".

The house was packed with people, all of whom knew a huge storm was in the making, and that the heat was out, and the electricity might soon also be interrupted. Clearly, the whole group antici-pated that this Christmas party and the accompanying opportuni-ties to learn about hypnosis were well worth the inconvenience of the travel conditions.

I remember being engrossed in conversation for a long time before realizing that no one had come up to greet me or to probe, to present the questions they had wondered about for years, or, especially, to ask the inevitable, "What was it like to be the daughter of Milton Erickson?" For at least an hour I huddled under the blankets with the rest of the students and professionals, listening to the ordinary conversation, making my own remarks, being listened to, and even discounted by other's opinions.

After a while, I noticed that my key maiden name had been omitted on my name tag. My memory hearkened back to the conversation in which I had told Kay about my wish to be anonymous in a crowd of interested students of hypnosis. And there I was—just another person. Without my request Kay had taken me more seriously than I realized. Her sensitivity to my wishes was a real gift.

The impact of the whole situation hit me after someone made an erroneous comment about Erickson, a simple mistake. I corrected the remark and this sparked an inquiry as to how I was so certain my facts were correct. When I divulged the truth, I turned and saw Kay smiling a Cheshire cat look of satisfaction. We kept each other's gaze as we heard the murmuring and the realignment of energy, then the beginning of the "inquisition"—the to-be-expected questions about my family life. It was very affirming for me to share that experience with Kay.

Her gift, the taste of normalcy, allowed me to explore the unnamed portion of my identity. Kay's actions gave me a greater sense of comfort and balance of who I am as an individual who has come from an exceptional home. Since that time, I have never felt the need to hide or fade, but now have a real comfort with who I actually am.

Kay had an outstanding ability to nurture students, colleagues, and friends and help them grow past limitations. She had a special skill of making the inept feel adequate, of turning social blunders into moments of comic relief and of inspiring ongoing self-improvement and refinement. Communicating with her easy laugh, knowing smile, a glint in her eye with a perfectly timed glance or a perplexed look, Kay was a friend and a mentor to a multitude.

Kay's friendship helped me to grow into the person I am today. Her enthusiasm and joy of life, coupled with trustworthiness, dignity and elegance gave me a model that I think back on every time I am faced with a tough situation. She still guides me.

Actively Tuning In

Arnold Freedman

"It's not a matter of actively doing something to change the situation so much as it is listening to ourselves. Because we get signals from the patient all the time. And we need to learn to do what Erickson was so famous for, and that was to go where the patient is and see the situation from the client's point of view. And that is a very different perspective and one that too few are willing to pay attention to. The idea that we can accomplish this through words is a major responsibility." (Kay Thompson, Chapter Six.)

I was hooked during my first phone call with Kay over 30 years ago. I had a negative view of university faculty at the time, but she changed that. She was enthusiastic and encouraging, and connected with me. She seemed genuinely interested in my work and my patients and was always supportive. I would periodically call her about difficult cases and she always had something helpful to offer and encouraged me to continue and persist. I shared the successes I had with hypnosis, since it was not understood in my work environment, and her encouragement was powerfully reinforcing for me.

One of the most noteworthy characteristics about Kay was her ability to tune in to the client. She was really connecting with them and being where they were. Stacie Murrer, a friend of both mine and Kay's, explained this by saying, "Kay is not above you. She is right there side by side with you. She is not trying to impose anything on you."

Kay brought me to Phoenix to meet Erickson. When I walked into his house, Kay introduced me to him. He looked up at me intently from his wheelchair, like my dog looks at me. It was very physical, as if he was taking me in and seeking to understand me. I think Kay was doing the same thing, but she wasn't as obvious as Dr. Erickson. That sense of tuning in and being where the person is struck me as very powerful.

Kay worked with a couple of my patients. One had a tic, which was more like a social phobia. Kay agreed to see him with me. The way she worked with him at that time was characteristic of this "tuning in". She was both in her trance and was tuning in with him. She would speak very deliberately and work off her connection with the person. Although she had some favorite stories and metaphors which she used frequently, wherever she went was from her unconscious and the connection with the person. This was awfully important. You get into a kind of sync with the person. And you don't look like you are struggling, or overinvolved with the patient.

Before meeting Kay, I tended to jump ahead of the client and offer an assessment and treatment that the client was not necessarily ready to accept. Kay's emphasis was to connect with the client and stay with him. I learned that if you are with a client and you empathize with them and communicate as exactly as you can what they intended to say to you, they know it. As you establish a connection with the client, you get in touch with a deeper sense inside yourself and the client seems more connected to his own inner self as well. And you can offer ideas that are probably more relevant to the client's needs.

It took me a long time to develop the ability to connect with the client and stay with him. A few years after Kay's death, I think I am just beginning to fully appreciate what she demonstrated and taught. When I am "off the mark" with a client, it is likely because I haven't really connected with them.

Through learning to really join the client, I became more willing to see clients whom I would never have agreed to see before. I would have perceived them as too difficult, if not impossible. One example was a case in which a woman called me and asked if I could use hypnosis to help her daughter. I am usually on guard when people call me asking for hypnosis because there is so much misinformation and unrealistic expectations about it. She described her daughter's problems and told me that she had seen psychiatrists, been on several different medications, and had even been hospitalized. She was persistent and pleaded with me to call her daughter.

My first reaction was to turn her down. There were all the usual "professional" reasons not to see her daughter. As I thought about it, I could hear what Kay would have done. I decided to take on the challenge and see what I could find out. I called the young woman and she told me that she was very depressed because she had a compulsion, about which she was ashamed, and which controlled her life. She described a physical condition for which she was hospitalized at an early age, and which created a great deal of dependency on her parents and other caregivers. She also said that when she was young, she was overweight and the kids picked on her.

I felt Kay's influence very powerfully and listened to this young woman who was in pain. I could hear the anxiety and apprehension that she had lived with. I told her that I could help her deal with the anxiety in a way that she had not done before. She made an appointment and we did some formal hypnosis. She said she could never remember being that relaxed and comfortable. She had a job that was far below her capacities and education and hoped eventually to make a living through her music. She loved to play music, but although she was very good when she would practice alone, she froze up when she was playing professionally. She applied the hypnosis immediately to her music. At first, she tried to relax right when she was performing but that didn't work. She realized on her own that she needed to relax before each song. She said when she made that adjustment, her performances improved.

With that boost in confidence, she expressed an interest in finding a better job and seeking new friends. Staying with her as Kay would have done, I helped her to see that she was also anxious about changing her job and interacting socially. When I suggested she could apply her self-hypnotic skills to these other tasks, she agreed and started to implement changes in those areas also. I could not have done the work I did with that client without Kay's pervasive influence on me. As strange and even bizarre as a client may seem, if you really tune in and hear them, and let them know that you are there where they are, you have the possibility of movement. For me, I feel if I have some grasp of their problem, I can communicate with them about it, no matter what they are saying. I can communicate with them in terms that make sense to me and then to them, so they can begin to accept suggestions.

And Kay certainly gave suggestions. She always offered a better way for the client to cope with their problems. She was constantly encouraging and reinforcing to everybody, her patients, students and colleagues. Kay made a lasting impact on all of us. She gave us a legacy that we can pass on to those whom we serve. She provided a bridge from Milton Erickson to us and future generations of care-givers. For me, it is a great honor and responsibility to carry on this tradition.

How Do You Thank Someone for Giving You Yourself?

Ronald Havens

Kay, I barely knew you, yet you changed my life and thereby changed the life of my clients as well. I cherish this opportunity to thank you.

When, in the early 1970s, I began attending hypnosis workshops sponsored by the American Society of Clinical Hypnosis, Kay was a dominant force on the training team. She spoke eloquently and pre-cisely about hypnosis, offered clear direction and guidance to par-ticipants, and obviously was in charge of coordinating and directing the entire workshop. In other words, she filled the role of past president of the organization quite effectively. Her manner was professional, yet collegial and friendly. Mostly she was rather serious and businesslike, but she could be funny and lighthearted at times.

She and the other presenters rarely strayed from the standard ASCH script, whose information and techniques were quite typical for the time. We were taught typical induction procedures like the eye-closure induction or the hand-levitation induction along with counting backwards from 10 to 1 to deepen the trance. Hypnotic suggestions were to be elicited just by asking (or directing) subjects to experience the phenomenon desired, such as a heavy arm or a numb hand.

Once I discovered Erickson's concepts and hypnotic techniques, through reading *Hypnotic Realities* by Erickson, Rossi and Rossi (1976), the standard ASCH approach seemed shallow, ineffective, and a bit misguided. Given the structure and goals of the ASCH workshops, it is probably to Kay's credit that she rarely mentioned Erickson and did not attempt to teach us the complexities of his approach. It must have taken some restraint to offer the scientifically and professionally "acceptable" point of view, rather than expound on the things Erickson had taught her. After *Hypnotic Realities* was published, however, the cat was out of the bag. There was a new hypnotherapeutic reality and the training ASCH offered no longer interested me.

I attended the first International Congress on Ericksonian Approaches to Hypnosis and Psychotherapy held in Phoenix, Arizona, in 1980, where several thousand professionals mourned his recent death and celebrated his work. Kay gave an eloquent and emotional address about her relationship with Dr. Erickson and what she learned from him. She ended it with a poem by Roy Croft, the first stanza of which is:

"I love you, not only for what you are,/But for what I am when I am with you."

There was not a dry eye in the place by the time she was finished.

The next time I saw Kay was in 1983 at the second International Congress of Ericksonian Approaches. She led a workshop there entitled "The Language of Hypnosis". By 1983, I had read almost everything Milton Erickson had ever written and had listened to many tape recordings of his teaching sessions as well. I was steeped in the Ericksonian approach. As I entered the conference room that day I thought I knew what an Ericksonian hypnotic approach was and I thought I knew what was involved in learning how to do it. But Kay had something else in mind. Although the brief blurb about her presentation in the conference schedule mentioned "utilizing apparently innocuous word plays, and using appropriate and meaningful themes as a focus for accomplishing change", I had no idea what this meant to her.

She began the workshop with a lecture, the content of which I have forgotten entirely. After that she told us a few sample metaphors that were full of puns and plays on words, and then she set about teaching us how to construct such metaphorical anecdotes on our own. "Pick out a topic related to the client or the client's problem." In my case, I picked trains, because the person I was thinking of kept moving from one university to another looking for the perfect education. "Think of all the words that relate to that topic." I obediently listed track, engine, engineer, whistle, ticket, seats, conductor etc. "What other meanings do those words have?" A one-track mind, stay on track, keep track of things, etc. "Now, use all of that in a story." I felt confused, but probably no more confused than many of the others there. I thought I had the basic idea, but was not sure what to do with it.

Shortly thereafter I had another opportunity to attend a workshop that Kay was leading. Immediately after her introductory lecture she conducted a dual induction with Eric Greenleaf. As I sat with my eyes closed, completely absorbed by the sound of her voice and the meaning of her words, something clicked into place. I heard the multiple meanings of words in her rhymes, associations, and word play. I understood what she was saying and how she was saying it. I "knew" that this was what she had been teaching us to do several years before, and I knew I now knew how to do it. In fact, I could not wait to get home to do it with my clients.

Prior to that moment, my hypnotic approach consisted largely of mimicry of things Milton Erickson had done. After that moment, my interventions took on a life and style all their own. They became an outlet for a poetic form of communication I had not used since a poetry course during my undergraduate days. Every hypnotic induction became an opportunity to create a new poetic metaphor designed to captivate and entertain that particular person, to communicate several messages at the same time, and to stimulate that individual's own creative healing energies. Eventually, I coauthored two books (*Hypnotherapy Scripts* and *Hypnotherapy for Health, Harmony and Peak Performance*), each of which contains numerous examples of these poetic productions, most of them constructed using the instructions and suggestions given by Kay Thompson during her workshop in 1983, and later demonstrated powerfully by her during that group induction process. They are not particularly good poems at all, but they are surprisingly effective nonetheless. And it is a joy to create and use them.

Although I like to think that Kay would recognize her influence on the way I conduct my hypnosis sessions now and perhaps even approve of them, I also know that what I am doing is nothing at all like what she would say or do under the same circumstances. She did not teach me to imitate her. Kay fostered the individuality and growth of others. She encouraged her students to recognize and fulfill their fullest potentials, use their own abilities in whatever way worked best for them, and trust their own unconscious, just as Erickson had done with her. She modeled mental and verbal playfulness, demonstrated humor and spontaneity, provided gentle but firm direction, and approached everyone with a warmth and encouragement that enabled others to blossom.

Somehow she gave me permission to be myself, to release and rely upon a part of me that had been overlooked and ignored up to that point. After all, my father was an amateur artist, my aunt was a professional artist, and my youngest son has just finished his degree in fine arts. Before Kay, this side of me was in cold storage, and now it is out in the open, an integral part of my professional and personal life.

How do you thank someone for giving you yourself? Perhaps the only way you can is by doing the same for others. We cannot all do it as well as she did, but if everyone she touched did it for just one or two others, the world would be a better place indeed. Thank you, Kay. I hardly knew you at all, but few people have a bigger place in my heart or in my life.

The Rose: Awakening Potential

Saralee Kane

Even though I only knew Kay for several years, her profound teaching continues to reverberate in every aspect of my life. Her poignant address, "The Curiosity of Milton Erickson", at the First International Congress on Ericksonian Therapy in 1980, made a lasting impression on me. Years later, when I developed a pain condition related to a herniated cervical disc, I contacted her for help. Even though we hadn't met and it was during the Christmas holidays, she generously made time to see me.

At the end of our session, Kay gave me a tape of our work together with an unusual suggestion: "Don't listen more than once a day!" She also gave me her e-mail address and asked me to contact her. In several weeks, I was surprised and pleased to find an increasing sense of control over my pain, and at the same time a lessening interest in my pain and increasing interest in hypnosis. I carefully reviewed Kay's tape, transcribing every word and noting every suggestion I thought she was making. Through this process, I began to understand the profound depth and mastery of her interventions and became determined to learn everything I could from her. We began to correspond by e-mail and periodic telephone calls and I returned to the United States several times a year to meet with her.

The topics of our correspondence and discussions immediately expanded to cover my personal explorations with hypnosis as well as my clinical work with clients. During our discussions, she frequently interspersed metaphors or stories and she was clearly pleased when I told her that I found myself thinking about her stories more often than the questions I had formulated for our meetings.

However, I remained vigilantly attentive to the profound implications of her casual, indirect, and brief comments during all of our interactions. Subtle communications, both verbal and nonverbal were an integral part of the weave of Kay's everyday conversations.

In order to share some aspects of Kay's inimitable teaching presence which are not already represented in this section, I have chosen to reconstruct from my tapes and notes, what I remember of our discussion during one of these sessions. This particular vignette combines two very brief, yet related conversations during our meeting.

"You have challenged everything I have known, Kay," I declared with the deepest respect. After a pause, passed in reflection, Kay and I spoke simultaneously: "Everything I(You) *thought* I(You) knew!" We broke into laughter. I laughed at the surprise of our simultaneous response and the important understanding that it reflected. Talking with Kay was a wonderful mixture of pleasure, challenge and encouragement, and laughter was one of the important ingredients we shared often.

I added, "Everything I have believed has been turned upside down." I paused in thought, searching for any remaining beliefs. "There is one belief, just one that I still hold onto. I believe in coincidence; it is basic to my perception of reality." Kay didn't respond verbally and simply nodded her head, clearly in recognition of my comment, but not necessarily in agreement.

Later during our conversation, I shared a recent experience. "I was going through some very old papers in the attic and came across my notes from the First International Congress on Ericksonian Therapy, and I was surprised to find notes from a lecture by you." "Wow! That's neat," Kay exclaimed. Her tone and gaze were warm and engaging. We both paused in silence. "Pure coincidence!" she exclaimed, her tone decisive and authoritative, as was her changed posture.

Confused and almost disoriented by her challenge, I felt trapped in a powerful bind. The difficult moment expanded well beyond my comfort level. Kay spoke again, "As I get older," and she paused, "I'm beginning to think that there is no such thing as coincidence." Her tone and posture changed again. She was pensive and open and her tone was soft and understanding. I felt her joining, "as I get" and "I'm beginning" just as I was just beginning to understand something different about coincidence.

Curiosity about a recent experience had in fact been percolating in my consciousness and the association to coincidence brought my memory to the surface. "This makes me wonder. When I was visiting a relative recently, I woke up early and couldn't figure out how to use the shower. So I ended up taking a bath, something I hadn't done in years." We both laughed. "As I lay in the tub, I looked at my stretched out body and felt an intense appreciation of the wonder and beauty of the human body. At that moment, I realized that my relative, who was quite heavy did not have a positive feeling about her body and was not taking care of her body. During the remainder of my visit, I made several indirect comments about the miracle of the human body.

"I know that this might sound strange, but I have been wondering about my inability to use the shower that morning. I don't know if I have ever not eventually figured out how to use a shower!" We laughed again. "I'm wondering now about unconscious awareness and how much it affects one's perceptions and actions, perhaps even in a situation like this?"

Kay answered decisively: "Yes! I firmly believe that your unconscious may have wanted you to have that experience. And purposely kept you from figuring out how to use the shower." Even though I had asked the question, I was shocked. I often secretly hoped that Kay would contradict my hypotheses, not confirm them, and reinstate the reality I had thought I had known before meeting her. I was only wondering about a connection, but she had expanded my suggestion well beyond anything I had even considered.

"It's tuning in and interacting with the environment and affecting my actions and organizing my learning. That's amazing! My consciousness is also outside of my body?" I asked incredulously. "Yes!" she affirmed emphatically.

I remember entering a period of reflection, perhaps reorientation. During these moments Kay would often speak to me, confirming my learning, and sometimes sharing a similar experiential understanding.

Over the years I have pondered and reflected on our correspondence and discussions. Those sessions were profoundly meaningful in my life, and years later, I still feel that I have only begun to understand them. One word, thought, in the phrase, "I thought I knew," gave me a fundamentally new perspective in my understanding of the challenges Kay offered. Each and every word could be significant and have multiple implications. I continue to explore the space between what I think I know and what I can learn in any situation.

Kay was fierce and relentless, the ultimate teacher and therapist. Perhaps coincidence was an important belief to challenge, because of the importance of understanding unconscious awareness in my life and work. Or perhaps she understood that any belief or construct could restrict one's ability to remain open to experience. I realized that nothing would or could impede Kay's determination to teach me what she thought I needed to learn. When discussing my work, she often asked me if my response had been conscious or unconscious, and it was clear she trusted experiential learning and unconscious responses.

She was tuning in to me, evaluating what I could handle, challenging me and encouraging me; it almost felt as if I was "dough" in her hands and she was kneading me in the directions I needed to grow.

She was phenomenally patient and would wait until the perfect moment and then, *Pow!*, she would deliver her message. Her timing and understanding of my emotional state and thus receptivity was as important as any communication she was giving. Her awareness of the subtlety of my "personality energies", reflected by a delicate inflection, sigh, or slight movement was something she was attending to and using, with or without my conscious awareness. She was constantly working in a subtle field of awareness that I was just beginning to follow. And her subtle movements and responses were fundamental in my learning.

Her entire energy, attention, and capacities were directly and completely focused on awakening the client's potential. "I hold everything they can become, not just who they are now; otherwise how will they grow?" she told me. Her focused energy created an integrity of presence, including her intention, actions, body movements, language and all aspect of her communication, both verbal and nonverbal. In a sense, this integrity felt like a "field", which was following and leading, entraining and communicating on multiple levels of consciousness.

I also was amazed by the fluidity and expertise with which she was able to shift positions. She was loving and accepting and had a unique capacity to "hold" others with loving presence. And yet she could instantly become firm, fierce, and challenging, as with this bind. She was mischievous and playful as we engaged together and was deeply supporting and encouraging when appropriate. She could take all the positions, all of the archetypal positions, and within a very brief period of time.

And I haven't even mentioned the content of our interaction. Kay's teaching about the pliability of reality constructs continues to be fundamental in my learning. Utilizing and trusting unconscious awareness, and listening to and respecting its organizing activities, has become one of the most significant aspects of my hypnotic work and personal journey.

I feel in awe when I reflect on the complexity of Kay's therapeutic communications, and yet she used the simplest language to convey understandings, and was very open and willing to share her own vulnerabilities, when appropriate. "Your clients can identify with you when you share that you are also on this journey," she told me. I am certain that Kay would have wanted to extend her loving and generous wishes to all. Her last words to me were, "Have a good journey, take your time, and enjoy your journey."

The Power of Her Gifts

Dan Kohen

I am reminded of the power of Kay's gifts on a daily level as I join colleagues in meetings, participate in groups, teach and work with children, youth and their parents in clinical sessions. When people speak I listen to their words on multiple levels, and when I am most appropriately and effectively paying attention, I am able to understand and respond much more effectively and in a much more therapeutic manner to all of their communications.

This evening I was preparing my medical records notes of my encounters with patients earlier this afternoon. It occurred to me that this day, as on most of my days when I am teaching pediatric residents or seeing children and adolescents in our Behavioral Pediatrics Clinic, was replete with examples of how Kay's influence, tutelage and wisdom permeates my work at most if not all turns.

While meeting with first year pediatric residents about preparing clinical presentations, I find myself providing reframing comments, queries, challenges not so much to their discoveries or conclusions, but to the way in which they talk about what it is they have learned;

and how they propose they would *talk about stuff with their patients and their parents*. Actually, residents often say they would talk "to" their patients, and I regularly suggest it would be preferable to talk "with" them. I feel Kay smiling and imagine her saying "that's right …" perhaps the way Milton Erickson might have analogously modeled for her learning.

Today one of the residents said, "Well, in getting more of their history I'd want to know what they had *tried* so far to help the problem." When I then asked him what he meant, he said "Well, I'd want to know more of the history, like what they had *done* so far to help the problem." I asked the other resident if she had *heard* what her colleague had just said. She said she had but she had not. I asked if he had—he wasn't sure. I repeated what he'd said, and we had a discussion about the difference between "trying" and "doing". I explained that I tell patients, even the first day that I meet them, that when that word *try* is used, I call "time-out" and inform them that the word *try* is no longer allowed in my office. And, I suggest "Just do …" instead. I believe I was saying it before I relearned it, again, from a second-generation Kay Thompson disciple, Yoda, the Jedi-Master of *Star Wars* fame. In *The Empire Strikes Back*, he said, "Luke, there is no try, just do …"

Later this afternoon, a young man with *previously* "intractable" migraine, came in for a follow-up visit. Since his second hypnosis session, he had been almost pain free for over a month. But, with the anticipation of school restarting, he had not been doing as well. When asked what works best in helping him, he was very clear in saying that, "Self-hypnosis is better than Lorazepam."

I noted myself asking him, "Did you ever wonder if you are doing self-hypnosis even when you're not doing self-hypnosis. You know, that other kind of doing?" And he smiled. (And I felt Kay smiling again.) He was eager to practice self-hypnosis and went into trance quickly with the very formal induction technique frequently used for young people (i.e. something on the order of "go ahead and begin"[23]). I heard Kay in my mind again as I said, "That's right, you

---

[23] Of course, this is said with tongue firmly planted in cheek; that is, children rarely require any formal hypnotic induction "ceremony", and commonly a simple invitation to begin or to imagine/daydream about a favorite activity is all that is needed to "officially" initiate a more focused hypnotic state.

can follow your breath, and just pay attention to it as you breathe in comfort and as you breathe out tension. Just pay attention to the way that tension goes away and to the way you do that. That's right." (And there was a sense of Kay's presence.)

And a few moments later:

"It's nice to know that you can remember to forget what wasn't important to remember any way, the way you know how to do that, either by forgetting to remember it, or instead by remembering to forget it, or alternatively, perhaps you'll decide somewhere inside to remember to forget to remember or to forget to remember to forget. Either way is fine, just let your mind do the work. I know you won't mind letting your mind do that. The mind knows by itself how to mind, that's right."

After this brief practice, he alerted, smiled broadly, reported that the headache he had come in with was now down to a one. I congratulated him on having done so. I'm proud of him.

Kay was the guest faculty teacher on several occasions for our annual workshops of the Minnesota Society of Clinical Hypnosis. During one of these workshops, after running around attending to administrative matters, I thought I'd treat myself to at least half of Kay's afternoon workshop with the advanced group.

As she was putting on her microphone I asked her what she was going to be teaching this afternoon. "Oh, you'll see. You'll like it. You'll be surprised." I was. She began by observing aloud that there were three vacant chairs and that the middle chair was waiting for someone (from the advanced group) who would learn the most. Moments later a medical resident in family practice took the chair.

Directing her remarks to the group, she then announced, "Dr. Kohen and I will shortly be demonstrating the phenomena of dual induction." I was indeed surprised. I had never done this before. She had not asked me. Later she told me she thought that asking me in advance would have perhaps evoked more anxiety than was necessary so she just purposely skipped that step! However, she knew, of course, that I would do it. She smiled. She whispered something on the order of, "Just start wherever you want and I'll follow and catch up." I sat down on one side of the volunteer and she sat down on the other.

I began talking with something on the order of, "Just go ahead and close your eyes and take your mind back. That's good." I have little recollection of what precisely followed except that I remember talking a lot about ego-strengthening kinds of things such as "being surprised how much you learned as a child", and then interspersing other metaphorical suggestions for regression, like: "A and how much you retained. B and how curious it is. C how effortless. D than can be. C D, so you see, D." Sometime—who knows how long—perhaps 15 to 20 minutes later, we finished and I was (and still am!) quite astonished that the last 8 or 10 words out of my mouth were identical to and simultaneous with the last 8 or10 words that Kay spoke into the volunteer's other ear. He was the only one more astonished than I was. And Kay just smiled. I feel her smile now.

And she is the clear inspiration (for all of its multiple levels of meaning, clearly) that in every hypnosis teaching I do, I give some version or another of a presentation called "How We Talk is How We Think, What We Believe, What We Come to Expect and What We Teach."

The Importance of Rapport

Marion P. Kostka and Penny Kostka

It is often asked, "Where does one begin?" And frequently the most common answer is, "At the beginning." When and how does one begin the hypnotherapeutic process? As with any therapeutic relationship, it begins with building rapport. Dr. Kay Thompson was a master of this essential skill. She used verbal and nonverbal approaches to connect with her subjects and to put them at ease. Building rapport was not only the beginning of the relationship but, in effect, was the beginning of the hypnotic intervention.

For more than 20 years, Kay was a mentor for members of the West Virginia University Hypnosis Study Group. During that time, one of our most powerful learning experiences was to observe her demonstrate hypnotic approaches with volunteer subjects, all of whom had identifiable concerns. More often than not, she had little or no background information about the individual before this initial meeting. As with many initial meetings, "small talk" might most aptly describe these initial interactions. But small talk is not necessarily nonimportant talk.

Kay was very adept in using this opportunity to "connect" with the client. When we analyze Kay's work, it is evident that the rapport she established was a critical element in her success with patients. She was able to communicate a genuine interest in her patients and their condition and this strengthened the therapeutic alliance. Trance is intensely focused attention and no doubt Kay was as intensely focused on her subject as they were on her. This frequently resulted in a spontaneous trance experience in both and further established that she was "with them". She acknowledged that this allowed her to dissociate from the audience and to use her unconscious. She felt that she did her best work when trusting in her unconscious abilities.

On one occasion, while working with a woman with a seven-year history of TMJ pain, she was discussing the role of stress in her condition. She said, "I really wouldn't care how you dealt with stress except for the fact that it's hurting your mouth and that's what gets *me* upset." This response appeared to solidify the relationship, as she became an ally in this woman's quest for pain relief.

While this initial "small talk" appears to be casual, it is very purposeful. Kay intended to put the subject at ease and acknowledged that it had the same effect on her. In addition to this calming effect, she was gathering essential information that she would later utilize in her hypnotic work. A classic example of this was a demonstration with a woman who had suffered for 21 years from chronic disabling headaches. She had consulted numerous physicians and therapists, and she had been medicated by some and trained in biofeedback by others, but with little success. Kay remarked that she had been subjected to E-T-K-T-M (Every Test Known to Man). The client agreed and stated that there was rarely a day that she did not experience some type of headache.

During their "small talk," Kay commented on a butterfly broach that the woman was wearing and how that kind of jewelry was

made. The discussion included the beauty of the pin and the butterfly itself. Later in the 90-minute session that followed, Kay utilized
the butterfly in a metaphor to communicate a number of concepts.
She described how the butterfly's cocoon held it prisoner with its
beautiful silk threads and, when it finally broke free, it developed
into the beautiful butterfly we all know. This metaphor was woven
into others related to issues of control.

At a six-month follow-up, the client was symptom free. When the
client was asked what contributed to the rapport she apparently felt
with Kay, after some thought, she acknowledged that she perceived
Kay as being totally focused on her as if no one else was in the
room. She "knew" that Kay understood her and was determined to
help in any way she could.

Kay drew upon a wide range of life experiences—from spelunking
and mountain climbing to the trimming of pine trees—all activities
that she shared with her husband Ralph. These experiences were
often the basis of the many therapeutic metaphors that she used
with patients. Kay cautioned us to be careful and respectful when
working with a client who is more knowledgeable in a subject than
the therapist. Since trust is such an essential ingredient in building
rapport, inaccuracies could actually inhibit the establishment of
rapport.

Kay emphasized this point during a demonstration of pain management with a paralyzed racecar driver. She admitted knowing little about NASCAR and used her ignorance about his profession as
a way of establishing rapport by acknowledging his expertise.
Asking for information and learning from the subject is another
way to strengthen the bond between therapist and client. She
demonstrated her interest in his work and as the session progressed, verbally expressed her concern for his current situation
and how she might be of assistance to him. Her eye contact, her verbal intonation, as well as her reassuring touch of his hand, reflected
this genuine concern for his condition with no hint of pity. She was
willing to share her expertise as part of "his team" in dealing with
the pain.

Kay's subjects frequently experienced spontaneous trances early
in their interactions with her. While this demonstrated her skill in

conversational trance induction, she valued formal induction techniques and utilized them in her work with patients. She demanded that her students use and understand the value of formal inductions.

Kay continually emphasized that hypnosis, whether verbal or non-verbal, is a form of communication. She loved to play with the sounds of language and frequently used homonyms in her conversational trance inductions. She would mix the sounds and meanings of words in building indirect suggestions for her clients. When working on a weight control issue, she would imbed a message with homonyms, suggesting that the client "wait for the right time to weigh the reasons to begin to lose weight along the way". She might continue with similar sounds (i.e. sway, hey, hay, say, may) as she moved to other parts of the message. She loved oxymorons, and when appropriate, double entendre.

As with so many aspects of Kay's work, underlying this "fun" had a serious purpose: to connect with her clients on a number of levels of consciousness. She emphasized the intentional use of language due to the many meanings implicit in a word and the various levels of consciousness at which it will be perceived. "Every word can and will mean everything." Nowhere is this more important than in these beginning stages of the relationship. She taught that when rapport is successfully established, reaching the other levels of consciousness through trance is a relatively easy process.

Kay loved working with children. Children squirm and wiggle and frequently do not even keep eye contact with the facilitator and thus do not exhibit the features that we expect as part of the hypnotic experience. She knew this and most importantly accepted this behavior. This acceptance was crucial to developing the rapport necessary for the work that followed. For some children, this acceptance was a unique experience and as they sensed that her interest in them was genuine, the most interesting information would frequently be divulged—information that she would weave into their work together.

As she did with adults, Kay utilized whatever they gave her. Kay emphasized that children were especially sensitive to the issue of acceptance. In demonstrations with children, Kay always seemed to have a supply of silver dollars. She would sometimes use them as a focus of attention and frequently would allow them to keep one as a "thank you" for their help. I don't know how many children every actually spent their dollar, but I suspect that most kept it as a remembrance of a unique experience with a woman who talked with them and genuinely listened to what they said. No matter what the age, building rapport is the key that opens the door to everything therapeutic.

Kay established herself as an ally with her subjects by helping them discover what they were capable of achieving. She never promised what she couldn't deliver. Many years ago she made us a promise that as we learned more about hypnosis, it would affect our every therapeutic interaction. She suggested that we would never speak or listen in quite the same way. She was right! While an outside observer might identify a small portion of our clinical work as being hypnotic in nature, it actually permeates everything we do. It extends far beyond the early but critical stages of building rapport. We're acutely aware of all the levels of communication that occur in therapy. We are consciously aware of the words we choose and all their meanings. We listen and thus hear on all levels and we utilize not only what our clients bring to us but also how it's delivered. It's all about communicating.

Loving Presence

Peter Letarte

I'm lucky enough to be married to Kay's niece, Kate. I work in academic medicine and it always seemed to me that Kay's family never really got how important she was professionally. I thought they just didn't get it: a woman of that intelligence, drive, and accomplishment. But the fact is they got it better than I did. They never defined Kay in those terms. The reason was that she never defined herself that way.

I hadn't been dating Kate very long before I heard about this marvelous woman and I heard about those things that are so easy to be seduced by, her academic achievements, her accomplishments, the power of her life.

I heard about a woman who had been a mentor to her nieces and nephew, not just by example, but actively teaching them to aspire to what they could be, to get in touch with their motivation. The children would go to Pittsburgh to get dental work done by her. She used her craft as her bridge to be connected with her family. I thought this was impressive. I thought I understood.

When I met her, Kate told me that her aunt was coming to Chicago. We hadn't been dating very long. As I was walking into Kate's apartment and Kay was sitting on her couch, she turned and looked at me with that deep penetrating gaze that I was later to learn was a very kind gaze. There was a presence in the room, a palpable intelligence.

There was something more there. There was a feeling that you were at once instantly understood. When meeting your girl friend's relatives, this isn't necessarily a good thing! But that presence was to be with me through the remainder of my relationship with Kay.

On Thanksgiving, when there were point papers to be reviewed, talks to be given, courses to be put together, she came to Cambridge to be with her family. It wasn't hard to figure out her priorities. While she was there, she would talk to us. You could talk to her. Yes, she appeared stern and there was this piercing gaze. But if you talked to her, she understood, not only because of her intelligence but also because she was listening with her heart. You felt understood.

When it was time to be married, my family, which was not an easy family, and which to intellectuals and the more proper people of the world was a troublesome family, had to meet and get together with Kate's family. As we walked into the house, Kay and I talked. It was clear that she viewed my family from a very different point of view, with empathy and with an understanding I have never seen in anyone else.

When it came time for children, well, children are irritating, especially to people who are as busy and involved as Kay was. But Kate and I were not reprimanded for our children being annoying. We were reprimanded for not understanding them, for not understanding the child in them, and for not embracing that child.

There was a presence there. You see, I guess I expected her to respond as the academic, the accomplished woman. And to do that is to get her all wrong. It's to come at her backwards. She did not define herself that way. She was not centered in that.

Kay was centered in love, a strong colorful love that gave her a driving passion for life, and her accomplishments were the fruit of that love. It gave her the passion that led her to climb mountains, to go hiking, to go camping with Tom and Julia, our children. It was the passion that yielded all these other accomplishments. To understand Kay you have to realize that that is what was at her foundation. That foundation gave her a heart that allowed her to see into the hearts of other people. It allowed her to understand things, not for their superficiality but for their foundation. The Apostle Paul warned us that to speak with the tongues of men and angels and to have not love is to be merely a sounding gong. That was not a problem for Kay. And one other thing. People who are founded in love tend to have a presence. They tend to be palpable when you walk in the room. It wasn't until years later that I understood that was what I felt that time when I first met Kay. That presence is gone from us now and we will all miss it very, very much.

Helping People Achieve Unusual Events

Stacie Murrer

Dr. Kay F. Thompson was my mentor for over 18 years. I was one of her many "students" whom she coached. She guided each one of us down our own path and made us feel very special.

Kay delighted in teaching, whether it was hypnosis, dentistry, cooking, or life. It didn't matter what it was we needed, she was always showing the way. I remember time after time she would say, "Here is your one," with that twinkle in her eyes. That "one" would be something that I didn't know.

Kay taught me that "pain is a warning signal and once everything that could be done and should be done, has been done, then there is no reason to have anymore pain". She also taught me hypnosis. She allowed me to show up at advanced hypnosis training, and then never cashed my checks. Kay knew. It seemed she always had an answer that fit and that is why we kept asking.

A patient of mine was diagnosed with probable Stargardt disease, which is an autosomal recessive retinal disorder. Vision acuity is often reduced to 20/200. When her mom called me saying that she was going blind, I knew that Kay would and could help.

Kay met with her two times to make hypnosis tapes. Every night her mom would play the tapes while she was sleeping. When her doctor, a pediatric ophthalmologist, reexamined her eyes, he found that her corrected visual acuity was now 20/20. This ophthalmologist described her situation as "truly an unusual course of events". Kay was involved daily in helping people achieve unusual events.

The first time I was pregnant, I was very nauseous and sick and this was a serious problem for my dental practice. One evening as I was finishing work, Kay and her close friend and colleague, Russell Scott, stopped by. They sat me down and did a dual induction. I never got sick again then or during my other three pregnancies.

In Kay's obituary there was a story about an 8-year-old who was afraid of dentists. This little girl sat in Kay's dental chair and her body was very tight and tense. Kay looked at her and said, "You're sitting like a tin soldier. Why don't you pretend you're Raggedy Ann?" Kay repeatedly taught us to pay attention to our patients' psychological states and this is one of the fundamental things I have utilized in my work.

Kay believed in hypnosis and saw it work in her life and in others' lives, and she worked hard to make it work, continually practicing her skills. She taught and lectured internationally, coached and mentored her students and colleagues, and was extraordinarily generous.

Kay cared about people of all sizes and shapes; she made no distinctions when people were in need. She believed that hypnosis helps give people "quality to the end" and felt it was her responsibility to share what she knew could help others. She taught and gave from her heart. Her kind words and encouragement made a significant difference in my life.

Kay Thompson, DDS, Genius of the Heart

Jane A. Parsons-Fein

Before I met Kay I was told that she was a fierce and frightening woman who didn't particularly like social workers. Later I heard that she had been in an automobile accident and was confined to a wheelchair. While visiting my family in Pittsburgh, I telephoned her. I was a social worker; she was warm and engaging. So much for hearsay. That was the beginning of our long and close friendship.

Several years later, I was told by a fancy Fifth Avenue dentist that I needed a year's work of periodontal scraping. I called Kay. She said, "Come to Pittsburgh." I was scared, but I had seen a film of her own rhinoplasty-dermabrasion surgery in which she had used self-hypnosis and I trusted her. You could not *not* trust Kay Thompson. I knew how completely she trusted herself when she told me the following story about her own surgery.

When she decided to use self-hypnosis without anesthesia for these two complicated medical procedures, she lay on the gurney in the hall for a long time because the surgeon was late. She became anxious and wanted to leave. She said to herself in trance, "Legs, if this is a mistake, get off the gurney and let's leave." She waited. Her legs didn't move. She trusted them.

I learned a lot about myself from Kay during my procedure; it took four hours to complete, not the New York dentist's suggested 12 months. A Pittsburgh periodontist, who was a hypnosis student of Kay's, did the root scraping, Kay did the hypnosis. I had no anesthesia, felt no pain, there was no swelling, and I healed in half the time. I had my personal lesson in pain control and I learned how important it was to trust my own unconscious (with a little help from my friend).

Kay became my trusted mentor. She pushed me to be politically active in hypnotherapy organizations and was very supportive during my husband's long illness.

Kay said: "The dreamer is the true realist," speaking to our conscious sense of reality and at the same time to our unconscious, where our dreams come from and where we have a different experience of what we know. She used words to unlock the doors of these vast creative areas in people's minds which they can tap into, but which they rarely define consciously. It is a special kind of knowing which Kay taught me how to trust. She used her understanding of this kind of knowing, this dream world of the unconscious to motivate people and to help them cope successfully with their reality. In those awful days after my husband's death, Kay anchored me to the resources of my unconscious dream world which helped me deal with the reality of my loss.

Kay was a staunch and challenging friend. Working with her was always an adventure, a trip into one's own mysterious self. You could discover playfulness again and you could find yourself catapulting into an internal space that went beyond thrilling. It was the wonder world of the child. It was easy to trust yourself around her.

Kay was as authentic in her work as she was in her relationships. She skillfully set up the flow of communication between her own unconscious and the unconscious of her clients. The integrity of her trust in her own unconscious, her trust in herself, and in her trust in the abilities of others, could bring their dreams into their reality.

Kay blended conscious and unconscious so elegantly that people around her could discover ranges of thought and feeling they didn't know they had. She was always with you on your journey into yourself because she was also in her therapeutic trance. My first experience of her doing a group induction was when she said, "I couldn't stand up in front of all of you and do this if I weren't in trance myself."

She could artfully join her subject's metaphor on many levels: pacing language, body shifting, voice tone and rhythms, shifting to challenging questions such as, "Do you *really* think that is what you think?" She had a quick wit and was a master of pattern interruption, distraction, and playful banter. When a demonstration subject spoke of flying, she asked, "People talk about autopilot. Is that what you are doing in your unconscious?"

At the onset of trance she established the pattern of expecting the subject to listen on at least two levels simultaneously. Her sentence structure, changes of tense, use of double negatives and meaningful delivery of phrases were designed to confuse the conscious mind, while on an unconscious level the meaning was very clear. Erickson said that the mind abhors a vacuum and when it is confused, it will immediately latch onto a clear statement. In the midst of the following confusing sequencing, the unconscious can hear "entranced", "really knowing", "make the meaning", "listening learning" and "change":

"And you can become so entranced with really knowing all there is you need to know about how to make the meaning of this listening learning change into something that it wasn't when it began, only because you had not thought about it as being what you didn't think it was."

She amplified the confusion of the meaning of the words, emphasizing superficial coherence while conveying a clear meaning that the unconscious can hear, that you *can* know what you don't know that you know. Kay stressed that this message to the unconscious be emotionally recognizable; confusion for the sake of confusion is not the point. Confusion is used to distract the conscious mind so that the unconscious can be free to hear the message.

The last time I saw Kay was at the ASCH meeting in April 1998. I think I knew on some level how ill she was, but didn't let myself know clearly. We were all dancing. Then I looked over to where she had been sitting and she was gone. She died May 26, 1998. We dedicated a blue spruce evergreen to Kay in Central Park, near where she had stood 15 years before, dedicating 15 smoke bushes to Dr. Erickson. There had been tornado warnings that evening and the wind blew hard through the trees as we walked back to where we celebrated her life with music, singing, food and wine.

Kay was tough minded, uncompromising and honest, but what really guided her was her humanity and her connection to her own heart. Anyone who worked with her would be touched by the lines of poetry that she brought into her inductions, often at surprising times, almost like a pattern interruption to bring you deeper into yourself. But it shouldn't be surprising; Kay herself was a pattern interruption which always left you more of who you were, than who you were when she found you. "The Rose" was one of her favorite songs. She thought every line of it was a beautiful meta-phor for the dream and the reality of life, as in the second stanza:

It's the heart afraid of breaking that never learns to dance

It's the dream afraid of waking that never takes the chance

It's the one who won't be taken who cannot seem to give

And the soul afraid of dying that never learns to live.

Kay dreamed her life awake with exquisite elegance. Her humanity, humor and depth of trust in herself are always with me. I learned to trust myself (not easy for any of us) because of her. I think what I miss the most is the light and the intelligence that flickered in her eyes from one moment to the next. There will never be another Kay Thompson and aren't we grateful that we knew her.

Doing the Right Thing

S. Timothy Rose

Kay Thompson was a friend of mine. I first met her in 1984 on the floor of the House of Delegates of the American Dental Association. We were on the same side of an issue, to formalize a continuing education process for the dental profession. Although we did not prevail then, the process ultimately became ADA policy, largely due to Kay Thompson's belief that it was "the right thing to do". She had a strong belief in doing the "Right Thing".

We became better friends several years later when we were elected to the Board of Trustees for the American Dental Association. Along with Drs. Bill Finigan and Ray Kline, we spent significant amounts of time together during the next four years. Kay was "one of the boys". She contributed to the process and added an insight on issues that was unique and broadened our collective perspective on those issues. She possessed the human touch, which had clearly been developed during her years of private dental practice. While we did not talk a great deal about our clinical practices, it was evident that she had some unique experiences and possessed insights and gifts when it came to treating the unique patient population that was her practice.

Her interest in hypnosis always fascinated me. We talked about it on several occasions, and she agreed to "educate me" after we had completed our term on the Board of Trustees. Circumstances change, and this of course never happened, which I still regret.

Kay was an individual; highly intelligent, unconventional, insightful, informed, opinionated, compassionate and a tenacious person who, though usually lively, was basically shy. She was a good listener and an excellent conversationalist, often witty and always interested. She was generous with both her time and her talents helping and encouraging many people to pursue their dreams. Toward the end of her professional career, she was particularly concerned that other women become involved in the politics of dentistry. She spent a considerable period of time encouraging and pushing women into leadership roles in the dental profession. She was one of the early women leaders of our profession.

Kay had the ability to cut right through a conversation to the important issues. On the day that I became president-elect of the American Dental Association, she was one of the first people to congratulate me. While she gave me a big hug, she whispered in my ear that it was my job and she expected me to give it my best effort. She did not condone anything but the best effort in anything she did in her life. She is missed and her contributions to our profession will be remembered.

Appendix II
Accompanying CD

Kay Thompson utilized every part of her self in her work, using her voice to embody her messages by means of changes of tone, inflection, emphasis, phrasing and rhythm, engaging audiences worldwide. Hypnosis is an oral art and Thompson's performances were among the most sophisticated in the field.

Her "live" presentation was such an important part of her teaching, that we have created a CD as an accompaniment to this volume. It would be impossible to claim that this was a collected works without having also collected her spoken voice. Some of her most memorable "performances" have been included for the readers' learning and enjoyment.

List of Tracks

1. Highly personal interrelationship   03:41

In this selection, Kay Thompson shares a fascinating clinical vignette about teaching anesthesia and emphasizes the importance of the interpersonal relationship for achieving trance.

2. Motivating the Anxious Patient   02:20

Thompson demonstrates how she motivates the patient who is anxious and uptight to learn hypnosis.

3. Doing the Unexpected   07:00

In this intriguing clinical vignette with a midbrain stroke patient, Thompson demonstrates eliciting anger to generate the energy for change.

4. Dealing with Acute Pain   09:11

Kay Thompson demonstrates her clinical approach with clients in acute pain, including differentiation, making the pain worse, using a hypnotic induction and intervening, as appropriate. This is a wonderful example of Thompson's unique use of inflections, changes in tone and rhythm.

5. Acknowledging and Supporting Patient's Hard Work   04:22

In this selection, Kay Thompson discusses how easy it is for families or support systems to take for granted the enormous effort involved in change, and illustrates the importance of the therapist's continuing support for the patient's hard work.

6. Abreaction and Control of Trance   03:20

In this important vignette, Thompson discusses how she works with clients who abreact and how she challenges clients to accept the control they have in trance.

7. Hypnoanesthesia during Surgery   05:56

Kay Thompson discusses an extraordinary surgical film of a patient having both rhinoplasty (breaking nose bones and reconstructing nose structure) and dermabrasion (facial skin removed) while using hypnosis as the only anesthesia.

8. Tantrum   03:07

In this amusing example, Thompson illustrates how to work with children in a panic or tantrum.

9. Dealing with Pain 10.37

In this poignant vignette, Thompson demonstrates the importance of helping patients believe that their lives have been worthwhile and discusses the amazing control people can have over letting go.

10. Hiking 12:11

A wonderful collection of some of Kay's metaphors—using a hiking story, she discusses mountain climbing, reducing tension through visualizing releasing lactic acid, relaxing like a marshmallow and putting down unnecessary burdens.

Source Notes

We list below the sources for each chapter included in this book. Special thanks are due to the copyright holders for permission to reproduce previously published material:

Chapter One. "An Introduction to Hypnosis" is from the following workshop of that same title, with additions from the article, "Hypnosis in Dentistry". The workshop, "Introduction to Hypnosis", was first presented during the 24th Annual Advanced Workshops in Clinical Hypnosis, cosponsored by the Minnesota Society of Clinical Hypnosis, the Behavioral Pediatrics Program, Department of Pediatrics, Medical School, and Department of Continuing Medical Education, University of Minnesota, St. Paul, Minnesota, June 1995. "Hypnosis in Dentistry" was first published in Clinical Dentistry, 1982, Vol. 1, pp. 1–10.

Chapter Two. "The Curiosity of Milton H. Erickson, MD" was first published in *Ericksonian Approaches to Hypnosis and Psychotherapy*, edited by Jeffrey K. Zeig. Brunner/Mazel, New York, 1982, pp. 413–21.

Chapter Three. "Almost 1984" was first published in *Ericksonian Psychotherapy: Vol. 1, Structures*, edited by Jeffrey K. Zeig. Brunner/Mazel, New York, 1985, pp. 89–99. Question–answer segment at the end of the article is from the original lecture, "Almost 1984", which was first presented during the Second Erickson Congress, Phoenix, AZ, December 1983. (Tapes No. P320-42A&B.)

Chapter Four. "Metaphor: A Myth with a Method" is from the article by that name with additions from the original lecture of the same title. The article was first published in *Brief Therapy, Myths, Methods, and Metaphors*, edited by Jeffrey K. Zeig and Stephen G. Gilligan. Brunner/Mazel, Inc., New York, 1990, pp. 247–57. The original lecture was presented at the Brief Therapy Conference, sponsored by the Milton Erickson Foundation, San Francisco, December, 1988.

Chapter Five. "Motivation and the Multiple Levels of Trance" was first published in *Developing Ericksonian Therapy: State of the Art*, edited by Jeffrey K. Zeig and S. Lankton. Brunner/Mazel, Inc., New York, 1988, pp. 150–63.

Chapter Six. "Language to Effect Change" was presented at an advanced workshop at the Seminar on Ericksonian Approaches to Hypnosis and Psychotherapy, Phoenix, AZ, December 1997.

Chapter Seven. "Metaphor, Analogy, and Word Play Development" was presented at the 24th Annual Advanced Workshops in Clinical Hypnosis, cosponsored by the Minnesota Society of Clinical Hypnosis, the Behavioral Pediatrics Program, Department of Pediatrics, Medical School, and Department of Continuing Medical Education, University of Minnesota, St. Paul, Minnesota, June 1995.

Part III Commentary. "And Her Words Will Go On" contains lyrics from "The Rose" by Amanda McBroom. Copyright Warner-Tamerlane Publishing Corp. and Third Story Music Inc. All Rights Reserved. Used by Permission of Warner Brothers Publications U.S. Inc., Miami, Florida.

Chapter Eight. "The Case Against Relaxation" was first published in *Hypnosis*, edited by Graham Burrows, D. R. Collison and L. Dennerstein, Elsevier/North Holland Biomedical Press, Amsterdam, 1979, pp. 41–5.

Chapter Nine. "Whose Story is This, Anyway? A History of His-Story" was first published in *Ericksonian Methods, The Essence of the Story*, edited by Jeffrey K. Zeig, Brunner/Mazel, Inc., New York, 1994, pp. 136–46.

Chapter Ten. "Autohypnosis" was first presented at a workshop, "Clinical Hypnosis: Strategies in (Hypnotic) Communication", sponsored by the Ontario Society of Clinical Hypnosis, Toronto, Canada, May 1983, and recorded by the Content Management Corporation (formerly Audio Archives of Canada).

Chapter Eleven. "The Mythical Trance: The First Conversational Induction" was first published in *Theoretical and Clinical Aspects of Hypnosis*, edited by Harold Wain, PhD, Miami: Symposia Specialists, 1981.

Chapter Twelve. "Dual Induction" was presented at a workshop, entitled "Group Induction", during the Fifth Erickson Congress, December 1992, by Kay Thompson and James Auld. (Tape No. E297-98.) Special thanks are due to James Auld for his introduction and for transcribing the simultaneous part of the dual induction.

Chapter Thirteen. "Posthypnotic Suggestion" was presented at a workshop during the Second Erickson Congress, Phoenix, AZ, December 1983. (Tapes No.P320-32A&B.)

Chapter Fourteen. "Utilization" contains three selections of excerpts from workshops. The first workshop, "Utilization Techniques", was presented during the 24th Annual Advanced Workshops in Clinical Hypnosis, cosponsored by the Minnesota Society of Clinical Hypnosis, the Behavioral Pediatrics Program, Department of Pediatrics, Medical School, and Department of Continuing Medical Education, University of Minnesota, St. Paul, Minnesota, June 1995. The second selection, *"Clinical Utilization"*, was first presented during the workshop, "Therapeutic Uses of Language", sponsored by the New York Society for Ericksonian Psychotherapy and Hypnosis (NYSEPH), 1987. (Set of 8 tapes: Excerpts from Tape Nos. 1, 4 and 7.) The third selection, "Balance and Control", was presented during the workshop, "Pain Control in Traumatic Situations", during the Second Erickson Congress, Phoenix, AZ, December, 1983. (Tape No. P320-24B.)

Chapter Fifteen. "Patient Management and Pain Control" was presented at a workshop during the 24th Annual Advanced Workshops in Clinical Hypnosis, cosponsored by the Minnesota Society of Clinical Hypnosis, the Behavioral Pediatrics Program, Department of Pediatrics, Medical School, and Department of Continuing Medical Education, University of Minnesota, St. Paul, Minnesota, June 1995.

Chapter Sixteen. "Pain Control in Traumatic Situations" was presented at a workshop during the Second Erickson Congress, Phoenix, AZ, December 1983. (Tape No. P320-24A.)

Chapter Seventeen. "Pain Control: Selections from Panel Discussions". The first selection is from discussions during a meeting of the Society for Clinical and Experimental Hypnosis, 1972. Following are excerpts from a series of panel discussions and workshops: (1) "Panel Discussion on Pain Control", Sixth Erickson Congress, Tracking Ericksonian Methods, 1994. (G 264-131. #TP-4.) (Other participants were: David Cheek, MD, Ronald Havens, PhD, Philip Baretta, MA.); (2) "Panel on Pain Control", Fourth Erickson Congress, Brief Therapy, 1988. (Other panel members were: Jeff Feldman, PhD, Les Kadis, MD, and Sandra Sylvester, PhD.) (W332-89.); (3) "Intermediate Language Workshop" at the Seminar on Erickson Methods, December 1997.

Chapter Eighteen. "Creative Problem Solving" contains excerpts which were selected from the following workshops: (1) Workshop on "Therapeutic Uses of Language", sponsored by the New York Society for Ericksonian Psychotherapy and Hypnosis (NYSEPH), 1987. (Set of 8 tapes. Tape Nos. 4, 5 and 6); and (2) "Creative Problem Solving", which was presented at a workshop during the 24th Annual Advanced Workshops in Clinical Hypnosis, cosponsored by the Minnesota Society of Clinical Hypnosis, the Behavioral Pediatrics Program, Department of Pediatrics, Medical School, and Department of Continuing Medical Education, University of Minnesota, St. Paul, Minnesota, June 1995.

Chapter Nineteen. "The Oral Cavity: The Emotional Learning Center of the Body—The Dentist is a Therapist Too!" is from Dr. Thompson's private papers with additions from her plenary address (of the same title) at the seminar on Ericksonian Approaches to Hypnosis and Psychotherapy, Phoeniz, AZ, December 1997.

Chapter Twenty. "Hypnosis in Dentistry" was first published in *Clinical Dentistry*, edited by James W. Clark, DDS, J. B. Lippincott, New York, 1982, Vol. 1, pp. 1–10. (Portions of this article, from the section about the history of hypnosis, have been deleted and integrated into the first chapter, "Introduction to Hypnosis".)

Chapter Twenty-one. "Conversational Induction with Utilization of Spontaneous Trance" was presented at the Second Erickson Congress, Phoenix, AZ, December 1983. (Tape P 320–87.)

Chapter Twenty-two. "Strategies of Hypnotic Utilization" contains selections from the Southern California Society for Ericksonian Psychotherapy and Hypnosis Classics Series: *The Hypnotic Language and Metaphors of Kay Thompson*, 1994. (Set of 8 Tapes. Selections from Tape Nos. 2, 3, and 6.)

Chapter Twenty-three. "Pain Control and Healing Enhancement" was Clinical Presentation No. 3 at the Seminar on Ericksonian Approches to Hypnosis and Psychotherapy, Phoenix, AZ, December 1997. (Tape No. AS97-CP No. 3.)

Chapter Twenty-four. "Clinical Posthypnotic Suggestion" contains demonstrations from a workshop, "Post-Hypnotic Suggestion" during the Second Erickson Congress, Phoenix, AZ, December 1983. (Tape No.P320-32 A&B.)

Chapter Twenty-five. "Ethics in Caring" contains excerpts that were selected from the following workshops: (1) "Case Presentations/ Discussion/Ethics Supervision Panel", Sixth Erickson Congress, Tracking Ericksonian Methods, 1994a. (Other panel member was Betty Alice Erickson, MS.); (2) "Ethical Issues in Ericksonian Therapy", Sixth Erickson Congress, Tracking Ericksonian Method, 1994b. (Other panel member was James Keim, MSW.); (3) "Pain Control in Traumatic Situations", Second Erickson Congress, 1983; (4) "Patient Management and Pain Control" was presented during the 24th Annual Advanced Workshops in Clinical Hypnosis, cosponsored by the Minnesota Society of Clinical Hypnosis, the Behavioral Pediatrics Program, Department of Pediatrics, Medical School, and Department of Continuing Medical Education, University of Minnesota, St. Paul, Minnesota, June 1995b; (5) "Introduction to Hyponosis" was presented during the 24th Annual Advanced Workshops in Clinical Hypnosis, cosponsored by the Minnesota Society of Clinical Hypnosis, the Behavioral Pediatrics Program, Department of Pediatrics, Medical School, and Department of Continuing Medical Education, University of Minnesota, St. Paul, Minnesota, June 1995a; (6) Additional remarks are from Dr. Thompson's private papers for an address which she gave to the Pennsylvania Dental Association 130th Annual Session, May 1998.

Chapter Twenty-six. "How I Got to Be What I Am Becoming" is from Dr Thompson's private papers, for an address she gave to the American Society for Clinical Hypnosis in March 1998.

Chapter Twenty-seven. "Why Do We Learn Hypnosis?" is a selection of excerpts from "Creative Problem Solving", presented at a workshop during the 24th Annual Advanced Workshops in Clinical Hypnosis, cosponsored by the Minnesota Society of Clinical Hypnosis, the Behavioral Pediatrics Program, Department of Pediatrics, Medical School, and Department of Continuing Medical Education, University of Minnesota, St. Paul, Minnesota, June 1995. Comment-and-answer passage is from "Conversational Induction with Utilization of Spontaneous Trance", which was presented at the Second Erickson Congress, Phoenix, AZ, December 1983. (Tape P 320–87.)

Vignette entitled "Kay Thompson: Genius of the Heart" contains lyrics from "The Rose" by Amanda McBroom. Copyright Warner-Tamerlane Publishing Corp. and Third Story Music Inc. All Rights Reserved. Used by Permission of Warner Brothers Publications. U.S. Inc., Miami, Florida.

Sources for accompanying CD

We list below the sources for each audio selection included on the accompanying CD. Special thanks are due to the copyright holders for permission to reproduce previously recorded material:

1. "Highly Personal Interrelationship" is from the Workshop on Therapeutic Uses of Language, sponsored by the New York Society for Ericksonian Psychotherapy and Hypnosis (NYSEPH), 1987 (Tape #1).

2. "Motivating the Anxious Patient" is from Clinical Hypnosis: Strategies in Hypnotic Communication, sponsored by the Ontario Society of Clinical Hypnosis, Toronto, Canada, May 1983, and recorded by the Content Management Corporation (formerly Audio Archives of Canada) (Tape #22).

3. "Doing the Unexpected" is from the workshop "Patient Management and Pain Control" from the 24th Annual Advanced Workshops in Clinical Hypnosis, cosponsored by the Minnesota Society of Clinical Hypnosis, the Behavioral Pediatrics Program, Department of Pediatrics, Medical School, and Department of Continuing Medical Education, University of Minnesota, St. Paul, Minnesota, June 1995.

4. "Dealing with Acute Pain" is from the workshop "Patient Management and Pain Control" from the 24th Annual Advanced Workshops in Clinical Hypnosis, cosponsored by the Minnesota Society of Clinical Hypnosis, the Behavioral Pediatrics Program, Department of Pediatrics, Medical School, and Department of Continuing Medical Education, University of Minnesota, St. Paul, Minnesota, June 1995.

5. "Acknowledging and Supporting Patient's Hard Work" is from the workshop on "Therapeutic Uses of Language", sponsored by the New York Society for Ericksonian Psychotherapy and Hypnosis (NYSEPH), 1987 (Tape #5).

6. "Abreaction and Control of Trance" is from "Clinical Hypnosis: Strategies in Hypnotic Communication", sponsored by the Ontario Society of Clinical Hypnosis, Toronto, Canada, May 1983, and recorded by the Content Management Corporation (formerly Audio Archives of Canada) (Tape #22).

7. "Hypnoanesthesia during Surgery" is from the workshop, "Patient Management and Pain Control" from the 24th Annual Advanced Workshops in Clinical Hypnosis, cosponsored by The Minnesota Society of Clinical Hypnosis, the Behavioral Pediatrics Program, Department of Pediatrics, Medical School, and Department of Continuing Medical Education, University of Minnesota, St. Paul, Minnesota, June 1995.

8. "Tantrum" is from the workshop on "Therapeutic Uses of Language", sponsored by the New York Society for Ericksonian Psychotherapy and Hypnosis (NYSEPH), 1987 (Tape #7).

9. "Dealing with Pain" is from the workshop "Patient Management and Pain Control" from the 24th Annual Advanced

Workshops in Clinical Hypnosis, cosponsored by the Minnesota Society of Clinical Hypnosis, the Behavioral Pediatrics Program, Department of Pediatrics, Medical School, and Department of Continuing Medical Education, University of Minnesota, St. Paul, Minnesota, June 1995.

10. "Hiking" is from "Strategies of Hypnotic Utilization", Southern California Society for Ericksonian Psychotherapy and Hypnosis Classics Series: *The Hypnotic Language and Metaphors of Kay Thompson*, 1994, Tape #3).

Bibliography

1963

"A rationale for suggestion in dentistry", *American Journal of Clinical Hypnosis*, 3, pp. 181–6.

1964

Thompson, K. F., Weyandt, J. A. and Irwin, F. D., "The clinical teaching of hypnosis: Illustrative procedures", *American Journal of Clinical Hypnosis*, 6(4), pp. 337–9.

1966

"Communicate to motivate", *American Journal of Clinical Hypnosis*, 9, pp. 22–30.

1969

Woody, R. H., Houck, J. J. and Thompson, K. F., "Proposals for education and training in clinical hypnosis", *American Journal of Clinical Hypnosis*, 12, pp. 95–9.

1970

Pearson, R. E., Thompson, K. F. and Edmonston, W. E., "Clinical and experimental trance: What's the difference?", *American Journal of Clinical Hypnosis*, 13, pp. 1–7.

1976

"A clinical view of the effectiveness of hypnosis in pain control", in M. Weisenberg (ed.), *Pain: New Perspectives in Therapy and Research*, (pp. 67–73), New York: Plenum.

1978

"The role of suggestion in pain and anxiety control", in C. R. Bennet (ed.), *Conscious Sedation in Dental Practice* (2nd ed., pp. 58-72), St. Louis, MO: C. V. Mosby, (original work published 1974).

1979

"The case against relaxation", in G. Burrows, D. R. Collison and L. Dennerstein (eds), *Hypnosis*, (pp. 41–5).

"Cognitive factors in the control of pain" (Discussion), in L. I. Grossman (ed.), *Mechanism and Control of Pain* (pp. 229–33), Issy les Molineaux, France: Masson.

1980

"Hypnose en pijnbeatrijding", *Nederlands Tijdachrift voor Tandheelkunde*, March, 88–0.

1981

"The mythical trance", in H.J. Wain (ed.), *Theoretical and Clinical Aspects of Hypnosis* (pp. 55–65), Miami, FL: Symposia Specialists.

1982

"The curiosity of Milton H. Erickson", in J. K. Zeig (ed.), *Ericksonian Approaches to Hypnosis and Psychotherapy* (pp. 413–21), New York: Brunner/Mazel.

"Hypnosis in dentistry", in J. W. Clark (ed.), *Clinical Dentistry* (pp. 1–10), New York: J. B. Lippincott.

1985

"Almost 1984", in J. K. Zeig (ed.), *Ericksonian Psychotherapy: Vol. 1. Structures* (pp. 89–99), New York: Brunner/Mazel.

1988

"Motivation and the multiple states of trance", in J. K. Zeig (ed.), *Developing Ericksonian Therapy: State of the Art* (pp. 150–163), New York: Brunner/Mazel.

1990

"Metaphor, a myth with a method", in J. K. Zeig and S. G. Gilligan (eds), *Brief Therapy, Myths, Methods, and Metaphors* (pp. 247–57), New York: Brunner/Mazel.

1994

"Whose story is this, anyway—A history of his-story", in J. K. Zeig (ed.), *Ericksonian Methods, the Essence of the Story* (pp. 136–46), New York: Brunner/Mazel.

Films

Kay Thompson made several teaching films relating to hypnotherapy. The three listed below are the best known. She was the subject of the third film.

Hypnoanesthesia and Bleeding Control for Dental Surgery in the Hemophiliac.

Removal of Impacted Maxillary Third Molar Utilizing Hypnoanesthesia and the Alert Trance.

Rhinoplasty, Submucous Resection and Dermabrasion Utilizing Hypnosis.

A Sampling of Kay Thompson's Oral Presentations

Kay Thompson was a very active participant in professional meetings throughout her working life, whether she was teaching in workshops or taking part in seminars or presenting papers at meetings. The listing below includes samples of her most notable work.

1982
Dental advanced workshop. Ninth International Congress of Hypnosis and Psychosomatic Medicine. Glasgow, Scotland. August.

Basic and advanced workshops on hypnosis utilization. Department of Psychology, University of Kansas, Lawrence, KS. September.

Patient management and pain control utilizing hypnosis, presented at the School of Dental Medicine, University of Pennsylvania, Philadelphia, PA. November.

Hypnosis: A practical skill for caring dentists. All-day registered clinic, American Dental Asssociation meeting, Las Vegas, NV. November.

Language of hypnosis; Autohypnosis workshops. Erickson Congress on Hypnosis and Psychotherapy, Dallas, TX. December.

1983

Hypnosis and suggestion: Practical aids in dentistry, presented at the School of Dental Medicine, Department of Continuing Education, University of Pittsburgh, Titusville, PA. January.

Patient management and pain control, presented at the Pacific Medical Center, San Francisco Academy of Hypnosis. January.

Hypnosis: An alternative to drugs for the dental patient. presented at the School of Medicine, University of California, San Francisco. January.

Hypnosis applications for physicians, presented at the School of Medicine, Department of Continuing Education, University of Pittsburgh, Titusville, PA. April.

Ideal marketing tools: Patient management and pain control. Paper presented at the California Dental Association Scientific Session, Anaheim, CA. April.

Clinical hypnosis: Strategies in (hypnotic) communication. Workshop presented to the Ontario Society of Clinical Hypnosis, Toronto, Canada. May.

Verbal and nonverbal communication of meaning during hypnosis. Paper presented at the British Society for Clinical and Experimental Hypnosis, Churchill College, Cambridge, U.K. September.

Language of hypnosis. Workshop presented at the 2nd International Congress on Hypnosis and Psychosomatic Medicine, Phoenix, AZ. December

Communication for patient management and pain control. Paper presented at the European Society of Hypnosis, Vienna, Austria. August.

1984

Language of hypnosis, presented at the School of Medicine, West Virginia University, Morgantown, WV.

1994

Using the problem as solution; Verbal and nonverbal communication, presented to the Mind-Body Connection Hypnosis Workshop, West Virginia graduate College, Charleston, WV. June.

Language for patient management and pain control, presented at the Yankee Dental Congress, Boston. January.

1995

Language for physiological pain control and healing, presented to the Frontiers of Hypnosis meeting, Federation of Canadian Societies of Clinical Hypnosis, Banff, Alberta, Canada. May.

1996

Breaking the trance of pain; Why and how the language of hypnosis develops, presented at the Deutsche Gesellschaft fur Hypnose e.V., Badlippspringe, Germany. October.

1997

The emotional learning center of the body, presented at the International Society of Hypnosis, San Diego, CA. June.

The dentist as therapist; Quintessence of dental hypnosis, presented at the Deutsche Gesellschaft fur Zahnarztliche Hypnose, e.V., Munich, Germany. September.

Contributors

James M. Auld, BDS, is a dentist in country general practice, Australia. He is Past President of the Australian Society for Hypnosis (ASH).

Betty Alice Erickson, MS, is in private practice in Dallas, Texas. She is an international teacher of Ericksonian Psychotherapy and Hypnotherapy and the author of numerous book chapters and articles. She has served in many editorial capacities, including Executive Editor, *Milton H. Erickson Foundation Newsletter*. She is a daughter of Dr. Erickson.

Arnold Freedman, PhD, is in private practice in Pittsburgh, Pennsylvania. He was formerly Chief of the Psychology Service at the VA Medical Center in Pittsburgh, Pennsylvania.

Harold Golan, DMD,* was Past-Assistant Clinical Professor, Department of Oral and Maxillofacial Surgery at Tufts University School of Dental Medicine. He was Past President of the American Society for Clinical Hypnosis (ASCH) and the American Board of Hypnosis in Dentistry.

Ronald Havens, PhD, is Professor of Psychology at the University of Illinois at Springfield. He is in private practice in Springfield, Illinois.

Roxanna Erickson Klein, RN, PhD, is a clinical nurse in home settings with hospice patients. She is on the Board of Directors of the Milton H. Erickson Foundation in Phoenix and Milton H. Erickson Institute of Dallas. She is a daughter of Dr. Erickson.

Daniel P. Kohen, MD, is Director of the Behavioral Pediatrics Program and Professor in the Departments of Pediatrics and Family Practice and Community Health at the University of Minnesota.

Marion P. Kostka, EdD, is a psychologist at the Carruth Center for Counseling and Psychological Services at West Virginia University and also has a private practice in Morgantown, WV.

Penny Kostka, MA, shares a private practice with her husband in Morgantown, WV and is employed as a counselor at the Garrett County Mental Health Center in Oakland, MD.

Ralph Krichbaum was Kay Thompson's husband.

Peter Letarte, MD, was a nephew of Kay Thompson.

Alexander Levitan, MD, is Emeritus Clinical Associate Professor of Medicine in the Department of Family Practice and Community Health at the University of Minnesota. He was Past President of ASCH.

Camillo Loriedo, MD, is director of the Italian Institute for Relational Therapy and Professor of Psychiatry at the University of Rome. He is president of the European Society for Hypnosis and on the Board of Directors of the Milton Erickson Foundation.

Stacie A. Murrer, DDS, is a dentist in private practice in Monroeville, Pennsylvania.

Akira Otani, EdD, is a psychologist at the University of Maryland Counseling Center in College Park, Maryland.

Jane A. Parsons-Fein, MSW, is in private practice in New York City. She is President, American Hypnosis Board for Clinical Social Work and President Emeritus, New York Milton H. Erickson Society for Clinical Social Work. She is Fellow and Consultant of the American Society of Clinical Hypnosis.

S. Timothy Rose, DDS, is a dentist in private practice. He is Past President of the American Dental Association.

Sidney Rosen, MD, is in private practice in New York City. He was Founding President, The New York Milton H. Erickson Society for Psychotherapy and Hypnosis (NYSEPH). He is the author of *My Voice Will Go With You: The Teaching Tales of Milton Erickson*.

Russell Scott, PhD,* was in private practice in Pittsburgh, Pennsylvania. He was Past Director of Planning, City of Pittsburgh and former professor, University of Pittsburgh.

Bernhard Trenkle, Dipl. Psych., is Director of the Milton Erickson Institute, Rottweil, Germany, and member of the Board of Directors of the Milton Erickson Foundation. He is Past President of Milton Erickson Society of Clinical Hypnosis, Germany.

Peo Wikström, DDS, is Founding President of the European Society of Hypnosis (ESH). He is a Past Editor of *HYPNOS*, Journal of SCEH, and the Journal of ESH. He is a fellow of ASCH.

*We regret to inform readers that Dr. Golan passed away in January 2000 and Dr. Russ Scott passed away in February 2004.

Index

USA & Canada orders to:
Crown House Publishing
P.O. Box 2223, Williston, VT 05495-2223, USA
Tel: 877-925-1213, Fax: 802-864-7626
E-mail: info@CHPUS.com
www.CHPUS.com

UK & Rest of World orders to:
The Anglo American Book Company Ltd.
Crown Buildings, Bancyfelin, Carmarthen, Wales SA33 5ND
Tel: +44 (0)1267 211880/211886, Fax: +44 (0)1267 211882
E-mail: books@anglo-american.co.uk
www.anglo-american.co.uk

Australasia orders to:
Footprint Books Pty Ltd.
Unit 4/92A Mona Vale Road, Mona Vale NSW 2103, Australia
Tel: +61 (0) 2 9997 3973, Fax: +61 (0) 2 9997 3185
E-mail: info@footprint.com.au
www.footprint.com.au

Singapore orders to:
Publishers Marketing Services Pte Ltd.
10-C Jalan Ampas #07-01
Ho Seng Lee Flatted Warehouse, Singapore 329513
Tel: +65 6256 5166, Fax: +65 6253 0008
E-mail: info@pms.com.sg
www.pms.com.sg

Malaysia orders to:
Publishers Marketing Services Pte Ltd
Unit 509, Block E, Phileo Damansara 1, Jalan 16/11
46350 Petaling Jaya, Selangor, Malaysia
Tel : 03 7955 3588, Fax : 03 7955 3017
E-mail: pmsmal@po.jaring.my
www.pms.com.sg

South Africa orders to:
Everybody's Books
PO Box 201321, Durban North, 4016, RSA
Tel: +27 (0) 31 569 2229, Fax: +27 (0) 31 569 2234
E-mail: warren@ebbooks.co.za